W9-CEH-520

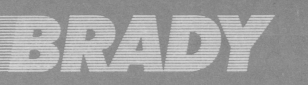

BEING A
LONG-TERM CARE
NURSING ASSISTANT

Third Edition

Connie A. Will, RN, BSN

Judith B. Eighmy, RN, BSN

BRADY
REGENTS/PRENTICE HALL
Englewood Cliffs, New Jersey 07632

Will, Connie A.
   Being a long-term care nursing assistant / Connie A. Will, Judith B. Eighmy. — 3rd ed.
      p. cm.
   Includes index.
   ISBN 0-89303-101-1
   1. Long-term care of the sick.   2. Nursing.   3. Nurses' aides.   I. Eighmy, Judith B.   II. Title.
    [DNLM: 1. Long Term Care—methods—nurses' instruction.
   2. Nurses' Aides. WY 193 W6896b]
RT120.L64W54 1991
610.73 '61—dc20
DNLM/DLC
for Library of Congress   90-15105
                                                                                        CIP

Editorial/production and supervision: Ed Jones
Page layout: Maureen Eide
Cover design: Suzanne Behnke
Cover photo: George Dodson
Manufacturing buyers: Mary McCartney and Ed O'Dougherty

© 1991, 1988, 1983 by Prentice-Hall, Inc.
A Simon & Schuster Company
Englewood Cliffs, New Jersey 07632

*All rights reserved. No part of this book may be
reproduced, in any form or by any means,
without permission in writing from the publisher.*

Printed in the United States of America
10 9 8 7 6 5 4 3 2 1

ISBN 0-89303-101-1

Prentice-Hall International (UK) Limited, *London*
Prentice-Hall of Australia Pty. Limited, *Sydney*
Prentice-Hall Canada Inc., *Toronto*
Prentice-Hall Hispanoamericana, S.A., *Mexico*
Prentice-Hall of India Private Limited, *New Delhi*
Prentice-Hall of Japan, Inc., *Tokyo*
Simon & Schuster Asia Pte. Ltd., *Singapore*
Editora Prentice-Hall do Brasil, Ltda., *Rio de Janeiro*

Dedication

We dedicate this book to those concerned and caring individuals who serve residents in long-term care facilities. We believe that only through increased knowledge, awareness, and understanding of the unique needs of long-term care residents will the highest quality of life be achieved.

Now Available from

BRADY

Being A Long-Term Care Nursing Assistant, 3/e
Pocket Guide

Connie A. Will, RN, BSN
Judith B. Eighmy, RN, BSN

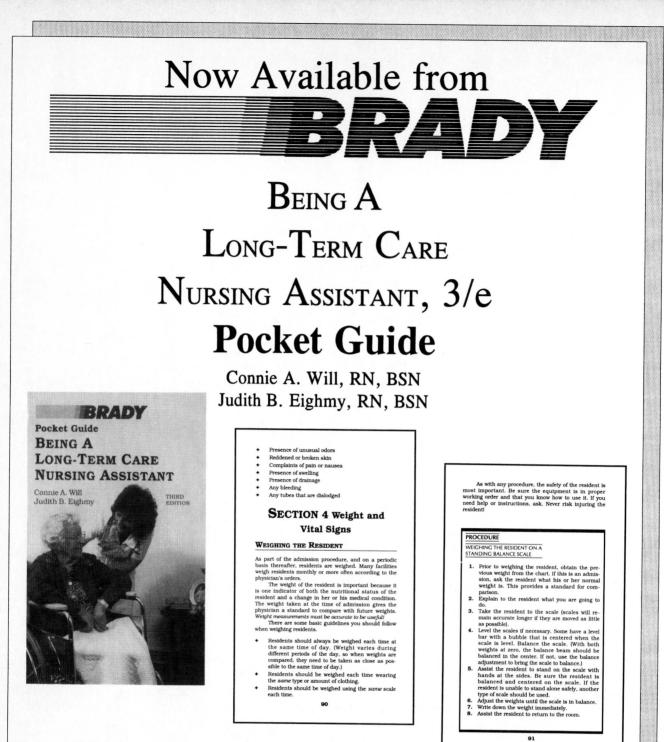

'Handy compact pocket size

'Large, clear type for easy reading

'Keyed to **Being a Long-Term Care Nursing Assistant**, 3rd edition

© 1991, 394 pp., (D1305-4)

To order your copy, call (201) 767-5937
Instructors inquiring about multiple copies and classroom adoptions call: 1 (800) 638-0220
25% discount for classroom sets

■ Contents

1 INTRODUCTION TO LONG-TERM CARE

2 YOUR WORKING ENVIRONMENT

3 SPECIAL NEEDS OF THE ELDERLY AND CHRONICALLY ILL

4 BASIC NURSING CARE

■ Procedures

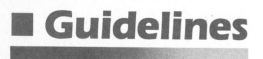

■ Guidelines

■ Preface

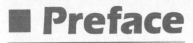

Being a Long-Term Care Nursing Assistant, 3rd edition, has been compiled to fill the long existing need for a text specifically designed for the nursing assistant who is or will be employed in a long-term care facility. It is authored by nurses currently practicing and teaching in the long-term care (LTC) field who recognize the unique knowledge and skill needed to provide care and service to the LTC resident. It is designed to teach the nursing assistant to become an efficient, caring member of the health-care team.

The text provides a simple, clear, and concise framework for learning. It can be used as a primary learning tool for beginning students and as a resource text for expanding the knowledge and skill of the experienced nursing assistant. This comprehensive training text has been designed to include specific subjects required by states that mandate nursing assistant certification or training programs. All concepts presented are adapted for the long-term care facility and the unique needs of the residents.

The text has been organized in a systems approach to the learning process. Students are first given a basic introduction to the anatomy and physiology of each body system at the beginning of those chapters that deal with a specific system. Once the normal system has been studied, the age-related changes and common abnormalities are presented, along with nursing care guidelines and step-by-step procedures. Students are able to establish a direct relationship between the reason care is given and their role in providing that care.

The third edition has been updated to reflect the ongoing changes in long-term care facilities. Many facilities now provide more complex and technical kinds of care requiring more sophisticated knowledge and skills from the nursing assistant. Knowledge in other areas has also developed and new information on such topics as Alzheimer's disease, AIDS, and hospice care have been expanded in this edition.

The restorative nursing chapter has been revised and expanded to assist in developing a restorative program and to provide the restorative nursing assistant with a higher level of skill. The chapter on developmental disabilities is included in recognition of the need for basic information to meet the needs of those employed in this unique long-term care setting.

Throughout the text the authors have integrated these basic concepts:

- Resident welfare and safety
- Psychosocial needs
- Physical needs
- Rehabilitation
- Legal and ethical responsibilities
- Resident Rights

Feedback from residents regarding enhancement of the quality of life has been integrated and reinforced throughout the text. For example, the concept of choice and its impact on resident morale is stressed. Other quality-of-life issues such as touch, communication, and privacy are integrated throughout.

Each chapter is divided into short manageable sections. The sections include:

- Objectives that are achievable, understandable, behavioral, and measurable.
- Guidelines that present a logical sequential narrative to providing many aspects of care where a rote, step-by-step procedure is not practical.
- Procedures that give a step-by-step approach to tasks most commonly performed in the long-term care facility. Procedures have been modified to include types of supplies and equipment commonly used. All procedures are highlighted in color for added emphasis. Universal precautions are incorporated in each procedure as appropriate.
- Information tables that provide ready reference materials for the student and instructor.

New terms are printed in boldface and defined in the text to facilitate learning and expand the student's health-care vocabulary. Abbreviations are included early to familiarize students with commonly used medical abbreviations.

The glossary defines all new words presented in the text as well as other care-related terms.

The student workbook has been revised to enhance learning. The workbook contains numerous activities that not only are measures of the objectives, but are also instructional in themselves.

An instructor's guide is available that contains complete lesson plans, answers to workbook activities, supplemental material on principles of adult learning, and teaching strategies. The lesson plans include numerous suggestions to enhance student learning and add interest.

The authors, reviewers, and advisors have endeavored to produce a uniquely comprehensive and thorough text to meet the educational needs of the long-term care nursing assistant.

The addition of four-color photos and new line drawings, along with a new book design, greatly enhances and updates the appearance of the book.

■ Acknowledgments

With deepest gratitude the authors acknowledge the considerable contributions, assistance and support of family, friends, and associates. We sincerely thank our families for their advice, support, and endurance during this revision.

We thank our husbands Vernon Will, President of Extended Care Enterprises, and Nicholas Eighmy, President of SNF Forms, for their invaluable assistance and support, as well as for their contribution of time and resources during this revision.

We thank David Juberg, President of Hallmark Health Services, for his support and Eldon Teper for his friendship and expertise as well as his willingness to pick up many duties left undone.

For technical assistance in the use and programming of the computer input, special thanks to Ralph and Kelli Lockhart of ADD-On Health Systems, Inc., of Laguna Hills, CA.

For sharing their clinical expertise in the chapter on developmental disabilities, we acknowledge Adrienne Appleton, Rachel Bennet, and Terry Henry.

For sharing expertise in hospice care we thank Dennis Rezendes of Community Hospice Care of Orange County.

Grateful acknowledgment is made to the Prentice Hall staff, Natalie Anderson and Ed Jones, editors, and Louise Fullam for her support.

We recognize the talents of George Dodson, photographer, whose skills have made an invaluable contribution to this revision.

We thank Extended Care of Anaheim; Extended Care of Riverside; Manor Care Nursing Center, Silver Spring, MD; Holy Cross Hospital, Silver Spring, MD; and Centers for the Handicapped, Inc., Silver Spring, MD, for their cooperation in providing facilities, staff, and residents to be used in several photographs in this edition.

We continue to be thankful for the encouragement and ongoing support of those who teach nursing assistants across the country. We appreciate their sharing of positive feedback and know they will find this third edition even better.

ART CREDITS

Figure 2-18:   Courtesy Burroughs Wellcome Co.

Figure 3-14:   Courtesy Cremation Association of North America.

Figure 5-11:   Courtesy American Cancer Society.

■ About the Authors

Connie A. Will, RN, BSN, PHN, is a graduate of California State University at Long Beach and has been active in long-term care as a nursing consultant, educator, and owner for the past fourteen years. Ms. Will owns and operates long-term care facilities in Anaheim and Riverside, California. Ms. Will's teaching experience includes providing nursing education in both the acute and long-term care settings as well as being a professor of nursing in the community college RN program. Ms. Will has planned and developed special care units for residents suffering from Alzheimer's disease and for terminally ill residents. Ms. Will designed and implemented a Medicare certified in-patient hospice unit in Arizona as well as a successful home-care hospice program which provides care to terminally ill residents in long-term care facilities. Ms. Will has provided consultation for facilities in interior design of environments for the elderly and chronically ill. Ms. Will along with Ms. Eighmy pioneered the Nurse Assistant Certification Program in California through the California Association of Health Facilities.

Judith B. Eighmy, RN, BSN, PHN, is a graduate of Texas Woman's University and has completed coursework for a Master's degree at California State University at Los Angeles. Ms. Eighmy has been a nursing consultant and educator in long-term care for the past fourteen years. In addition to teaching many continuing education courses in the community and university settings, she has experience in nursing education in both the acute-care hospital and nursing school. She has taught review classes for foreign nurses, preparing them for the NCLEX-RN examination. She has developed and monitored Quality Assurance Programs for long-term care facilities and is widely recognized for her expertise in rehabilitation programs for the elderly and chronically ill. Ms. Eighmy recently provided consultation for a series of nurse assistant educational videos developed by Medcom, Inc., of Garden Grove, California. Ms. Eighmy along with Ms. Will pioneered the Nurse Assistant Certification Program in California through the California Association of Health Facilities. Ms. Eighmy is currently the Vice President of Quality Assurance for Hallmark Health Services.

Ms. Will and Ms. Eighmy are currently completing an innovative system of resident care planning and management which will be available in both a computerized soft-ware program as well as a reference text to be published in association with ADD-On Health Systems, Inc., in 1990.

CHAPTER 1

Introduction to Long-Term Care

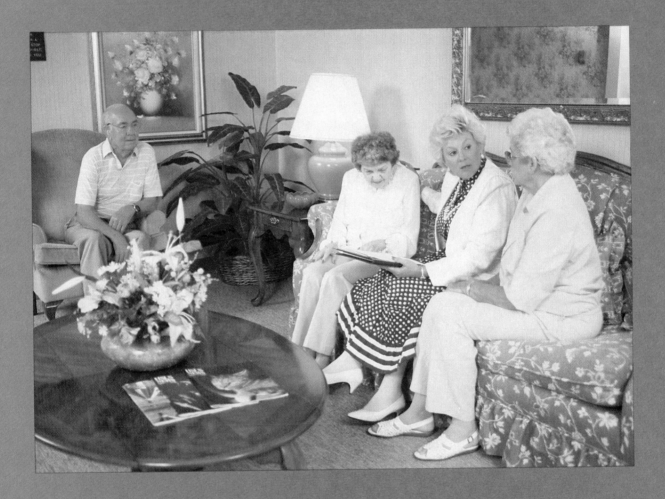

OBJECTIVES/WHAT YOU WILL LEARN

When you have completed this section, you will be able to:
- Identify four basic purposes of long-term care facilities
- Describe the functions within the long-term care facility
- List the three most common reasons residents require long-term care

LONG-TERM CARE FACILITIES

The **long-term care (LTC)** facility is an integral part of the nation's health-care system. Census bureau statistics reflect the dramatic increase in the over-65 population and the expected continuing growth during the next decade (Fig. 1-1). As life expectancy increases, the need for LTC services also increases — one out of every five persons over the age of 75 will require LTC services. After age 85, 23 percent will require LTC services.

The General Accounting Office has identified the three major reasons our elderly require LTC services:

- Inability to perform **activities of daily living** (ADL) such as eating, bathing, toileting, and dressing (Fig. 1-2)
- Decreased mental abilities with various dementias causing confusion and difficult behaviors as well as common medical problems such as heart disease, stroke, hypertension, hip fracture, and arthritis
- Absence of a caregiver, spouse, immediate family member, or friend

The LTC facility is both a hospital with hospital-like services and the residents' home. The majority of people admitted to LTC facilities reside there permanently. The average length of stay in a LTC facility exceeds two and one-half years. Its primary functions are as follows:

Four Basic Functions and Purposes of the Long-term Care Facility

1. To provide care to residents based on their identified needs
2. To utilize a multidisciplinary health-care team to plan care and provide services
3. To prevent illness, injury, or loss of function
4. To promote recovery and health through maintaining existing abilities and restoring residents' former abilities

---

Some common terms used to describe LTC facilities are:

- Skilled nursing facility
- Nursing home
- Convalescent hospital
- Rehabilitation center
- Extended care hospital
- Nursing care center

TYPES OF LTC FACILITIES

Some LTC facilities offer specialized care. They provide services to residents with special needs or problems, such as:

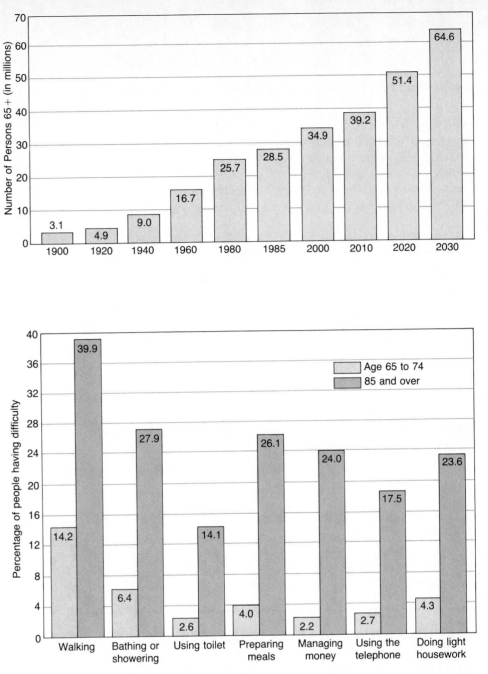

FIGURE 1-1
Increases in life expectancy, 1900 to 2030.

FIGURE 1-2
Percentage of elderly people who have difficulty performing seven ordinary tasks.

Facilities for the Developmentally Disabled Client

A **developmental disability** is a condition closely related to mental retardation — the client is often seriously handicapped. Clients who have cerebral palsy, autism, and various seizure disorders are often residents in the developmentally disabled (DD) facility. There are common goals in providing care to the DD client:

- Maintaining good physical health (many DD clients have severe physical disabilities)
- Creating as normal and homelike an environment as possible while teaching the client to become as independent as possible
- Managing behavior and teaching the client to control unacceptable behaviors

Care of the DD individual requires unique knowledge and training. A special chapter is devoted to this subject.

Facilities That Provide Special Rehabilitation Services

These facilities are often called extended care hospitals or rehabilitation care centers. This type of facility offers specialized care to assist residents in restoring normal levels of functioning following a stroke, fracture, or accident. There are physical therapists, speech therapists, occupational therapists, and licensed nurses available to provide specialized care and services on a daily basis. Residents in these facilities usually have a good potential for recovery and will remain in the facility only during the recovery phase of their illness.

Facilities That Specialize in Caring for Patients with the Same Problems

- Alcoholic rehabilitation treatment centers
- Drug abuse units
- Psychiatric/mental-health units
- **Hospice** inpatient centers (a facility that provides care to residents who have a limited life expectancy)
- Centers that deal with Alzheimer's and similar dementias

Facilities That Provide Subacute and Skilled Nursing Care

These facilities care for the seriously ill as well as chronically ill, recuperating, and dying residents. This type of facility generally offers the following services:

- Physician
- Twenty-four-hour nursing care
- Pharmacy
- Dietary
- Recreational
- Social
- Physical therapy
- Speech therapy
- Occupational therapy
- Audiology
- Psychological
- Podiatry

Facilities That Provide Other Levels of Care

These facilities offer care to residents who have special needs for supportive services but do not require as much direct nursing care as that provided by a skilled nursing or subacute facility. Other levels of care you may hear about are personal and supervisory. Some facilities provide several levels of care.

State and federal programs support more than 50 percent of the residents in LTC facilities through Medicare, Medicaid, or local programs. The payment system is directly related to the level of care that residents require.

ORGANIZATION OF THE LTC FACILITY

Most LTC facilities are organized in a similar way, and the easiest way to understand the lines of authority and responsibility is to understand the organizational chart of a typical facility (Fig. 1-3). This helps establish appropriate lines of communication with facility management. Communication is always smoother when the chain of command is followed and understood.

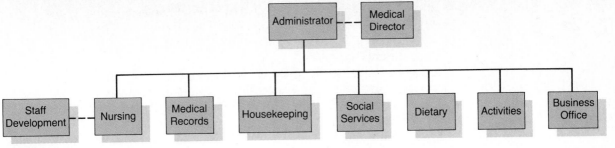

FIGURE 1-3
Organization of a long-term care facility.

TABLE 1-1. COMPARISON OF ACUTE CARE AND LONG-TERM CARE

Acute Care Hospital	Long-Term Care Facility
The patient/resident is:	
• more dependent	• more independent
• in a passive role	• in an active role
• acutely ill or in need of special services	• chronically ill or in need of skilled nursing care
• seen daily by a physician	• seen occasionally by a physician (usually monthly)
• admitted for days	• admitted for weeks, months, years
• less concerned with social and recreational needs	• more concerned with social and recreational needs
The treatment is:	
• related to the reason for admission (injury, disease, etc.)	• related to multiple problems, including psychosocial
• "cure oriented"	• aimed at rehabilitation — restoring and maintaining well-being
Nursing assistants:	
• have responsibility for fewer patients	• have responsibility for more residents
• have less freedom to help plan patient care	• have more freedom to help plan resident care
• perform many technical skills	• perform fewer technical skills
• give limited rehabilitative nursing care, little to do with patients' personal life and psychosocial problems	• give more rehabilitative nursing care and deal more with residents' personal life and emotional problems
• usually not required to have special training/certification for acute care hospitals	• required to have special training/certification for LTC facilities

LONG-TERM CARE VERSUS ACUTE CARE

Long-term care facilities differ from acute and general hospitals in many ways. Some of these differences are shown in Table 1-1.

There are alternatives to placement of residents in LTC facilities. Some apartment complexes, for example, offer supportive services for elderly residents, such as providing meals, housekeeping, transportation, and recreational programs. This is often referred to as *congregate living*. These options, along with services provided by home health-care agencies, allow elderly residents to remain independent longer.

Home health-care agencies provide services to the chronically ill, disabled, or recuperating patient in the home. These services may be provided by any of the following:

- Public health nurse
- Registered nurse
- Physical therapist
- Occupational therapist
- Speech therapist
- Dietician
- Social worker
- Home health aide

This program is often very acceptable to patients because there is little disruption in their lifestyle. Only patients whose medical needs can be adequately met at home are provided with home-care services. If the care is to be funded by Medicare or Medicaid, the patient must meet certain requirements to be eligible for covered services.

Adult day-care centers provide care for those who cannot or do not want to be alone during the day. These centers provide social and recreational activities as well as meals and snacks. Many include a place for resting or napping. Medical care is not provided unless the center is part of a licensed LTC facility. Many people are able to remain home with family longer because of the part-time assistance that adult day-care centers provide.

SECTION 2 THE NURSING ASSISTANT AS AN EMPLOYEE

OBJECTIVES/WHAT YOU WILL LEARN

When you have completed this section, you will be able to:
- Define the terms *policy, procedure,* and *job description*
- Explain where the employer's "rules" for employees can be found
- Compare your own job description with the sample job description provided

POLICIES, PROCEDURES, AND JOB DESCRIPTIONS

All LTC facilities must provide care and services according to established state and federal laws and regulations. The facilities are inspected regularly to ensure that these regulations are followed. If facilities fail to meet the established standards, they may lose their license to operate as well as state and federal payment for services.

As you learn about the LTC facility, you will become familiar with the specific state and federal regulations you will be expected to follow as you provide nursing care. Facilities establish written policies, procedures, and job descriptions to help them comply with regulations and to make their employees more efficient in the delivery of services to residents (Fig. 1-4).

These policies, procedures, and job descriptions are very important "tools" you will need to help you become successful as a nursing assistant.

- A **policy** describes what will be done.
- A **procedure** describes how something is to be done.
- A **job description** describes who is to do what.

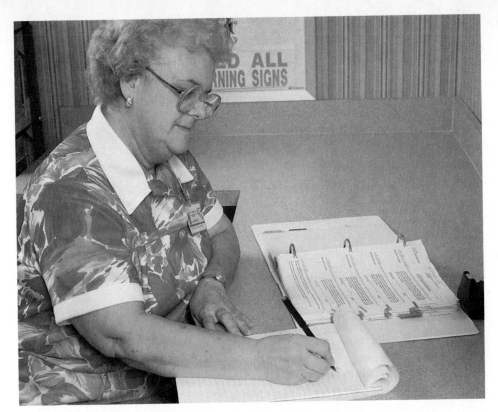

FIGURE 1-4
Using the *Policies and Procedures* manual.

A sample job description for a nursing assistant is included here. It is easy to see that the role of the nursing assistant is a responsible one that requires both knowledge and skill.

SAMPLE JOB DESCRIPTION

Nursing Service:	Nursing Assistant
Position Summary:	The Nursing Assistant is responsible for providing direct resident care under supervision of the Charge Nurse. The Nursing Assistant follows established facility policies and procedures while providing care, and coordinates resident care with other facility personnel and families.
Position Relationships	
Responsible to:	Charge Nurse
	Treatment Nurse
	Nurse Supervisor
	Director of Nursing
Workers Supervised:	None
Interrelationships:	Director of Nursing
	Nurse Supervisor
	Charge Nurse
	Treatment Nurse
	Other Department Supervisors
	Physicians
	Families
	Consultant Personnel
	Ancillary Service Purveyors
Qualifications	
Education:	High school diploma desirable
Personal:	Presents a neat, well-groomed appearance
	Good physical and emotional health

1. Follows established performance standards and performs duties according to nursing service policies and procedures.
2. Requests clarification and/or training for policies and procedures that are not clearly understood.
3. Assists new employees in following established hospital policies and procedures.
4. Provides direct resident care as assigned, completing assignments accurately and in a timely manner.
5. Identifies special resident problems and reports immediately to the charge nurse.
6. Conducts resident rounds daily and initiates corrective action immediately.
7. Identifies safety hazards and emergency situations and initiates corrective action immediately.
8. Provides nursing care to residents without violating the "Resident's Bill of Rights."
9. Participates in hospital education programs as assigned (i.e., orientation, inservice, and precertification) and coordinates training needs with the Director of Staff Development.
10. Attends all classes as assigned and completes assignments accurately and on time.
11. Demonstrates an attitude of cooperation and enthusiasm in classroom and resident care activities.
12. Assumes personal responsibility for following hospital procedures related to control of equipment and supplies within the unit.
13. Assumes accountability for compliance to federal, state, and local regulations within the unit assigned and within the span of control of the nursing assistant.
14. Reports to the charge nurse or nurse supervisor unusual problems or incidents as well as failure of fellow employees to adhere to established policies and procedures.
15. Accurately documents incidents and/or unusual problems following established hospital procedures.
16. Demonstrates consistent ability to work cooperatively with residents, charge nurses, treatment nurses, restorative assistants, other nursing assistants, physicians, families, consulting personnel, and ancillary service purveyors.
17. Participates in resident care conferences and other hospital meetings as assigned.
18. Participates in the development of an individualized plan of resident care for residents assigned. Reviews care plan daily and performs nursing care as outlined.
19. Provides nursing care as outlined by the charge nurse and the resident care plan.
20. Documents, in the nurse assistant notes on each shift of duty, care and treatment provided to the resident and resident's response or lack of response to care provided.
21. Reports changes in resident condition immediately to the charge nurse or nurse supervisor.
22. Seeks assistance when confronted with a resident problem that requires special assessment.
23. Performs basic nursing skills as outlined in hospital education program, demonstrating knowledge and competence.
24. Follows hospital procedures for admission and discharge/transfer of residents — completes all documentation accurately.
25. Greets residents by name and speaks to resident and family members in a kind and thoughtful manner.
26. Listens to resident and family complaints attentively and reports problems promptly to the charge nurse.
27. Responds appropriately to the feelings of others by listening attentively and taking follow-up action.
28. Controls angry feelings and only expresses anger in appropriate areas.
29. Demonstrates concern for all residents' welfare by rendering immediate assistance to *any* resident in need.
30. Answers call lights promptly.
31. Demonstrates warm, caring feelings about residents by responding appropriately to the needs expressed.
32. Works wherever assigned with a cooperative spirit.
33. Comes to work as scheduled and consistently demonstrates dependability.
34. Comes to work on time and consistently demonstrates punctuality.
35. Comes to work in clean, neat uniform and consistently adheres to dress code.

Now review your own job description carefully and make sure that you understand it. Your job description should:

- Clearly define your responsibilities
- Describe the duties you will be expected to carry out
- Describe your relationships with other departments as well as the department of nursing

PERSONNEL POLICIES

Personnel policies describe both the benefits provided to employees and the expectations of the employer. Included are guidelines for acceptable employee behavior. Just as we all must follow the "rules of the road" to avoid chaos on the streets, employees must follow the "rules to work by" to have order within a facility. Review the sample standards of conduct that follow.

Standards of Conduct

The following actions are never tolerated in facilities. Any instances of the following behavior will result in disciplinary and/or legal action.

1. Verbal and/or physical abuse to a resident, visitor, or supervisory personnel.
2. Inefficiency, inability, and/or gross or repeated negligence in performance of assigned duties.
3. Stealing or willfully destroying or damaging any property of the facility, its residents, visitors, or other personnel.
4. Disobedience or insubordination to supervisors.
5. Disorderly, immoral, or indecent conduct.
6. Reporting for work, or attempting to work, while under the influence of/or addicted to alcohol, drugs, or narcotics.
7. Borrowing money or other possessions from residents and/or accepting gratuities or tips from patients and/or their families.
8. Unauthorized possession of firearms or other weapons on facility property.
9. Absence without notifying the supervisor or admininstrator.
10. Smoking in an unauthorized area.
11. Selling tickets, pools, raffles, or soliciting of any kind on hospital premises.
12. Using the facility business phone for personal calls.
13. Altering, falsifying, or making a willful misstatement of facts on any resident record or chart, job, or work report.
14. Failure to provide care to residents in such a way as to guarantee them their right to be treated with respect and dignity.
15. Failure to protect confidentiality of resident records, information, and so on, or disclosing anything of a personal nature concerning a resident at any time either inside or outside the facility.
16. Punching another person's time card or requesting that another person punch your time card.
17. Refusal to work where assigned.

ORGANIZATION OF THE DEPARTMENT OF NURSING

Generally, each department of the LTC facility will have additional policies and procedures specifically related to that department. Make sure you understand what these are and where they are located for the department of nursing.

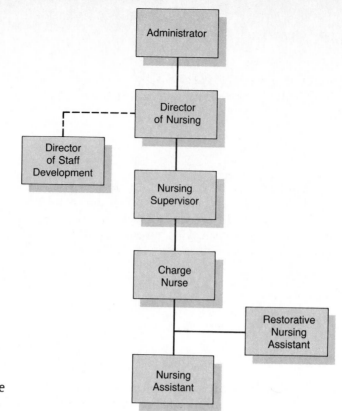

FIGURE 1-5
Organizational chart for the department of nursing.

The department of nursing is organized similarly in most LTC facilities (Fig. 1-5). The lines of responsibility and authority are dictated by state and federal regulations.

- The **director of nursing** must be a registered nurse (RN). Most have specialized training and experience in caring for the elderly or the patient population served.
- The **nursing supervisor** is generally a registered nurse who is in charge of either an entire shift or a specific section of a facility.
- The **charge nurse** is responsible for or in charge of a specific unit on a specific shift. The charge nurse reports to the nursing supervisor. The charge nurse may be a **registered nurse** (RN), a **licensed vocational nurse** (LVN), or a **licensed practical nurse** (LPN).
- The **director of inservice training** or **staff development** is a licensed nurse (RN, LPN, LVN) who is responsible for orientation and training of nursing personnel. The director of inservice training or staff development may report to the director of nursing or to the facility administrator.
- The **nursing assistant** *always* works under the direct supervision of a licensed nurse (Fig. 1-6). The nursing assistant usually reports to the charge nurse.

Understanding the chain of command helps you establish appropriate lines of communication. Usually, the nursing assistant communicates information about a resident directly to the charge nurse. If others need to know, the charge nurse should pass on the information.

If you are not satisfied with a response you get, you can go to the next higher person on the organization chart. When a conflict with a person in another department arises, refer the problem to your immediate supervisor. Although

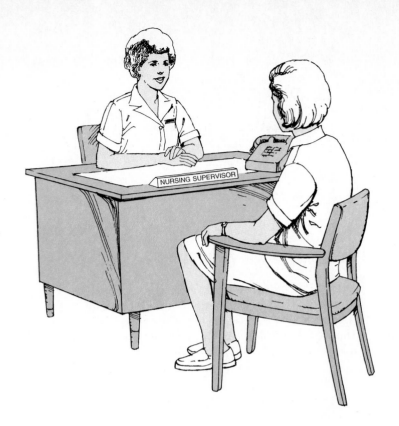

FIGURE 1-6
Nursing assistant working under the supervision of a licensed nurse.

"going all the way to the top" may bring faster results, the chain of communication is then broken and the entire structure of authority is undermined.

Providing care and service is a big responsibility, and doing a good job is often difficult. To be successful, a facility must have employees who work together and who are dedicated to their work (Fig. 1-7). To become a valued member of the health-care team, you need to thoroughly understand and accept the roles and responsibilities assigned to you as a nursing assistant.

FIGURE 1-7
Cooperating with fellow workers.

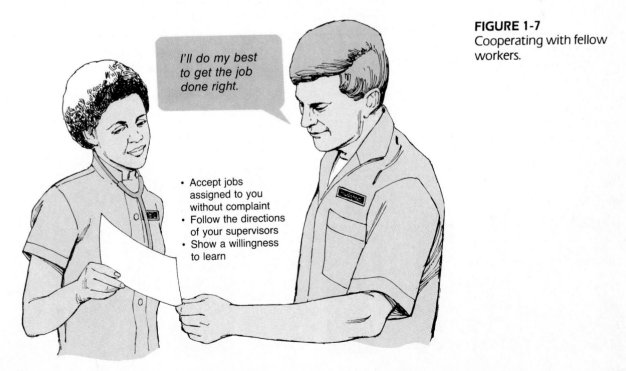

OBJECTIVES/WHAT YOU WILL LEARN

When you have completed this section, you will be able to:
- Identify actions that are unethical or illegal
- Point out situations that show a resident's rights are being violated
- Define the terms *libel* and *slander*
- List three ways the nursing assistant can help prevent theft and loss

RESPONSIBILITIES AS A NURSING ASSISTANT

As a nursing assistant, you must acquire knowledge and demonstrate the ability to perform nursing skills competently. The skills you will be able to perform when you have completed your course of study are included in the table of contents and in the workbook. Review these skills in order to understand those tasks that are within the role of the nursing assistant. You may acquire additional training according to the specific requirements of the state in which you work.

In the performance of your duties as a nursing assistant, you have a serious legal obligation both to the residents you care for and to your employer. **Legal** means according to the laws of the community, state, or nation. The public expects that those providing care to residents in LTC facilities are qualified to do so. They have the right to expect that those providing care will behave in a way that does not cause the resident any harm, emotional or physical. You are legally responsible for your actions and for your failure to act.

In 1987 a new law was passed by the U.S. Congress which expanded and strengthened the rights to be guaranteed all residents living in nursing facilities or long-term care facilities (Fig. 1-8). Each employee, resident, and family member must be informed of these rights on a regular basis. As you review the rights that follow, you will probably notice that these are rights to which you as a citizen are entitled. They may seem apparent and not necessary. However, two research studies indicated that in the past these rights had not been guaranteed each resident, so it became necessary to put them in writing and to hold long-term care facilities responsible for implementing them.

FIGURE 1-8
Resident's rights.

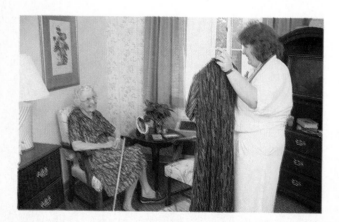
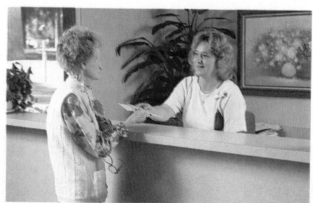

Resident Rights

The resident has a right to a dignified existence, self-determination, and communication with and access to persons and services inside and outside the facility. A facility must protect and promote the rights of each resident, including each of the following rights:

The resident has the right to exercise his or her rights as a resident of the facility and as a citizen or resident of the United States.

The resident has the right to be free of interference, coercion, discrimination, or reprisal from the facility in exercising his or her rights.

In the case of a resident adjudged incompetent under the laws of a state by a court of competent jurisdiction, the rights of the resident are exercised by the person appointed under state law to act on the resident's behalf.

The resident has the right to inspect and purchase photocopies of all records pertaining to the resident, upon written request and 48 hours' notice to the facility.

The resident has the right to be fully informed in language that he or she can understand of his or her total health status, including but not limited to his or her medical condition.

The resident has the right to refuse treatment, and to refuse to participate in experimental research.

The resident has the right to manage his or her financial affairs and the facility may not require residents to deposit their personal funds with the facility.

The resident has the right to choose a personal attending physician.

The resident has the right to be fully informed in advance about care and treatment and of treatment that may affect the resident's well-being.

The resident has the right, unless judged incompetent or otherwise found to be incapacitated under the laws of the state, to participate in planning care and treatment or changes in care and treatment.

The resident has the right to personal privacy and confidentiality of his or her personal and clinical records. Personal privacy includes accommodations, medical treatment, written and telephone communications, personal care, and visits and meetings with family and resident groups.

The resident has the right to voice grievances with respect to treatment or care that is or fails to be furnished, without discrimination or reprisal for voicing the grievances.

The resident has the right to prompt efforts by the facility to resolve grievances the resident may have, including those with respect to the behavior of other residents.

The resident has the right to examine the results of the most recent survey of the facility conducted by federal or state surveyors and any plan of correction in effect with respect to the facility.

The resident has the right to receive information from agencies acting as client advocates, and to be afforded the opportunity to contract agencies.

The resident has the right to refuse to perform services for the facility.

The resident has the right to perform services for the facility, if he or she chooses.

The resident has the right to privacy in written communications, including the right to send mail and to receive promptly mail that is unopened; and to have access to stationery, postage, and writing implements at the resident's own expense.

The resident has the right to have regular access to the private use of a telephone.

The resident has the right to be free from any physical restraints imposed, or psychoactive drugs administered for purposes of discipline or convenience and not required to treat the resident's medical symptoms.

The resident has the right to be free from verbal, sexual, physical, or mental abuse, corporal punishment, and involuntary seclusion.

The resident has the right to choose activities, schedules, and health care consistent with his or her interests, assessments, and plans of care.

The resident has the right to interact with members of the community both inside and outside the facility.

The resident has the right to make choices about aspects of his or her life in the facility that are significant to the resident.

The resident has the right to organize and participate in resident groups in the facility.

The resident has the right to participate in social, religious, and community activities that do not interfere with the rights of other residents in the facility.

The resident has the right to reside and receive services in the facility with reasonable accommodations of individual needs and preferences, except when the health or safety of the individual or other residents would be endangered.

The resident has the right to receive notice before the resident's room or roommate in the facility is changed.

Some states have adopted additional rights. Find out about the residents' rights established by your state. Both federal and state laws must be guaranteed to all residents. Disobeying these laws or denying residents these rights can result in fines, imprisonment, or both.

In addition to resident rights, civil rights are guaranteed to all residents. Civil rights refer to the freedom from discrimination guaranteed to all citizens. This includes discrimination because of:

- Age
- Sex
- Religion
- Race
- Ethnic origin
- Physical handicap

Just as your employer may not discriminate in hiring practices, you may not discriminate in providing care or services to residents. LTC facilities provide services and care to residents of vastly different backgrounds, ethnic groups, religions, and economic levels. Regardless of whether a resident is wealthy, a private-paying resident, or a resident whose care is funded through state and federal assistance programs, *all residents must receive equally good care!*

Many facilities utilize the services of an **ombudsman** (an impartial person who investigates complaints and acts as an advocate for residents and/or families). The ombudsman is provided access to the resident, resident records, and facility personnel, as well as any other information needed to gather information or facts related to a complaint.

LEGAL RESPONSIBILITIES

In addition to the residents' rights and civil rights, residents are protected by the laws that apply to everyone. Striking or handling a resident roughly or stealing from a resident are examples of crimes punishable by law.

As a nursing assistant, you also have legal responsibility regarding the accuracy or exactness of information you write in the resident's health record, which is a legal document.

A legal term related to providing care is **negligence.** This is the failure to act as an average nursing assistant would act under the same circumstances.

Gross negligence is more serious. Gross negligence occurs when the person responsible shows so little care that it appears that he or she is indifferent to the welfare of others.

Examples of negligence are:

- A nursing assistant fails to raise the side rails on the resident's bed, and the resident falls out of bed.
- A nursing assistant leaves a helpless resident unattended in the bathtub.
- A nursing assistant fails to perform assigned nursing care, such as repositioning or feeding a helpless resident.
- A nursing assistant takes a resident out-of-doors on a sunny day. The resident is left out too long and receives a sunburn.

Other important legal terms and definitions you should know are:

- **Assault** — A threat or an unsuccessful attempt to commit bodily harm
- **Battery** — An assault that is actually carried out (the person is actually harmed in some way)
- **False imprisonment** — Detaining or restraining a person without proper consent (placing a resident in restraints without the order of a physician, or using restraints for the wrong reasons)

In order to protect the rights of older people, many states have laws relating to **elder abuse.** These laws state that professionals (physicians, nurses, therapists, ministers, and so on) have a legal responsibility to report any suspected physical, mental, or financial abuse of older residents. This suspected abuse must be reported to the proper authorities. This means that any suspected abuse by staff must also be reported to the authorities. As a nursing assistant, you must report to your charge nurse any events you observe or hear about that might be considered elder abuse.

You can avoid involvement in legal actions by:

- Protecting the residents' personal and property rights
- Providing care according to facility policies and procedures
- Documenting care accurately
- Observing and reporting changes in a resident's condition
- Asking for help when you are unsure how to perform a task
- Reporting any suspected abuse of residents by anyone

ETHICAL CODE OF CONDUCT

In addition to following legal guidelines, a nursing assistant must also follow a **code of ethics.** This is a code of conduct for a particular group, the do's and don'ts for group members.

Some examples of ethical behavior for nursing assistants are:

- Assisting any resident in need whether or not you are assigned to that resident
- Reporting to work as scheduled
- Doing your best every day
- Avoiding gossip about residents and their families

Occasionally, a resident or family member may offer to pay or tip you to assure special treatment for their loved one. It is unethical to accept money under these circumstances.

When situations arise that involve ethical behavior, ask yourself these questions to help you make a decision. When you carefully consider your actions, you will make decisions that will not be harmful to yourself or others.

- How will my actions affect my residents?
- How will my actions affect my fellow workers?
- How will my actions affect my employer?
- How will my actions affect me?

CONFIDENTIALITY OF RESIDENT INFORMATION

An important legal and ethical responsibility is related to confidentiality of resident information. **Confidentiality** comes from two Latin words, *con* (with) and *fides* (faith or trust). Confidentiality, then, means "with trust."

Confidentiality guarantees the resident's right to privacy. It is based on the assumption that all information will remain private and will be used only as necessary to provide care or treatment. It is unethical and sometimes illegal to violate a resident's right to privacy.

Invasion of privacy is a legal term used to describe circumstances when personal information is exposed publicly that violates an individual's right to privacy. An example of invasion of privacy would be as follows: A resident receives a letter stating that her son is in jail. The nursing assistant reads the letter without permission and relates this information to others in the facility. This is an invasion of privacy.

The resident's **chart** (health record) is a legal document. It is the property of the health-care facility. As a nursing assistant, you are trusted to guard information contained in the chart. It is sometimes tempting to reveal information to your family or friends. This is always unethical and sometimes illegal and is punishable by law.

As a general rule, do not discuss personal information with:

- One resident about another resident
- Relatives and friends of the resident
- Visitors
- Representatives of news media
- Fellow workers, except when there is a need to know
- Your own relatives and friends

A legal and ethical problem closely related to confidentiality is **defamation of character,** which means to make false or damaging statements or misrepresentations about another person that defame or injure his or her reputation. There are two types of defamation of character: **slander** (a spoken statement) and **libel** (a written statement). Gossip is a type of slander.

THEFT AND LOSS

Theft and loss of a resident's personal items are problems that may occur in an LTC facility. A resident's personal belongings often represent all she or he has in the world. It may be difficult or impossible to replace these items if they are missing. It is your responsibility to protect residents from loss of items by using care in the handling of items and observing for and reporting any theft. Help create an atmosphere in your facility where theft is unacceptable. Usually, there is an inventory or list of items that catalogs the resident's belongings. Be sure that new items purchased or brought in by visitors are added to the list by reporting them to your supervisor. Remind visitors of the need to mark all items with the resident's name.

SECTION 4 PERSONAL QUALITIES

OBJECTIVES/WHAT YOU WILL LEARN

When you have completed this section, you will be able to:
- Evaluate yourself by completing the personal qualities assessment
- Determine if you are a good listener
- Explain how to tell the difference between information that should remain private and information that should be passed on to the charge nurse
- List five traits most beneficial in a helping relationship
- Give two examples of acceptable ways to control angry feelings
- Give three examples of what it means to be dependable

DESIRABLE PERSONAL QUALITIES OF THE NURSING ASSISTANT

As you can see, fulfilling the many responsibilities of a nursing assistant takes a special kind of person. What kind of person makes a good nursing assistant?

That question was asked of over four hundred nursing-home residents in a recent nationwide study regarding what makes up quality care and a quality environment. The *staff* was named as the number one factor in determining quality care. The residents said that they need a caring staff who are well trained and skilled. Good staff give the residents help when they need it. They give this help in a kind, courteous, and respectful manner. Residents also want staff to be friendly, cheerful, and pleasant as well as being patient and interested and taking time. Finally, they want staff who listen, take their complaints seriously, and talk to them.

Certain traits, habits, and attitudes are seen in people of all occupations who are successful in their work. Some of these traits are a part of one's personality. In other words, you have always had them. Others can be learned through practice until they become part of your personality. It's important to reflect and decide how you see yourself. How you feel about yourself really influences how you feel about others.

Sit in a quiet place and review the Personal Qualities Assessment contained in your workbook. Take time to think about these qualities and answer honestly. Place a check by the qualities you would like to develop further and describe in the space provided how you will begin. Set some time-limited goals. Review these each week and judge your progress. This is confidential information, so keep it in a private place where you can review and update it.

COMMUNICATION *Study 17-19 + 382*

In working through the Personal Qualities Assessment, did you notice how many elements dealt with some aspect of communication? One of the most important things you do as a nursing assistant is *communicate*. You communicate with residents, families, visitors, and other members of the health-care team. Most interpersonal problems that develop both at work and at home are due to a lack of communication. In order for communication to take place, three components are needed (Fig. 1.9):

- A sender
- A message
- A receiver

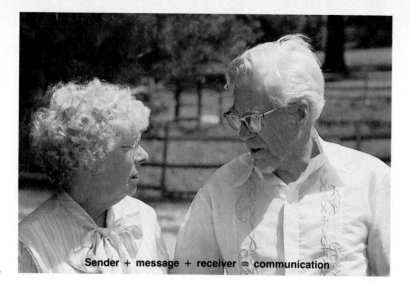

FIGURE 1-9
Elements of communication.

Sender + message + receiver = communication

If any of the three elements is missing, no communication can take place.

When communication takes place, the sender translates ideas into words. The sender also uses gestures, facial expressions, and body language to help the receiver understand the message. The receiver then translates the words and nonverbal observations back into ideas. Usually, the receiver understands what the sender wanted to convey.

Communication takes place with words as in speaking and writing or without words (nonverbal) through facial expressions, tone of voice, gestures, body position, and movement. We communicate all the time. Even as you read these words, you may be frowning with concentration, nodding with under-standing, or yawning with boredom. In fact, it is generally felt that nonverbal communication is more accurate than communicating with words because we have less ability to control our nonverbal communications.

Touch is another important form of communication. In all cultures, gentle touching conveys friendliness and affection. Studies about touch show that women are touched more than men and that the age group touched the least are persons age 66 to 100. Other studies have proved that people need to be touched. Those who are not develop both physical and emotional problems.

There is some risk involved in touching unfamiliar people for the first time. For some, touch is a sign of intimacy and closeness that is reserved for certain people. For this reason, when first meeting a new resident, ask permission or find out how the person feels about being touched. For most people, though, a warm handshake or a pat on the shoulder or the back are acceptable ways of communicating your acceptance and caring.

Communication with words is important, too. Words are symbols of ideas, objects, feelings, and actions. Unfortunately, many words have several mean-ings or mean different things to different people. Common words that teenagers use, for example, are either often misunderstood or not understood at all by their parents.

In the medical profession, words are often used that the general public does not understand. You will be learning some of this special language or jargon. Medical terminology must be used with care when communicating with resi-dents or in the presence of residents, family, and visitors. Misunderstanding could cause the resident unnecessary worry.

Another sensitive communication issue is talking in any language the resi-dent does not understand. It is improper for two staff members to speak another language in the presence or within the hearing of a resident. When the resident speaks a language the majority of the staff does not understand, it is important for the facility to locate a person who can translate and interpret for the resident.

Learn to communicate with your residents as you provide care. Avoid profanity or slang when you are in the health-care setting. Remember that your goal is to understand and to be understood.

There are some "golden rules" to help you to be a better communicator. Practice these skills at home and with friends as well as in your facility.

- Encourage the resident to express himself or herself more fully.
- Listen for the feelings being expressed, not just the words themselves.
- Avoid statements that negate the resident's feelings, such as "don't worry," "things aren't so bad," "you're really very lucky," and so on.
- Don't take away all hope but don't give false reassurances.
- When you are unsure about what a resident means, clarify by asking "Is this what you mean?" or "Do I understand you correctly?"
- Be courteous! Avoid rushing the resident, maintain good eye contact, and don't interrupt!

LISTENING SKILLS

Understanding requires good listening skills. In fact, communication can't take place without a listener or receiver. Test yourself with the questions that follow.

Are You a Good Listener?

Ask yourself if these statements apply to you.

1. I never interrupt when another person is speaking.
2. While the other person is talking, I plan what I'm going to say next.
3. I try to nod, smile, and say, "Yes, tell me more."
4. I keep a "poker face" when listening.
5. I don't judge whether a person is good or bad, right or wrong.
6. I maintain eye contact when a person is talking to me.
7. I give my complete attention to the person who is talking.
8. I usually finish the sentence when a person is unable to find the right word.

If you answered yes to 1, 3, 5, 6, and 7, you are a good listener. If you aren't satisfied with your score, improve your listening skills by practicing. In addition to understanding how to communicate, the nursing assistant needs to know when and to whom to communicate.

DEALING WITH PERSONAL INFORMATION

As you provide care, you will learn many personal and private things about the residents. Some of these are written in their health records, and some the resident, family, or visitors will reveal to you.

In addition to the legal and ethical considerations associated with confidentiality, there is a need to treat private or personal information as a gift entrusted to your care. A good rule is not to pass on any information to other people unless they have a need to know. To determine if someone has the need to know, ask yourself:

- Does the information need to be passed on because it would have some bearing on the resident's care?

- Does the person to whom I'll relate this information need it in order to plan or provide care?

Some residents will communicate information to you that no one needs to know. Gossiping about residents or their families is unethical. If what is confided to you needs to be passed on, explain to the resident, "What you've told me is very important. I must tell the charge nurse." If what you are told has no bearing on a resident's care or treatment, you will of course keep it confidential.

In an LTC facility, residents come to know each other very well. Frequently, one resident will ask you about the condition of another. Remember each resident's right to privacy and make only general comments. Do not discuss a resident's problems within hearing distance of other residents or visitors.

It is also unwise to share your personal or work-related problems with the residents. Complaints about co-workers, supervisors, or the employer are never appropriate. They may cause the resident needless worry, which affects his or her sense of safety and well-being.

COMMUNICATION WITH RESIDENTS WHO HAVE SPECIAL PROBLEMS

Some residents may seem not to hear or understand due to stroke, coma, deafness, or mental retardation, but never assume that you are not heard or understood. Treat all residents as if they can hear everything you say. Say nothing in the presence of a resident that you don't want to be heard. You may have to explain this tactfully to visitors also. Remember that at the time of death, hearing is the last sense to leave the body and may even be intensified. People who describe a "near-death" experience can often repeat every word spoken during the attempts to revive them.

In addition to not saying things you don't want the resident to hear, you must also communicate to each resident what you are going to do; for example, "I'm going to turn you on your right side now." Always explain what you are going to do, even when you aren't sure the resident understands. This may feel a little strange at first, but it's very important. You should talk to the resident as though he or she can understand and respond. In these situations, your tone of voice is also important. Never speak in a tone that would frighten the resident, and *never speak to the resident as though she or he were a child.* Terms such as "gramps," "pop," "mama," "baby," and the like should never be used unless the resident specifically asks to be addressed in that manner. All residents, regardless of their condition, need to feel that they are respected, valued members of society.

Even though the resident may not be able to communicate due to loss of hearing, stroke, or confusion, the need for communication still exists. There are some nursing measures designed to establish communication with residents who have these special problems, which you will study in another chapter.

ANSWERING THE CALL LIGHT

Answering the resident's call light is an important form of communication. It is a legal requirement that every resident have a mechanism that sends a signal, light, or bell to the nursing station. It is also necessary for residents to be able to reach the signal cord at all times. Most call systems operate so that when the button is pushed or the switch is turned on, a light flashes above the door of the resident's room and at the nursing station. The flashing light is accompanied by a signal at the nursing station such as a bell or buzzer.

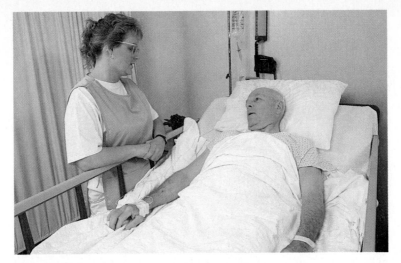

FIGURE 1-10
Answering the call light.

You must be alert and respond to the resident's call for help immediately (Fig. 1-10). To a waiting resident, every minute seems like forever. Failure to respond promptly sends a negative message to the resident.

Residents often express the fear that no one will respond if they have an emergency. In the nursing-home study conducted by interviewing nursing-home residents, the most important indicator of quality care was getting help when they need it. Answering the call light promptly is one of the most important ways you can show a resident that you care!

Caution: Some residents are unable or unwilling to use the signal cord. These residents must be checked frequently to see if they need assistance. It is a good habit to check with the resident before leaving the room and ask "Is there anything else I can do before I go?" Always be alert for cries of help or unusual sounds that would indicate that a resident is in trouble. Never ignore a cry for help.

Residents who have serious hearing or vision loss may use the signal cord differently. *Blind or visually handicapped residents always must be taught how to use the signal.* Help them locate the cord and assist them in practicing how to use it. If the signal is the kind that you push to turn on, you can call it a push button. If it works like a light switch, you can compare it to that.

Most facilities equip bathrooms and bathing areas with emergency call signals. These usually ring loudly and have a flashing red light. These indicate an emergency and must be answered *immediately* by any personnel in the area. Of course you must never jeopardize the safety of one resident to respond to the call of another. Always leave the resident in a safe place or position if you must go.

Communication is the foundation of any relationship. Relating to people means making a connection between yourself and another human being. The relationship between yourself, residents, visitors, and fellow workers depends on your approach to them. If you have a kind, courteous, tactful, sympathetic, and open manner, you will find it easier to form positive, rather than negative, relationships.

THE HELPING RELATIONSHIP

Research has been done to determine which traits are most beneficial in a helping relationship. The traits include empathy, respect, genuineness, warmth, and caring (Fig. 1-11).

Empathy is the ability to put yourself in another's place and to see things as he or she sees them.

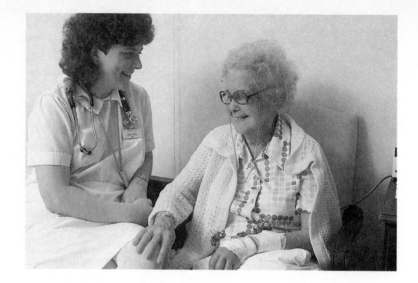

FIGURE 1-11
The helping relationship.

Respect is recognition of the worth of another person. When you respect others, you recognize their right to make up their own minds and to make good decisions.

Genuineness is simply being yourself. When your actions match what you say, you are genuine. Remember, actions speak louder than words.

Warmth is shown by demonstrating concern and affection. A nursing assistant shows warmth by the way care is given, demonstrating kindness, patience, and a gentle touch.

Caring is understanding the fears, problems, and distress of another person combined with concern and a desire to help. Caring requires action. As a nursing assistant, you can demonstrate caring in many ways: answering the call bell promptly, offering fluids to the resident, and being sure that the resident is clean and well groomed. Caring is *doing*, not just feeling.

Other personal qualities that enhance relationships with residents, visitors, and staff are courtesy, emotional control, and tact.

Behaving courteously means putting the needs of others before your own. It means cooperating, sharing, and giving. Being polite and considerate of others shows that you care about them. Putting the needs of others first may mean toning down your cheerfulness around a person who is in pain, very ill, or depressed. Or it may mean putting aside your own gloomy feelings to be more cheerful and positive. It is never appropriate to burden the residents with your personal problems. As you gain more experience in nursing, you will learn to "read" the feelings of others and to judge how you should respond.

EMOTIONAL CONTROL

Sometimes a resident, another staff member, or a visitor can upset you so much that you get angry. You may feel like making a rude or unkind remark. *Don't!* Stop and think. The resident or visitor may be worried, nervous, or tense. Fellow workers may be under extra stress because of a problem at home or on the job. Try to be understanding, and your anger will fade. Feeling angry is natural, but you should control the way anger is expressed. You have a serious obligation to control your temper. You may have to remove yourself from the situation to "cool off."

We all have different ways of "cooling off," depending on what we were taught as children and what we saw others doing. Physical activity is a common way to cope with anger. Another way that people control their anger is by talking.

Simply saying, "I am angry" really gives a great sense of relief. Both are acceptable, appropriate ways to express anger.

A nursing assistant must learn to accept criticism and constructive suggestions without becoming hurt or defensive. When your supervisor criticizes you or tells you to do something, you may feel like saying, "That is not my job," or "Why do you pick on me?" Stop, think, and examine your attitude!

Frequently, your supervisor has information that you may not be aware of. Sometimes decisions have to be based on what is best overall, not on what is best for just one person. Your understanding of that fact, as well as a cooperative attitude, will be admired and appreciated.

TACT

Tact is the ability to say or do the right thing at the right time. Every resident sees her or his own problems as being most important. Listen to their concerns. Don't judge or give advice. Everyone has a right to his or her feelings. They shouldn't be judged as right or wrong. You will learn how to help residents deal more effectively with their own feelings as you become more aware of residents' emotional needs.

All relationships are two-sided. Even though you communicate well and employ all the traits essential to a helping relationship, you may not get the response you desire. Many things influence the residents' behavior — their personality, physical health, emotional health, and life experiences. Understanding why residents respond as they do will help you accept their behavior and deal with it appropriately. You will learn more about dealing with difficult behavior in Chapter 3.

DEALING WITH FAMILIES AND VISITORS

Family and visitors often are the highlight of the day for residents. Knowing that one's family and friends are interested and concerned can relax tensions, ease feelings of loneliness and isolation, and reduce fears. Family members or visitors may be worried and upset over a resident's illness. They, too, need your kindness and patience.

You may find the following suggestions helpful when dealing with families and visitors.

- Listen to the visitor or family member. Whether it is a suggestion, a complaint, or just passing the time of day, listen! Some ideas or suggestions may be very helpful. Some complaints could be valid, others not. When a complaint is presented, try to obtain all the facts. Tell the visitor that you'll report it to the charge nurse. If it seems appropriate, take the visitor to the charge nurse so they can speak directly.
- Avoid involvement in family matters. Don't take sides in quarrels. Never give confidential information about the resident to family or visitors.
- Answer questions to the best of your ability. If you are unable or unsure of what to say, refer visitors to the charge nurse.

  Generally, there are certain rules that family and visitors are asked to follow:

- Family and visitors are not allowed to remove any facility property.
- Family and visitors are not permitted to bring food, beverages, or smoking materials to the resident without checking with the charge nurse.
- Family and visitors are not permitted to provide technical nursing services for residents.

Residents and visitors often attribute their own feelings of helplessness, anger, or guilt to others. You may have these feelings projected toward you. Try to understand and be patient, courteous, and professional, even when others are not.

ESTABLISHING A GOOD EMPLOYEE–EMPLOYER RELATIONSHIP

When you do your job to the best of your ability and work cooperatively with your fellow workers, you have taken the most important steps in establishing a good relationship with your employer (Fig. 1-12). All health-care facilities are organized to function efficiently with a certain number of people assigned to specific jobs. When employees are not dependable, everyone suffers, especially the residents.

Accuracy is part of being dependable. Accuracy means doing the right thing for the right resident at the right time in the right way. Always identify the resident before performing any nursing task. Check the resident's wrist band or photograph and verify accuracy by asking the resident his or her name (Fig. 1-13). If there is no wrist band, notify the charge nurse immediately.

Make sure you know how to do what you are assigned to do. Follow established policies and procedures to reduce errors or mistakes while providing care. If you are unsure of what to do, ask for help. Never take chances when your work deals with the welfare and safety of others.

FIGURE 1-12
What being dependable means:
- Report to work on time
- Keep absence to a minimum
- Keep promises
- Do an assigned task as well as you can, and finish it quickly, quietly, and efficiently
- Perform a task you know should be done without having to be told

FIGURE 1-13
Being accurate.

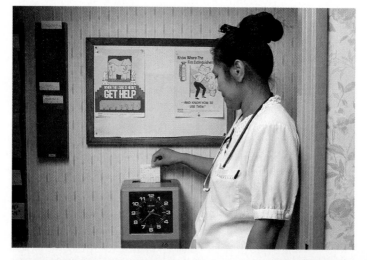

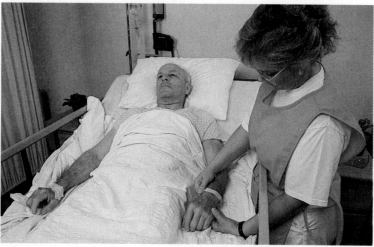

Should an error or mistake occur despite your best efforts, report the incident to your charge nurse immediately. No one is perfect, and mistakes do happen. An error becomes a serious legal issue if it is not reported and appropriate corrective actions are not taken.

SECTION 5 THE HEALTH-CARE TEAM

OBJECTIVES/WHAT YOU WILL LEARN

When you have completed this section, you will be able to:
- Describe your goal for higher or continuing education and list the steps necessary to reach that goal
- Match the members of the health-care team with their major responsibilities

THE HEALTH-CARE TEAM

The nursing assistant is an essential part of the health-care team (Fig. 1-14). You actually will provide more direct care than all the other members of the

FIGURE 1-14
Health care team.

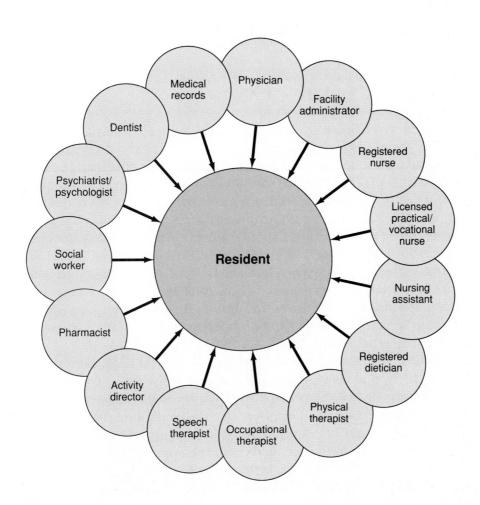

team. Teamwork is essential. Teamwork means that everyone knows what is to be done and does it to the best of her or his ability with a spirit of cooperation.

The health-care team is **multidisciplinary,** meaning that professionals with different educational backgrounds work together. They assess and evaluate the needs of the resident and together plan how to provide care and services that will meet these identified needs. The health-care plan becomes a written source of all these collected facts.

See the "Roles and Responsibilities of the Heath-Care Team" review chart provided in the workbook. You may be interested in learning more about some of the different professions. You can obtain additional information regarding educational requirements, prerequisites, and locations of programs by writing to the professional organizations listed. Request information specifically for the state in which you plan to continue your education since programs differ from state to state.

Being a nursing assistant is an important job in itself. However, if you find your work enjoyable and rewarding, consider continuing your education in the field of nursing. If you do not have a high school diploma, that should be your first goal. Local high schools offer basic education programs that lead to a high school equivalency diploma.

LTC facilities also have organized inservice education or staff development programs. In general, this department is responsible for:

- Orientation of new employees
- Providing continuing education for licensed and nonlicensed nursing personnel (often called inservice)
- Organizing, planning, and implementing nursing assistant training programs
- Bedside teaching, demonstrating nursing-care procedures, and supervising return demonstrations
- Classroom teaching and testing
- Providing instruction in the use of hospital equipment and supplies

Federal regulations now require special training for all nursing assistants employed in a LTC facility. Each state adopts and establishes its own nursing assistant certification program which meets the requirements of the federal program (OBRA). The program requires a specific number of hours of classroom or theory attendance and a specific number of hours of clinical or bedside practice. Some programs allow you to take a test and demonstrate skills instead of requiring hours. Training may be offered by the LTC facilities, public educational institutions, and private vocational schools. Some states also require nursing assistants to attend a certain number of hours of continuing education each year. Be sure you know what your state requires, and plan time to seek out new learning experiences.

The job of the nursing assistant carries with it great responsibility for the health, safety, and comfort of other human beings. When you fulfill this responsibility, you will enjoy many rewards. The satisfaction of giving your best, the appreciation of your employer, and the gratitude of the residents and their families all contribute to a positive feeling. It is a good feeling to help those who are sick, lonely, frightened, and confused toward a better quality of life. Knowing that even one person is better off because of your efforts means you have fulfilled your role and responsibilities as a nursing assistant.

CHAPTER 2

Your Working Environment

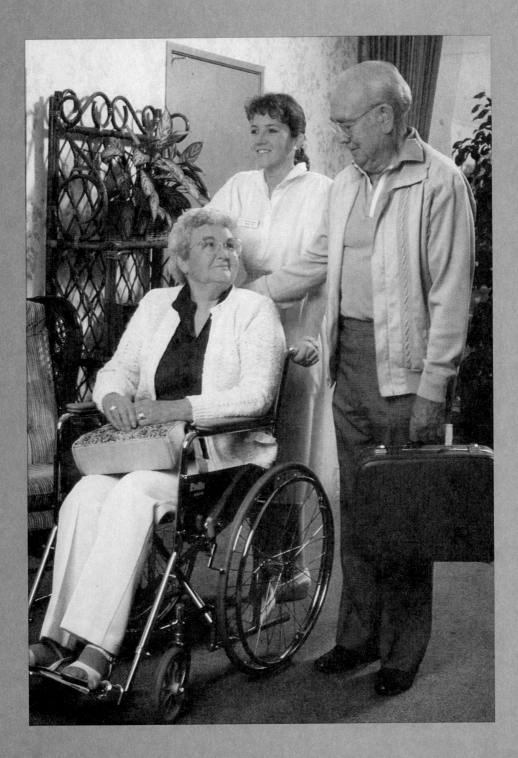

OBJECTIVES/WHAT YOU WILL LEARN

When you have completed this section you will be able to:

- Give four examples of the ways the nursing assistant helps to prevent residents from falling
- Select three ways the nursing assistant can help to prevent residents from being burned
- Demonstrate the application of a soft protective device
- Identify situations in which protective devices may be used
- Define *gravity, center of gravity,* and *base of support*
- Recognize safety hazards
- Demonstrate lifting an object using proper body mechanics

PROVIDING A SAFE ENVIRONMENT

Providing a safe environment is the responsibility of each facility employee (Fig. 2-1). You must always protect the welfare and safety of each resident. To do this, you must be alert to potential hazards and take appropriate action as necessary to prevent accidents and injuries.

Falls in health-care facilities account for almost 70 percent of all resident-related accidents! These falls occur most often at peak activity times such as mealtimes, bedtimes, and at change of shift. You can help prevent falls by:

- Answering the call light promptly so that residents who require assistance do not attempt to get out of bed without your help.
- Properly positioning residents in bed and wheelchairs, as well as using soft protective vests or seat belts when necessary.
- Following facility policies and procedures regarding the side rails. In general, side rails should be locked in the "up"position at night unless your charge nurse instructs you differently.
- Making sure that wheelchairs, beds, stretchers, and commodes have brakes locked when transferring residents.
- Keeping frequently needed articles within easy reach of the resident, such as water, bedpans, call signal cord, and TV control.
- Making sure that the bed adjustment **gatch** (handle) is positioned "in" to avoid tripping over it.
- Removing any obstacle from floors and seeing that spills are wiped up immediately to prevent slipping.
- Reporting to your charge nurse your observations that a resident is prone to falling, unsteady, dizzy, slides out of a wheelchair, or climbs out of bed.
- Reporting any building hazards immediately, such as loose floor tiles or carpeting, loose or broken hand rails, and leaks in bathroom and shower areas.
- Reporting broken or malfunctioning equipment immediately. Always use facility equipment according to written policies and procedures.

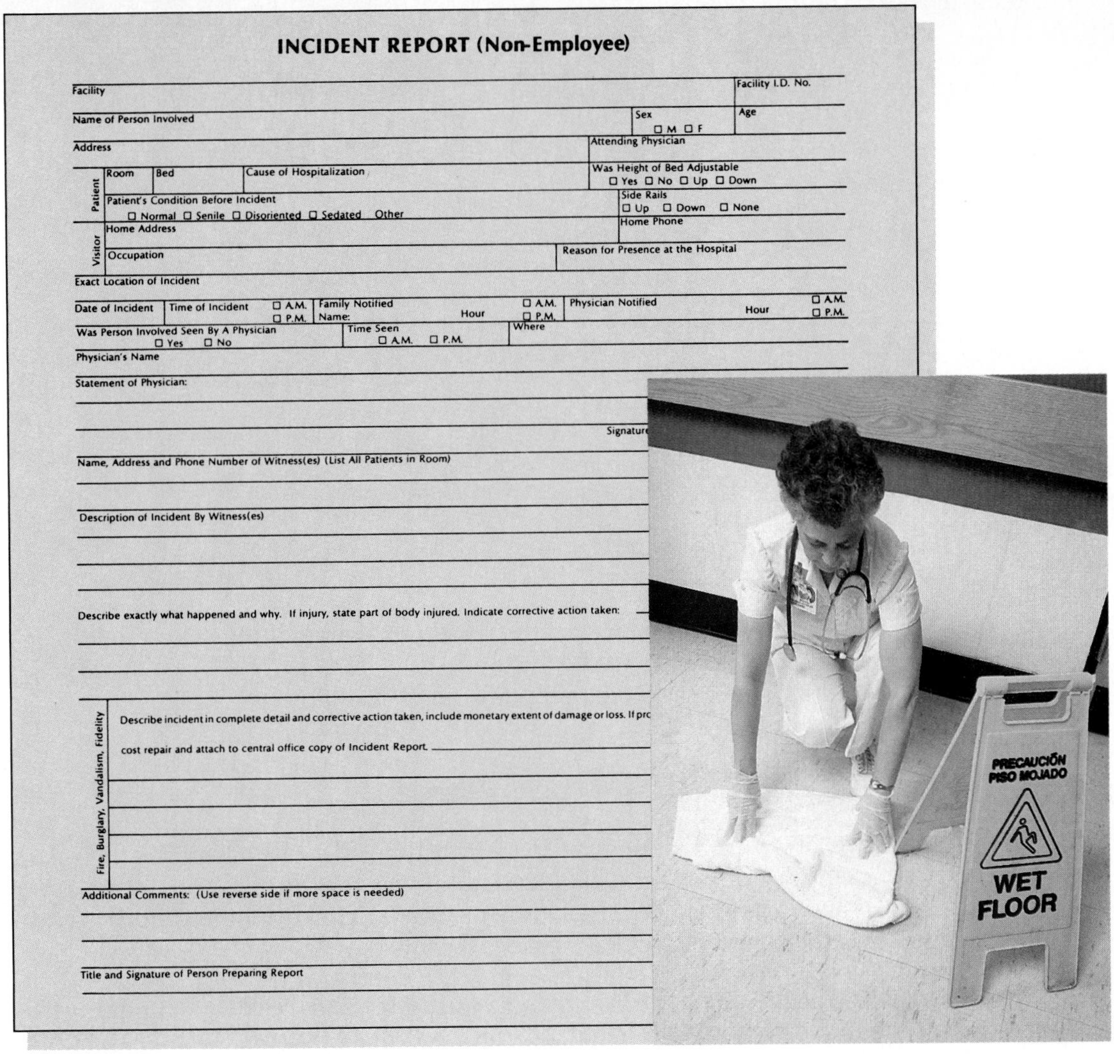

INCIDENT REPORT (Non-Employee)

Facility	Facility I.D. No.

Name of Person Involved	Sex ☐ M ☐ F	Age

Address	Attending Physician

Patient

Room	Bed	Cause of Hospitalization	Was Height of Bed Adjustable ☐ Yes ☐ No ☐ Up ☐ Down

Patient's Condition Before Incident
☐ Normal ☐ Senile ☐ Disoriented ☐ Sedated   Other
Side Rails ☐ Up ☐ Down ☐ None

Visitor

Home Address — Home Phone

Occupation — Reason for Presence at the Hospital

Exact Location of Incident

Date of Incident	Time of Incident ☐ A.M. ☐ P.M.	Family Notified Name: Hour ☐ A.M. ☐ P.M.	Physician Notified Hour ☐ A.M. ☐ P.M.

Was Person Involved Seen By A Physician ☐ Yes ☐ No | Time Seen ☐ A.M. ☐ P.M. | Where

Physician's Name

Statement of Physician:

Signature

Name, Address and Phone Number of Witness(es) (List All Patients in Room)

Description of Incident By Witness(es)

Describe exactly what happened and why. If injury, state part of body injured. Indicate corrective action taken:

Fire, Burglary, Vandalism, Fidelity
Describe incident in complete detail and corrective action taken, include monetary extent of damage or loss. If prc cost repair and attach to central office copy of Incident Report.

Additional Comments: (Use reverse side if more space is needed)

Title and Signature of Person Preparing Report

FIGURE 2-1
Being alert to potential hazards.

PREVENTING BURNS

Burns are the second most common hazard to residents in a health-care facility. Many residents have a decreased awareness of sensations of pain and temperature. The resident may not realize that the water is too hot. Some experience burns of the mouth from hot coffee without noticing. You can help prevent burns by:

- Checking water temperatures before placing residents in bath or shower.
- Reporting water temperatures that seem too hot in residents' rooms, showers, or bathing areas.
- Knowing the major causes of facility fires and practicing prevention.
- Constantly monitoring residents, visitors, and other employees to ensure safe smoking practices (Fig. 2-2). Report any violation of smoking rules to your charge nurse immediately. Remember, smoking is permitted only in designated smoking areas.
- Providing necessary assistance to residents with meals to avoid spilling hot liquids.

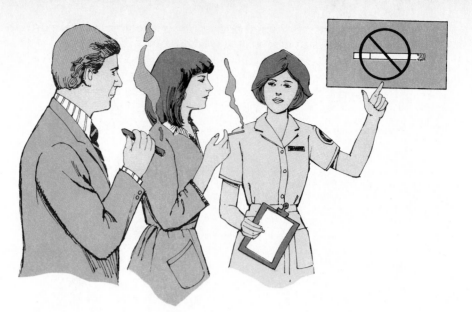

FIGURE 2-2
Ensuring safe smoking
practices.

- Using facility equipment (heating pads, heat lamps, hot packs, etc.) according to written policies.
- Protecting residents from overexposure to sunlight.

PREVENTING OTHER INJURIES

Residents of the LTC facility are frequently dependent on others for their care due to illness, confusion, disabilities, and even the effects of medication. For these reasons, you must be safety conscious at all times (Fig. 2-3). You can help prevent other types of accidents or injuries by:

- Making sure no harmful substances are left where residents might ingest them, for example, cleaning solutions, Clinitest/Acetest equipment, lighter fluids, fingernail polish remover, unauthorized medications, insect sprays, or powders.
- Being alert to the potential hazards of swinging doors or doors opening into rooms or corridors.
- Moving equipment, wheelchairs, food carts, scales, and stretchers safely around corners.

FIGURE 2-3
Being safety conscious at all
times.

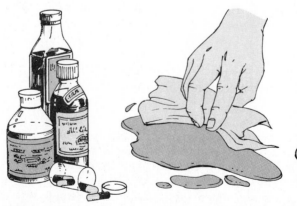

Keep harmful substances
away from residents

Wipe up spills immediately

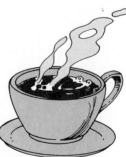

Use caution
when serving
hot foods
or liquids

- Being very careful of the feet when transporting residents in wheelchairs. Position feet on foot rests so that they are not in contact with the floor.
- Monitoring residents who may wander away. Special problems should be reported to the charge nurse immediately.
- Reporting immediately any observations that would lead you to believe that a resident is a danger to himself or others.
- Following the instructions of your charge nurse when providing care. Many times the physician gives special orders that must be carried out or harm could come to the resident:

> No weight bearing
> Keep head of bed elevated at all times
> Do not position resident on right side
> May be out of bed with assistance only

Failure to follow physician orders has *serious legal consequences* and could cause harm to the resident.

USE OF PROTECTIVE DEVICES

Many resident accidents can be avoided when soft protective devices are used and applied properly (Fig. 2-4). You will need to practice the correct application of these devices. A soft protective device is often called a **postural support** or restraint. A restraint holds back or limits a resident's movements. When you

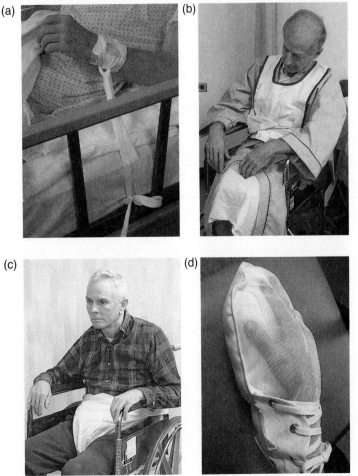

FIGURE 2-4
Soft protective devices:
(a) soft limb tie, (b) safety vest, (c) pelvic support, (d) soft cloth mitten.

restrain residents for any reason, you are infringing on their rights as individuals. For this reason, a protective device can be used *only under special conditions:*

- To protect residents from injury, such as falling from a wheelchair or out of bed
- To protect residents during treatment, such as tube feedings, intravenous therapy, or catheterization
- To keep residents from injuring themselves or others

Remember, when any type of protective device is used to restrain a resident, the physician must have given an order for its use. Postural supports include:

- Soft limb ties, used to keep a limb immobilized.
- Vest support or crossover jacket, put on like a jacket to provide postural support in a wheelchair and limit mobility of upper body in bed.
- Pelvic support, used between the thighs to keep a resident's hips from slipping forward. Special precautions must be used to prevent pressure on male genitalia.
- Soft cloth mittens, a mitt that limits mobility of hands and fingers. Used for residents who could harm themselves by pulling at dressings or scratching.
- Seat belts, a belt around a resident's waist to prevent falls from a wheelchair.

Residents who require restraints must be observed at least once every 1 to 2 hours. Check the restraint to be sure that it is not too tight and that proper circulation is maintained. Also check to see if the resident is comfortable and good body alignment is present. Make sure that the residents' special needs for hydration, toileting, and personal care are met.

A restraint *must* be released every 1 to 2 hours to allow a resident to change positions, exercise, and have periods of unrestricted movement. Gentle massage and application of lotion can help the resident relax before the restraint is reapplied.

No one likes to be confined or restrained! Restraints *must* only be used as a last resort to protect the welfare and safety of the resident or to protect others from a resident who poses a threat to them. Restraints must *never* be used as a form of punishment. Remember, use of a restraint takes away a resident's right to freedom and violates his or her right to be treated with respect and dignity.

When a resident is considered to be at high risk for falling or injury to self or others, various alternatives to the use of restraints need to be considered:

- Placing the resident in an area where he or she can be observed and monitored — near the nursing station or dining room.
- Encourage residents to participate in meaningful activities and social events.
- Pay close attention to residents' special needs and give them help when they need it (for example, answering the call light promptly).
- Establish a toileting routine for each resident, and follow it.
- Keep needed personal items within easy reach.
- Assist residents in changing positions and comfort measures often.
- Offer fluids and between-meal snacks and nourishments.
- Take extra time to give residents special attention.
- Encourage families and volunteers to take residents on outings.

When protective devices are used, follow these guidelines:

- Always approach the resident in a calm manner, regardless of his behavior.
- Explain to the resident (and family and visitors, if present) who you are and what you are going to do. Use terms that stress the protective nature of the restraint, such as "safety belt," and "postural support." In the case of restraints used for certain treatments, say, "This wrist tie is to help remind you not to pull the catheter out."
- Residents should never be restrained in chairs without wheels. In the event of fire or other emergency, you must be able to move and transport residents quickly.
- When restraining a resident in a chair, tie the restraint under the chair, out of the reach of the resident, rather than tying elaborate knots that are difficult to untie in an emergency.
- When you use any form of protective device, be sure the resident is properly aligned and comfortably positioned (see Chapter 8). Make sure the resident is protected from pressure caused by knots, wrinkles, or buckles.
- Pad bony prominences under the device to reduce pressure and prevent trauma (see Chapter 6).
- Protective devices should be applied snugly without binding. (You should be able to slip two fingers under the edges of the device after tying.) Never restrict movement, and never impair or stop circulation. Signs of restricted circulation include:

  Complaints of numbness or tingling
  Change in skin color (pale, blue)
  Change in skin temperature (cold)
  Swelling
  Complaints of pain

  Note: Never use a "slip knot." It can tighten with movement and restrict circulation.

- Never tie restraints to side rails or a part of the bed that would cause tightening when the position of the head or foot of the bed is changed.
- Always make sure the resident can reach and use the call light when restraints are in place.

Another way to help reduce falls is to assist residents with daily exercise designed to build muscle tone and increase strength — this will help with both walking balance and endurance. It is important to be sure that residents have properly fitted shoes with nonskid soles, and that the environment is free of obstacles and spills.

REPORTING RESIDENT INCIDENTS

Sometimes, despite our best efforts, accidents or incidents occur. Whenever an incident occurs involving a resident, an "incident report" must be written. This is true even if the resident was not injured. If you see a resident slip from a chair, find a resident on the floor, or observe any type of accident, you must report it to your charge nurse immediately so that emergency treatment and an incident report can be initiated.

BODY MECHANICS

Body mechanics refers to special ways of standing and moving one's body. The purpose of using good body mechanics is to maximize your strength, minimize fatigue, and, most important, avoid back strain and injury. When you understand basic principles of movement, you can make a conscious effort to use good body mechanics as you provide care.

Gravity is the attraction that the earth has for an object on or near the earth's surface. It is the force of gravity that keeps us on the ground instead of floating in space.

Everything has a **center of gravity** where the mass or the bulk of the object is concentrated (Fig. 2-5). Any object or person that is suspended from its center of gravity stays in balance without tipping or turning. The lower or closer the center of gravity is to earth, the more stable an object becomes.

Another term related to body mechanics is **base of support.** This is the base or foundation of an object or person. For example, when a person stands, the feet are the base of support. When the base of support is broadened, any object or person becomes better balanced and stabilized. If you stand with your feet very close together and someone tries to push you over, you can be pushed off balance very easily. As you spread your feet apart, your balance improves.

Rules to follow for good body mechanics are:

- When an action requires physical effort, try to use as many muscles or groups of muscles as possible. For example, use both hands rather than one hand to pick up a heavy object.
- Use good posture. Keep your body aligned properly. Keep your back straight. Have your knees bent. Keep your weight evenly balanced on both feet.

FIGURE 2-5
The line of gravity passes through the center of gravity and the base of support.

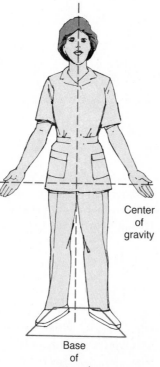

Center
of
gravity

Base
of
support

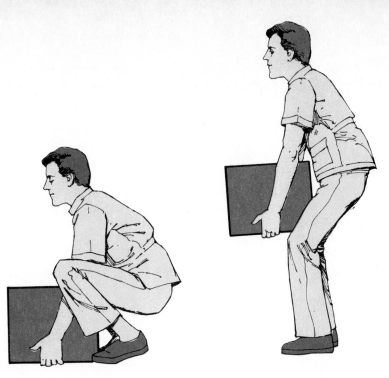

FIGURE 2-6
Lifting an object properly.

- Check your feet when you are going to lift something. They should be 12 inches apart. This will give you a broad base of support and good balance.
- When you have to move a heavy object, push or roll it rather than lifting and carrying it.
- Use your arms to support the object. The muscles of your legs actually do the job of lifting, not the muscles of your back (Fig. 2-6).
- When you are doing work such as giving a back rub, making the bed, or moving the patient, work with the direction of your efforts. Avoid twisting your body as much as you can.

GUIDELINES FOR LIFTING

When you lift an object, use good body mechanics:
- Bend your knees and get close to the load.
- Keep your back straight.
- Grip the object firmly with both hands.
- Lift by pushing up with your strong leg muscles.
- If you think you may not be able to lift the load or it seems too large or heavy, get help.
- Lift smoothly to avoid strain. Always count "one, two, three" with the person you are working with, or say "ready" and "go" so you work together. Do this with both the resident and with other nursing assistants.
- Pivot (turn) with your feet.
- Turn with short steps.
- Turn your whole body without twisting your back and neck

OBJECTIVES/WHAT YOU WILL LEARN

When you have completed this section, you will be able to:

- List the three things necessary to start a fire
- List four major causes of fires in LTC facilities
- Complete a fire prevention inspection checklist for the facility where you are working or receiving clinical instruction
- Given a situation in which there is a fire, describe the correct sequence of steps to be taken
- Explain why a nursing assistant needs to know disaster plans before a disaster occurs

MAJOR CAUSES OF FIRE

Most people are aware of the dangers of fire, yet every year thousands die from fire-related causes. This occurs, to some extent, because people are not well informed regarding the causes of fire.

The Major Causes of Fire

- Smoking and matches
- Defects in heating systems
- Improper rubbish disposal
- Misuse of electricity
- Spontaneous ignition

As a nursing assistant, you are responsible to see that residents, visitors, and employees follow the facility's smoking policies. Your facility has designated smoking areas. Know where they are and politely explain to residents and visitors where smoking is permitted or is not permitted. If the rules are not followed, report these violations to your charge nurse immediately. Obviously, you and your fellow employees must always adhere to the smoking rules.

The best way to handle a fire is to prevent it! Fire prevention is aimed at keeping three elements from coming together at the same time or place. These elements are: fuel, heat, and oxygen (Fig. 2-7). Because oxygen is always present, the other two elements must be controlled.

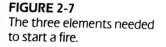

FIGURE 2-7
The three elements needed to start a fire.

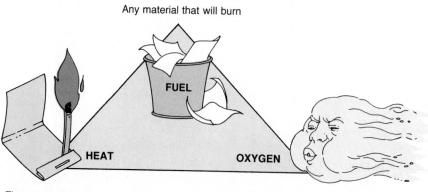

Any material that will burn

FUEL

HEAT

OXYGEN

Flame, sparks

Normal air

Ashtrays are potential fire hazards. A safe ashtray is made of a substance that will not burn. Never allow anyone to use paper cups or plates, trash containers, or plastic bags as ashtrays. Ashtrays must *never* be emptied into trash containers.

A resident's clothing may be ignited accidentally by a lighter, match, or hot ashes. Residents must be evaluated by licensed nurses to determine whether or not they are safely able to handle and keep smoking materials. For some residents, a "smoker's apron" may be needed. These fireproof aprons protect the resident and clothing from burns. Residents who are weak, confused, or taking certain medication may be dangerous to themselves and others and are not permitted to keep their own smoking materials. Sometimes families, visitors, or other residents will give smoking materials to residents. If the resident is not permitted to keep these items, explain politely, and ask them to give the materials to the charge nurse for safekeeping.

Misuse of electricity is the second most common cause of fire (Fig. 2-8). You can help prevent electrical fires by:

- Checking appliances for frayed wires, loose connections, or defective plugs before use. Report problems immediately.
- Not overloading circuits or overheating equipment.
- Using extension cords safely. Never place extension cords under rugs or drapes where they can become worn and cause a spark.
- Checking plugs to ensure that they have three plugs, for grounding.

Defects in heating systems represent the third most common cause of fires. It is generally the responsibility of the Maintenance Department to ensure that the heating system is operating safely. However, you must be alert and report dirty heating outlets, vents, or smoke coming from any vent immediately.

Spontaneous combustion (ignition of burnable materials caused by a chemical reaction) may occur when dirty, oily rags are placed in poorly ventilated spaces or closets. Be alert. If you smell something burning, investigate! If the door to a closet or storage area is hot, *never open it.* This would cause the fire to spread. Report this potential fire immediately!

When trash and rubbish are not properly disposed of, a fire hazard is created. Aerosol cans require special handling as they can rupture and create flying metal if incinerated. Aerosol cans should never be sprayed in the presence of an open flame or lighted cigarette. Make sure you understand how to dispose of trash in your facility.

OXYGEN SAFETY

Remember, oxygen is one of the three elements necessary to start a fire. Oxygen does not burn, but an oxygen-rich atmosphere will intensify the burning of ordinary combustibles. For this reason smoking is *never* permitted where oxygen is being administered or stored. Some facilities use oxygen concentrators

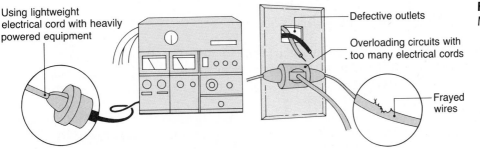

Using lightweight electrical cord with heavily powered equipment

Defective outlets

Overloading circuits with too many electrical cords

Frayed wires

FIGURE 2-8
Misuses of electricity.

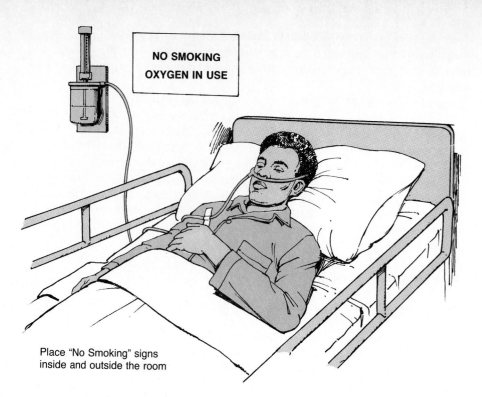

NO SMOKING
OXYGEN IN USE

FIGURE 2-9
Safety precautions for oxygen.

Place "No Smoking" signs inside and outside the room

which take room air and deliver concentrated oxygen to the resident. It is best to follow the same guidelines regardless of whether an oxygen cylinder is used or wall oxygen is administered:

- Post "NO SMOKING, Oxygen in Use" signs on the resident's door and at the bedside (Fig. 2-9).
- Check with your charge nurse before using any electrical equipment in the presence of oxygen. This includes electric razors, fans, radios, and TV sets.
- Never use flammable liquids such as alcohol, nail polish remover, or paint thinner in the oxygen-rich environment.
- Make sure the oxygen cylinder is secured with a chain to prevent it from falling to the floor.

As a nursing assistant, you have a serious responsibility to:

- Understand the nature of fire.
- Recognize fire hazards.
- Practice fire prevention as you provide care.

FIRE SAFETY PLANNING

When a fire occurs, you must act immediately. This is not the time to find out where the fire alarms are located or to learn how to use fire extinguishers or to review fire exit routes. You must be prepared through fire safety planning (Fig. 2-10).

In case of fire, you must decide: Do I start rescue or set off the alarm first? One way to help you remember the proper steps to follow is the word *RACE*. It stands for rescue, alert (or alarm), confine, and extinguish (put out the fire.)

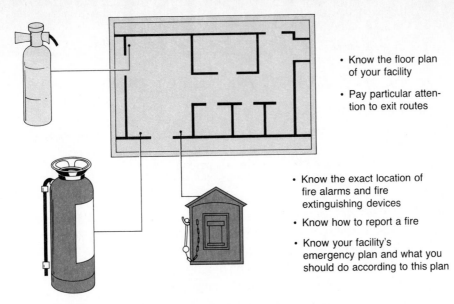

- Know the floor plan of your facility
- Pay particular attention to exit routes

- Know the exact location of fire alarms and fire extinguishing devices
- Know how to report a fire
- Know your facility's emergency plan and what you should do according to this plan

FIGURE 2-10
Fire safety planning.

Follow your facility's emergency fire procedures in a calm, efficient manner. Panic worsens any emergency. Follow the directions of your charge nurse. Lives can be lost if staff members fail to respond quickly and efficiently!

Your facility will hold special classes in fire safety, and you will participate in practice drills. Complete the fire prevention checklist provided in your workbook. Pay close attention so that if a fire emergency occurs, you will be prepared to respond appropriately.

The time to learn your facility's disaster plan is now. When a disaster occurs, it is too late! It is common to hear survivors of a disaster express regret and grief that they were not well enough prepared or informed to act efficiently. Every nursing assistant must know what to do in the event of a disaster!

GUIDELINES FOR DISASTER PREPAREDNESS

Facilities must always be prepared to cope with a disaster. A disaster is some type of catastrophe. It can be natural in origin, such as a flood, tornado, or earthquake, or it could be of human origin, such as an airplane crash, fire, or explosion. The threat of disaster is always present. Disasters don't just happen to others! Most facilities have disaster plans, and they practice disaster procedures on a regular basis. The most important points to remember in a disaster situation are:

- *First*, remove residents from immediate danger.
- Report to appropriate persons within the facility or other agencies, such as the fire department, police department, Red Cross, Civil Defense, nearest hospital, and so on.
- Follow the directions of the persons in charge.
- Evacuate the building, removing ambulatory, wheelchair, and bedfast residents, if instructed.
- Assist in organizing and monitoring residents when moving them to an appropriate shelter.
- Remove and secure necessary equipment, supplies, and records.
- Assist in the emergency record-keeping system.
- Think before you act. Make good use of your hands, feet, time, and energy. Don't be careless!
- Help lessen confusion by behaving in a calm, confident manner.

OBJECTIVES/WHAT YOU WILL LEARN

When you have completed this section, you will be able to:

- Define the terms *organism, microorganism, pathogenic, nonpathogenic,* and *aseptic*
- List five ways that microorganisms are spread
- List four signs of infection
- Define the terms *isolation, disinfection,* and *sterilization*
- Identify which areas are considered clean and which are considered dirty
- Give two examples of materials that are considered infectious waste
- Demonstrate proper handwashing technique
- Demonstrate proper linen-handling procedures
- Describe the three rules of universal precautions
- List the materials to which univeral precautions apply
- Explain when gloves are to be worn

INFECTION CONTROL

One of the most important aspects of environmental safety is infection control. All health-care facilities must establish infection-control programs. Each facility must have an infection-control committee to write and approve policies and procedures and to monitor the infection-control program. As a nursing assistant, you have responsibility to understand and to follow your facility's infection-control policies and procedures. By doing so, you protect the residents, yourself and your family, and your fellow workers from the possibility of acquiring an infection.

Some important terms related to infection control are:

- **Organism** — any living thing
- **Microorganisms** (commonly called germs) — tiny living things seen only with a microscope (Fig. 2-11)
- **Pathogenic** — causing disease
- **Nonpathogenic** — not capable of producing disease
- **Infection** — invasion of the body by a disease-producing (pathogenic) organism
- **Aseptic** — free of microorganisms

FIGURE 2-11
Microorganisms.

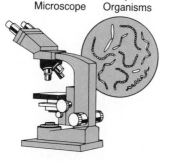

Micro Organisms

Microscope   Organisms

Microorganisms are everywhere — in the food we eat, the air we breathe, the water we drink, on objects we touch, and inside and outside our bodies. We are always in the presence of disease-producing microorganisms. Fortunately, the body has protective mechanisms to help us resist infection. The skin is one of the most important. If it is cut or injured, the person has a high risk of developing an infection. The mucous lining of the mouth and nose also helps to trap foreign substances and prevent infection. The body's immune system is designed to fight the invasion. Despite the body's defense system, all of us have experienced illness related to an infection:

- Common cold
- Influenza (flu)
- Infection of a cut or wound
- Mumps, measles, chickenpox
- Skin eruptions
- Athlete's foot

The microorganisms that produce disease in humans are classified as follows (Fig. 2-12):

- Bacteria
- Viruses
- Fungi (including yeast and mold)
- Protozoa
- Rickettsia
- Parasitic worms

BACTERIA

The most important (according to the frequency of occurrence) are the bacteria and viruses. However, each classification has groups that can cause acute illness.

Two types of *harmful* bacteria that are present in health-care facilities are *Staphylococcus* and *Streptococcus*. When these bacteria invade the body, they cause serious disease and illness. As a nursing assistant, you will come in contact with these and many other disease-producing microorganisms. When you understand how microorganisms are spread and what conditions affect the growth of bacteria, you will be better prepared to take special precautions (Fig. 2-13).

You can help reduce the **incidence** (number of occurrences) of bacterial infections when you pay careful attention to the resident's personal hygiene and skin care needs and when you help keep the residents' units clean and free from the conditions that promote bacterial growth.

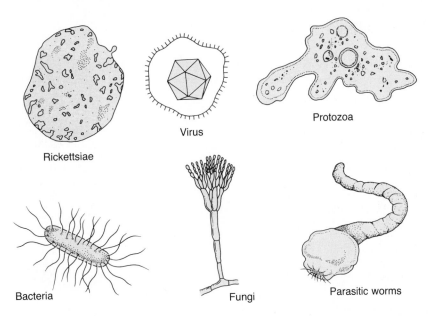

Rickettsiae

Virus

Protozoa

Bacteria

Fungi

Parasitic worms

FIGURE 2-12
Six major microorganisms known to cause diseases in humans.

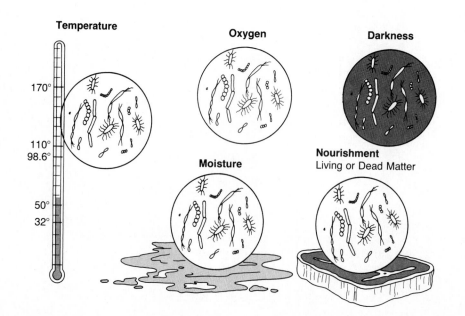

Direct contact	Touching the resident Rubbing the resident Bathing the resident Secretion from resident Urine from resident Feces from resident
Indirect contact	Touching objects Dishes Bed linen Clothing Instruments Belongings
Droplet spread within three feet	Sneezing Coughing Talking

Vehicle	Contaminated
	  Food
	  Drugs
	  Water or blood

Airborne transmission	Dust particles and moisture in the air

FIGURE 2-13
Ways that microorganisms are spread.

Bacteria are known to survive best in an environment that is warm, dark, and moist which contains both oxygen and nourishment (Fig. 2-14). Nourishment may be living or dead matter.

Specific drugs are known to kill specific bacteria. When infection occurs, the physician will order a sample of wound drainage or a scraping or swabbing of the infected area to be studied. This is called a **culture.** When the *bacterium* (singular of *bacteria*) is identified, the physician will order the proper drug known to kill that specific bacterium. These drugs are called *antibiotics*.

It is important to know that not all bacteria are harmful. For example, certain bacteria are responsible for the chemical changes that produce cheese,

FIGURE 2-14
Conditions that promote bacterial growth.

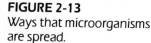

yogurt, sauerkraut, and alcohol. There are also "normal" or nonpathogenic bacteria that live and serve a necessary purpose in the human body. The bacterium called *Escherichia coli*, for example, is normally found in the intestinal tract. Here it assists in breaking down unused food particles, turning them into stool or **feces** (solid human waste). *E. coli* is **pathogenic** (disease producing), however, when it enters other areas of the body such as the urinary tract, as can happen when an individual wipes or cleans himself improperly, or when feces enter an open sore.

VIRUSES

Viruses generally are more difficult to treat because the drug must kill the virus without destroying the body cell in which the virus lives. For this reason, there are no drugs available to use against all viral infections. Vaccines have been developed that are effective against some specific viruses. Examples are measles, polio, and influenza vaccines.

Most disease-producing microorganisms release waste products known as **toxins** that act like poison in the body. The body's immune system tries to fight the toxins. When this occurs, the common signs and symptoms associated with infection are present:

- Drainage from wounds, eyes, ears, nose
- Reddened or inflamed areas
- Increased heat in an area
- Fever or chills
- Pain
- Swelling

Be alert for these signs and symptoms in your residents and report them promptly to the charge nurse. Elderly residents differ from children and adults in that they may not have a fever even though a serious infection is present. It is important to act upon the reported feelings and complaints of the resident.

PRINCIPLES OF INFECTION CONTROL

All infection-control programs are meant to:

- Protect residents, employees, families, and visitors from acquiring an infection from someone else (called **cross-infection**)
- Protect residents who have had an infection from becoming infected a second time (called **reinfection**)
- Provide residents, employees, and visitors with a safe environment that is as free as possible of pathogenic organisms (called **environmental control**)

Some basic terms associated with an infection-control program are:

- **Isolation** — to separate or set apart. Efforts are made to separate infectious residents and their belongings from others. Special procedures must be followed in handling these residents and their linen, trash, food trays, and personal belongings. There is a constant effort to avoid contact with infectious microorganisms by taking extra precautions. The kind of precautions necessary depend on the microorganisms causing the infection and how that type of infection is spread. For this reason, there are several different types of isolation. You will learn isolation procedures later in this chapter.
- **Disinfection** — the process of killing *most* microorganisms with a

6. The person standing at the door carefully secures the filled bag by tying or sealing and disposes of the contaminated trash, linen, or reusable equipment according to the facility's policies for disposal of infectious waste and handling of contaminated linens or equipment. The double-bagging procedure generally is done at the end of each shift.

• Place linen in laundry bag inside isolation unit

• Place any contaminated item in appropiate container inside isolation unit

• Seal bag

• Place sealed bag inside another bag, outside the isolation unit

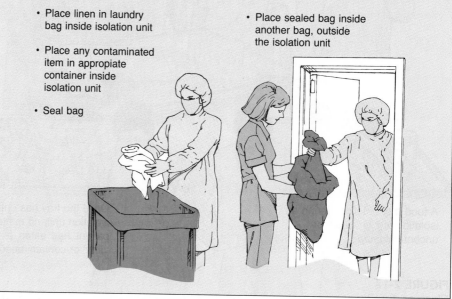

The double-bagging technique should always be used when removing specimens, linen, trash, and other contaminated articles from the isolation room.

Some residents in isolation require special precautions to be taken when handling articles contaminated with urine or feces. For example, it may be necessary to disinfect a bedpan each time the resident uses it. It is very important to clarify all instructions for isolation techniques with your charge nurse to ensure your own safety as well as that of the residents and personnel!

Remember, diseases are caused by microorganisms, and the spread of disease is greatly reduced by keeping everything clean. Being extra careful to avoid contamination is a way of keeping the environment safe. The most important measure you can take to reduce the chance of spreading disease and infection is to *wash your hands before and after contact with residents* and to *follow the isolation procedures carefully!*

SPECIAL NEEDS OF THE RESIDENT IN ISOLATION

The resident in isolation needs the same personal care as any other resident. It is very important to combine normal nursing care with good isolation technique. These tasks should be performed in your usual pleasant and supportive style. Make it clear that it is the disease-causing microorganisms that are unwanted, not the resident.

Residents in isolation may experience feelings of loneliness and anxiety. The entire staff must see that they are not deprived of contact with others. The need for touch, communication, and stimulation still exists. The resident should be provided with TV, radio, books, or magazines if appropriate. Visitors should be encouraged, although they must follow isolation techniques. Make a special effort to spend time with the isolated resident.

AIDS

One communicable disease that is a matter of great concern to the public and the health-care field is AIDS (acquired immune deficiency syndrome). AIDS is a condition in which the body's immune system is damaged by attack from a virus (HIV). When the immune system is damaged, the body cannot fight infection. This creates an opportunity for many other microorganisms to survive in the body. These organisms take advantage of a diseased immune system, resulting in the development of **opportunistic infections.** Examples of opportunistic infections include pneumocystis pneumonia, candidiasis, cryptococcosis, herpes, and cancers such as Kaposi's sarcoma and lymphomas (Fig. 2-18). AIDS is often first suspected because of the existence of one of these opportunistic infections.

At the present time the victim eventually dies as a result of one of the opportunistic infections. Because the disease is terminal, there has been an enormous amount of research on the subject. Every case that is identified is studied thoroughly. Independent research conducted throughout the world has resulted in consistent findings. Because of this research, the ways that AIDS is transmitted are well established.

AIDS is transmitted through sexual contact, needle and syringe sharing, from an infected mother to her unborn child, and blood transfusions (prior to the time the AIDS antibody test was developed and routinely used to screen blood). There must be some way for the virus to be passed from an infected person to the bloodstream of another person. AIDS is not transmitted through normal contact with strangers, family members, friends, or health-care workers — except if there is sexual or needle contact with an infected person. Current research shows that AIDS cannot be contracted from coughing, sneezing, touching, or using dishes and utensils in common. Health-care workers are considered to be at low risk for the disease. The only documented cases where health-care workers who were not part of a high-risk group were infected involved exposure to infected blood combined with breaks in the skin of the health-care worker.

There is a blood test that identifies those who have been exposed to the virus by measuring the presence of antibodies against the virus. Although the test is not 100 percent accurate, it has effectively protected the nation's blood supply by screening donors since 1985.

The blood test does not diagnose the disease itself or predict whether the person will actually develop AIDS. At present it is not known whether everyone who tests positive will develop the disease. The time between infection with the virus and onset of the first symptoms of AIDS is thought to be as much as five years, though it may be less.

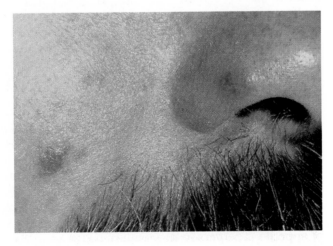

FIGURE 2-18
Lesions caused by Kaposis sarcoma on face of AIDS victim.

There are many different room sizes and arrangements, from private rooms to two, three, or more residents to a room. Regardless of the number of residents sharing a room, each needs his or her own "space."

For the majority of residents, the LTC facility is their home. Every effort should be made to create a homelike environment. Although certain items are basic, residents are encouraged to bring personal items, including pictures, furniture, and plants. A clock and a calendar will help the resident remain oriented to time and date. When you enter a resident's unit, try to imagine that you are entering their home. Ask permission, particularly if the door is closed or the curtain is drawn. "May I come in?" is a question that shows the residents you respect their privacy and recognize the unit as their own. You'll notice that when two or three residents share a room, they frequently draw imaginary lines to determine which space "belongs" to each. Some will become quite angry if another enters their space.

In most cases, the responsibility for the cleanliness and neatness of the resident's equipment is that of the Nursing Department. Housekeeping usually is responsible for the cleanliness of the floor, privacy curtains, windows, and the bathrooms as well as for emptying wastebaskets. You should be aware of your facility's policy on responsibility for the cleanliness of the unit.

There are certain health and safety rules regarding items that may be kept at the resident's bedside. For example, aerosol cans, razor blades, matches, medications, or food that is not in a closed container are items that may not be permitted at the bedside. If you observe any of these items within the resident's unit, report the information to the charge nurse immediately. Be sure you know what items are permitted at the bedside in your facility.

In addition to providing the resident with necessary furnishings and equipment, the unit should be arranged for the safety, comfort, and convenience of the resident.

Convenience is important in helping the resident to be as independent as possible. Many residents can do more for themselves if necessary items are placed within their reach (Fig. 2-20). For example, a resident who is paralyzed on one side may need to have the bedside table moved, depending on whatever side is easiest for the resident to use.

Independence is increased for the blind person if necessary items are always kept in the same place. You might even make a chart showing where the items belong. This chart could be kept at the bedside for easy reference by the staff.

FIGURE 2-20
Promoting independence.

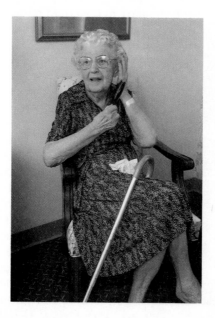

BEDMAKING

Although most residents spend a substantial portion of their time out of bed, the comfort and appearance of the bed is important. The nursing assistant must be able to make a bed that is neat and free of wrinkles. Wrinkles are uncomfortable and can lead to the development of pressure sores (see Chapter 6).

The bed may be made while the resident is in it (called an **occupied bed**) or when the resident is out of bed (called an **unoccupied bed**). The process is essentially the same, but both procedures will be included here. Review the guidelines for linen handling before you practice bedmaking. Although your facility may use fitted bottom sheets, this procedure includes making mitered corners using a flat bottom sheet.

In the LTC facility, you will not be changing the linens completely each day. Although each facility has its own policy, the usual routine is to change the bed completely on the days the resident is bathed or showered (twice weekly) and, of course, when soiled. On a daily basis, you may change only the pillowcase and draw sheet.

Each bed is made with a bottom sheet, top sheet, blanket and/or bedspread, pillow, and pillowcase. Additional bed linens depend upon the needs of the resident. For example, a resident who is **incontinent** (has no control over bowel and/or bladder function) will have a plastic draw sheet (a half sheet placed from knees to shoulders) covered with a cloth draw sheet and other protective pads or diapers. These additional pads may be cloth or disposable.

PROCEDURE

MAKING THE
UNOCCUPIED BED

1. Wash your hands.
2. Assemble linens.
3. Place linens on a chair near the bed in the order of use.
4. Adjust the bed to a comfortable working height.
5. Unfold the bottom sheet and place it lengthwise on the bed. Place the sheet so that the rough edges of the hem will be facing down, away from the resident.
6. Starting at the foot of the bed, open the sheet so that it hangs evenly on each side of the bed. The hem at the foot of the bed is placed so that it is even with the end of the mattress.
7. Raise the mattress and tuck in the sheet at the head of the bed.
8. Miter the corner. Face the head of the bed. With the hand closest to the bed, pick up the edge of the sheet about 12 inches from the edge of the mattress, making a triangle.
   (*Tip:* If you raise the sheet straight up rather than at an angle, you'll form a perfect triangle.)

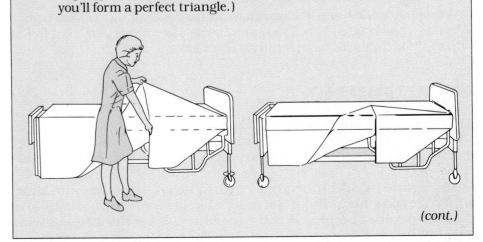

(cont.)

9. Lay the triangle on the top of the mattress.
10. Tuck the hanging portion of the sheet under the mattress.
11. Holding the fold at the edge of the mattress, bring the triangle down and tuck in.
12. Tuck the sheet in all the way to the foot of the bed.
13. Apply the plastic draw sheet, tuck in.
14. Cover the plastic draw sheet with the cloth draw sheet, tuck in. (Be sure the plastic is completely covered.)
15. Starting at the head of the bed, place the top sheet on the bed with the hem up (leave enough to fold over the edge of the blanket and/ or spread).
16. Place the blanket on top of the sheet, unless you are instructed otherwise.
17. Place the spread on top of the blanket.
18. Tuck in the top sheet, blanket, and spread together.
19. Miter the corner but do not tuck in on the side.
20. Move to the opposite side of the bed.
21. Beginning at the head of the bed, tuck in the bottom sheet, pulling tightly as you go.
22. Miter the top corner.
23. Tuck in the plastic draw sheet.
24. Tuck in the cloth draw sheet.
25. Miter the top covers (sheet, blanket, spread). Do not tuck in the sides. *Note:* To prevent pressure on the resident's toes from covers that are too tight, a "toe pleat" is made. Grasp both sides of the top covers at the mitered corner and gently pull the top covers toward the foot of the bed, making about a 3- to 4-inch fold across the foot of the bed.
26. Fold the hem of the top sheet over the blanket and spread.
27. Put the pillowcase on the pillow:
    - Hold the pillowcase at the center of the end seam.
    - With your hand outside of the case, turn the case back over your hand.
    - Grasp the pillow through the case at the center of one end of the pillow.
    - Bring the case down over the pillow.
    - Fit the corner of the pillow into the seamless corner of the case.

A properly made bed will enhance the appearance of the resident's unit. Stand back and look at the bed you've just made. Does it look neat? Is it free of wrinkles? Do the linens hang evenly on either side?

THE OCCUPIED BED

When a resident is unable to be out of bed, it will be necessary to change the linens with the resident in bed. The elements of bedmaking remain the same, with the additional need to protect the privacy, safety, and comfort of the resident.

Making an occupied bed frequently is part of giving incontinent care or caring for a resident whose bed is wet or soiled from perspiration, vomiting, or bleeding. You may change all or only part of the linens at this time. A partial bath may be part of the procedure as well as wiping off the mattress and plastic

- Fold the extra material from the side seam under the pillow.
28. Place the pillow on the bed with the open end away from the door.
29. Adjust the bed to its lowest position.

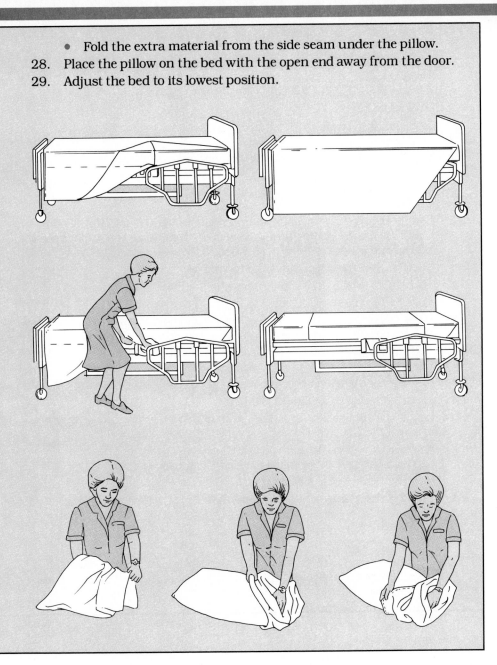

draw sheet. If the linens of an incontinent resident seem only damp, they should be changed anyway as the odor of urine will be present along with the potential for skin irritation.

PROCEDURE

MAKING THE
OCCUPIED BED

1. Wash your hands.
2. Assemble linens on a chair in order of use.
3. Inform the resident what you are going to do.
4. Provide privacy.
5. Adjust the bed to a comfortable working height with backrest and knee — rest flat, if allowed for that resident.

(cont.)

6. Loosen the sheets around the entire bed.
7. Raise the side rail on the opposite side from where you will be working.
8. Turn the resident to the side toward the raised rail, with the pillow under the head.
9. Roll the cloth draw sheet toward the resident, tucking it against the back.
10. Lay the plastic draw sheet over the resident, after wiping it off, if necessary.
11. Roll the bottom sheet toward the resident and tuck tightly under the back.
12. Unfold the clean bottom sheet and place the center fold in the center of the mattress. Position the sheet as in making the unoccupied bed with the hem even with the foot of the mattress.
13. Tuck in the sheet and miter the top corner.
14. Tuck in the sheet all the way down the bed.
15. Tuck in the plastic draw sheet.
16. Place the clean cloth draw sheet over the plastic draw sheet, tucking in the side closest to you.
17. Roll the cloth draw sheet toward the resident. Tuck the sheet under the back.
18. Raise the side rail on the side where you have been working.
19. Move to the opposite side of the bed.
20. Lower the side rail and roll the resident away from you, over the linens, onto the clean side.
21. Remove the soiled linens and place them at the foot of the bed, between the end of the mattress and the footboard.
22. Pull the clean linens toward you.
23. Tighten the sheets and tuck them in, moving from the head of the bed to the foot.
24. Raise the side rail so that you can leave the bedside briefly to dispose of the soiled linens.
25. Change the top sheet by placing it over the soiled sheet so that the resident remains covered. Have the resident hold the clean sheet as you pull the soiled sheet from below. Place at the foot of the bed.
26. Apply the blanket and/or spread.
27. Tuck in the top covers, mitering the corners.
28. Make the toe pleat.

As you practice bedmaking, strive to decrease the number of steps you take as well as the amount of time spent. An efficient nursing assistant can make a bed in 6 minutes!

Make this another opportunity to communicate with the resident. Encourage sharing of past and current events as well as feelings and ideas.

ADMISSION, TRANSFER, AND DISCHARGE

Admission of a resident to an LTC facility is often a time of great stress for both the new resident and the family. The admission process gives the resident and family their first impression of the facility, the staff, and the kind of care given (Fig. 2-21). When the admission is carried out properly and the resident

29. Change the pillowcase.
30. Position the resident comfortably with the bed in its lowest position.
31. Place the signal cord within reach.
32. Put soiled linens in the appropriate containers.
33. Wash your hands.

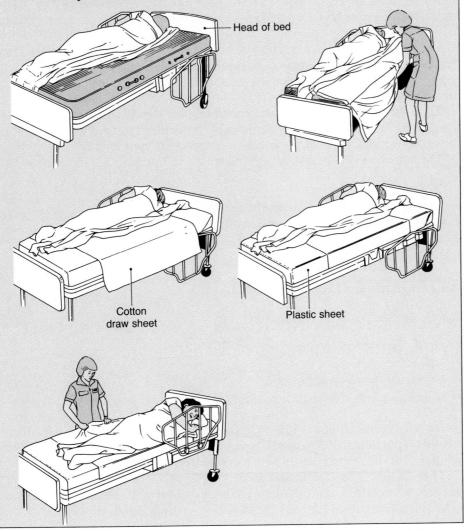

Head of bed

Cotton draw sheet

Plastic sheet

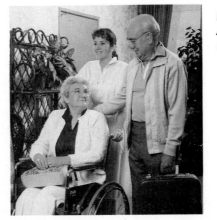

FIGURE 2-21
Admission: the first impression.

receives a favorable impression, the entire stay is more likely to be a positive one. The importance of this event cannot be overemphasized. If you take time to put yourself in the resident's place, you'll be better able to cope with the resident's feelings and behavior during this stressful experience.

One point of view is to look at the losses experienced by the average resident. These may include loss of a home, possessions, pets, a garden, loss of independence and freedom, loss of control over one's life, and loss of privacy. Although facilities make every effort to minimize these losses, to the resident they are highly significant. There indeed is "no place like home." Residents may grieve for the life they once had. Even if they accept the situation, they may never come to like it.

There are some residents who welcome admission to an LTC facility. They may have been lonely, frightened, or unable to meet their own needs. They will enjoy new companionship, good meals, a pleasant environment, and meaningful activities.

Each facility has policies and procedures for the admission of residents. Many procedures are similar regardless of the facility. Find out what the role of the nursing assistant is in the admission process of your facility.

The admission tasks generally include:

- Welcoming the resident
- Gathering information about the resident
- Orienting the resident to new surroundings
- Caring for the resident's personal belongings

WELCOMING THE RESIDENT

To welcome the resident, you should:

- Greet the resident by name
- Introduce yourself
- Explain what you will be doing
- Convey a warm welcome through your facial expression and tone of voice

Gathering information will be accomplished by many health-care team members, particularly during the first week. Each will be focusing on a different aspect of the new resident's needs and plans for care.

There is usually an admission form completed by the nursing department. You may be required to fill in all or parts of this form. It usually includes the following information:

- The resident's temperature, pulse, respiration, and blood pressure
- The resident's weight
- The resident's height
- Observation of the resident's:
  — Grooming and hygiene
  — Condition of hair and nails
  — Condition of skin (presence of scars, open areas, sores, bruises, growths, etc.)
  — Level of alertness, awareness of time and place
  — Sight, hearing, ability to move
  — Presence of any **prosthesis** (artificial limbs, eyes, etc.)

In addition to recording this information, any other usual observations, concerns, or complaints made by the new resident should be reported to the charge nurse.

ORIENTATION OF THE RESIDENT

While orienting the new resident to the facility, include any family members who are present. Begin the orientation in the immediate area and gradually include the entire facility. Be sure to emphasize use of the call signal whenever help is needed. Have the new resident practice using the signal once or twice.

A good orientation includes:

* An introduction to facility routines
* A review of facility policies and rules
* An introduction to roommate and staff
* A tour of the facility

It may be necessary to repeat the orientation several times. People who are anxious or frightened do not hear or remember information as well as they normally would.

CARE OF PERSONAL BELONGINGS

Care of residents' personal belongings begins at the time of admission. There is usually a personal-effects inventory made, and all items are listed and made a part of the health record. As a rule, residents should be discouraged from keeping valuable items in the facility. Such items should be placed in the facility safe or sent home with relatives. If the resident insists on keeping valuables, you should notify your charge nurse at once. When listing items brought in with residents, be accurate and complete.

Describe items objectively, without placing value on them. For example, if you describe a ring, say, "a gold-colored metal ring with a clear stone," rather than a "gold diamond ring."

In addition to listing items brought into the facility with a resident, the nursing assistant assists in marking items with the resident's name and in putting the items in the proper place. When possible, have residents assist and instruct you where they would like things kept. Allow them to make as many decisions as possible. This helps them feel more "in control" during this time.

Make a special effort during the early admission period to be warm, friendly, and attentive to the new resident. This helps to make the resident's first impression a positive one.

TRANSFERRING THE RESIDENT

The term **transfer** simply means to move from one place to another. You might transfer a resident from a bed to a wheelchair or from one room to another in the same facility or from the LTC facility to an acute care hospital.

There are some general principles to keep in mind when a resident is relocated. Regardless of the reason for the move, the resident should be informed of it as soon as possible. The reason and the destination should be given. Special care must be taken not to lose any of the resident's belongings. A careful check of the entire room and bathroom should be made.

Some residents may become disoriented as a result of a move. Familiar sights are no longer present to remind them of where they are. When moving residents, you may have to remind them frequently of the location of the new room. It may be weeks before they feel at home in their new environment. Because of this, moving residents should be kept to a minimum and done only when absolutely necessary.

Residents and families need to be informed in advance when a room change is planned, to allow them time to adjust to the idea. Helping residents who have formed close relationships with their roommates to remain together and/or introducing them to their new roommates in advance may reduce the anxiety that a room change may cause.

DISCHARGING THE RESIDENT

Residents sometimes may be moved to an acute care hospital. When the resident is expected to return soon, this move is referred to as a **transfer.** If the resident is gone for a long time or is not going to return at all, the move is called a **discharge.** Facility policy determines how long a resident may be out of the facility before being discharged. Usually, 72 hours is the deadline. At this point the records are closed. If the resident later returns, a new admission is made, and a new medical record is started.

If one of your residents is to be transferred, remember that the resident "represents" your facility. The kind of care you give will be judged by the appearance of the resident. Be sure the resident is clean and well-groomed and that the hair is combed and nails are trimmed and clean. Send any personal items needed such as dentures, glasses, or hearing aids with the resident. If the resident is to return shortly, personal items may be left in the room. Other times, personal items can be listed, packed, and put into storage. Items sent with the resident should be listed in the chart along with the time and method of transfer, such as by ambulance or by private car.

Residents who leave the facility permanently are considered discharged. They may be discharged to an acute care hospital, to home, or to another level of care, such as a residential care facility. Residents may be discharged only with a physician's order.

Just as the resident's first impressions are important to the relationship between facility and resident, last impressions are long remembered (Fig. 2-22). You should make a special effort to tell the resident good-bye and to extend good wishes for the future. Special care must be taken to see that no belongings are left behind. Usually, there is a personal-effects inventory list of items brought in with the resident. These items must be checked off at the time of discharge and the inventory form signed by the resident or a family member. Check your facility policy to see who is responsible for the various parts of the discharge procedure. The resident should be escorted from the facility by a staff member, who gives assistance with carrying belongings as needed.

FIGURE 2-22
Discharging the patient: the last impression.

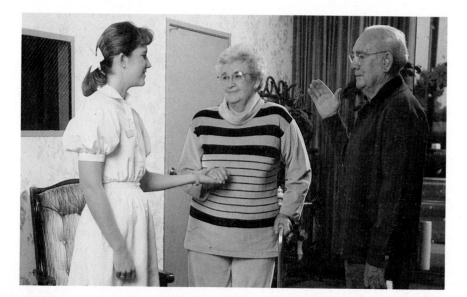

CHAPTER 3

Special Needs of the Elderly and Chronically Ill

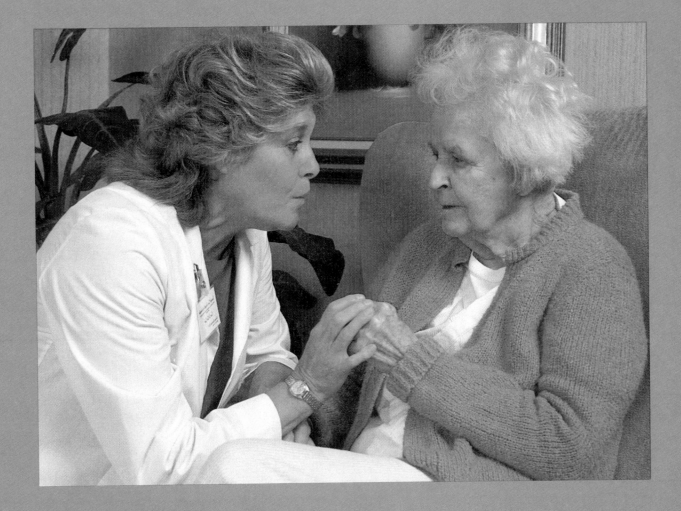

SECTION 1 PHILOSOPHY OF CARE AND REHABILITATION

OBJECTIVES/WHAT YOU WILL LEARN

When you have completed this section, you will be able to:
- Give three examples of ways the nursing assistant can encourage residents to be more independent
- List three observations you've made that reflect your facility's philosophy of care

PHILOSOPHY OF LONG-TERM CARE

The functions, purposes, and types of LTC facilities have been reviewed; however, the "philosophy of care" is something different. The study of **philosophy** is a search for a general understanding of values. It includes the most general beliefs, concepts, and attitudes of an individual or group.

REHABILITATION

Rehabilitation, or restorative care, is given to each resident. This means that efforts are directed to help each resident become as independent as possible. Rehabilitation includes prevention of complications, retraining in lost skills, and learning new skills. For example, care of a resident who is paralyzed on one side might be planned to prevent **contractures** (shortening of muscles from inactivity) in the affected limbs, to retrain the resident in walking, and to train the resident in the use of a cane.

Included in rehabilitation are all the tasks and skills needed for daily living. These skills are called **activities of daily living** (ADLs). ADLs include such things as communication, eating, grooming, dressing, bathing, walking, and toileting. The degree to which residents can become independent in ADLs depends on both their physical condition and desire to achieve independence. Very often this requires hard work.

The physician, as well as the rest of the health-care team, sets a goal (determines what is possible) and develops a plan for the resident to reach that goal (Fig. 3-1). Most residents can achieve a greater degree of independence when given the chance. As you acquire a rehabilitation philosophy, you will be able to

FIGURE 3-1
The health-care team.

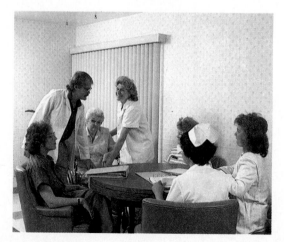

find ways that residents can be more independent. A rehabilitation philosophy includes learning to accept the accomplishment of small, simple goals. Although a cure may not be possible, you will come to enjoy the rewards from any progress the resident makes. Every resident should be encouraged to do as much as possible independently. Feeling good about oneself is increased by being independent. The best way to relearn old skills and to learn new skills is through repetition and practice.

Although the professionals on the health-care team are most qualified to teach the resident, the nursing assistant should help encourage the residents, praise their accomplishments, remind them of what has been taught, and report any need for further teaching.

Facilities accept the responsibility to assist the residents in meeting basic human needs. This means care must be provided to meet psychosocial (psychological and emotional) needs as well as physiological (body) needs. Care must be directed to both the mind and the body!

Philosophies, ideas, and goals are worthless unless they become deeds! In other words, a philosophy is of no value unless it is put into practice. You will know what kind of care philosophy your facility has by *what you see!*

The following are just a few examples of what you might see when a facility practices an accepted philosophy of care.

- The facility has a warm, homelike atmosphere.
- Residents are encouraged to make decisions about their care and do as much for themselves as possible.
- Residents take part in social and recreational activities.
- Residents are encouraged and assisted to wear their own clothing and to keep their own belongings.
- Residents are assisted to have good personal hygiene.
- Residents are always treated with respect and dignity.
- Residents are given choices and as much control as possible over their daily care and activities.

PROMOTING INDEPENDENCE

Helping the resident achieve greater independence is an essential component of the philosophy of care. Most residents can do something for themselves. Combing or brushing their own hair, holding the bread during a meal, or simply deciding what clothing they will wear for the day are examples. It may be difficult to stand by as a resident struggles to do a particular task. If so, you might either busy yourself with other activities that need to be done or simply leave the room for a few minutes. There should be an organized plan that identifies which tasks the resident is to perform for himself or herself. If not, you may identify those that seem possible for the resident to achieve. Never risk the safety of the resident by encouraging performance of dangerous tasks like bathing alone or transferring alone if not already approved by the health-care team. The nursing assistant plays a vital role in promoting independence because you are with the resident as the activities of daily living are being performed. As you carry out the daily care of your residents, review the "steps to independence" shown in Fig. 3-2.

Your efforts to carry out the philosophy of care will help you experience the rewards of seeing residents regain and maintain their independence.

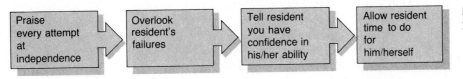

FIGURE 3-2
Steps to independence.

SECTION 2 PSYCHOLOGICAL ASPECTS OF AGING

OBJECTIVES/WHAT YOU WILL LEARN

When you have completed this section, you will be able to:

■ Define the term *psychosocial*

■ List the five basic human needs that Maslow described

■ Describe two additional ways you can help meet the residents':
  need for approval and acceptance
  need for recognition and respect
  need for self-esteem

■ List the three developmental tasks of aging

■ Complete a questionnaire about aging

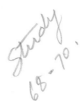

As the number of elderly persons continues to increase, society is becoming more and more aware of the needs and rights of the elderly. The problems of growing old in America are widely publicized. Common myths about aging are being dispelled through education and media programs. It is very important to understand the facts regarding the aging process and to remember that aging is not a disease. In order to measure your own attitudes and knowledge about aging and the aged, complete the "Attitudes About Aging" questionnaire included in your workbook. Most of the nation's elderly are active, productive people who live and function independently. Because of greater knowledge and emphasis on living a healthy life and preventing disease, more people are living longer than ever before.

Aging is an inevitable process and is as yet irreversible. We become old gradually. Most people meet the challenge of aging with imagination and success. America generally is a youth-oriented society. Our culture does not practice the kind of recognition and respect many other societies bestow upon their elderly. In addition, we are an industrial society where most people have to work outside of their homes, leaving no one at home to provide daily care for the elderly. The long-term care facility very often is the only practical way families can provide for the needs of their elderly. Contrary to the popular belief that families abandon their elderly in long-term facilities, studies show that most families continue to provide their elderly with loving support. When residents have no families, they often have longtime friends who visit and care for them.

When the elderly become ill and require the care and services of a long-term care facility, there are many adaptations necessary. Most important are the psychological and social changes that they experience. Care must be provided to meet their complex **psychosocial** needs.

● **psycho** — refers to mental or emotional processes
● **social** — refers to interactions and relationships with others

It is not easy to separate mental processes such as behavior and feelings from the social roles and relationships unique to each person. One of the most commonly accepted theories of aging suggests that personalities and their tendency toward certain kinds of behavior are consistent throughout life. A person who is a dynamic leader at age 30 will be a dynamic leader at age 70. When illness and hospitalization disrupt a person's life, role changes occur that make adaptation or adjustment necessary. The nursing assistant can help the resident successfully make these adaptations by understanding human motivation and behavior.

The effort to understand human personality began with Sigmund Freud, an Austrian physician who believed that the human mind has two levels: a conscious and an unconscious. Freud believed that by studying the conscious mind and behavior that we would better understand the unconscious mind.

As Freud's theories were examined and expanded, another branch of psychology developed based on the idea that all behavior is learned through a system of rewards and punishments. B. F. Skinner, a scientist, believed that "right" behaviors could be encouraged through a system of rewards and "wrong" behaviors could be eliminated through some types of punishment.

Another branch of psychology was introduced in the 1950's by Erik Erikson, Carl Jung, Abraham Maslow, and others called developmental psychology. They supported the idea that emotional well being, as well as each individual's personality development, depends on the successful completion of a series of developmental tasks at various stages in life. It is believed that successful aging and the completion of these developmental tasks result in wisdom.

The developmental tasks to be accomplished for the elderly resident include adjustments and adaptations to the biological, psychological, social, and cultural aspects of aging. These tasks are:

1. Adjustment to old age (accepting physical changes, role changes, and losses). The successful adjustment results in an acknowledgment of the realities of aging.
2. Belief that life is important and meaningful. The individual examines the meaning of his or her own life.
3. Review life's successes and failures and put them into perspective as they prepare for the end of life. The focus is how valuable life has been.
4. Acceptance that things in the past cannot be changed and letting go of feelings of disappointment and regret. The focus is on the present.
5. Adopting social roles that associate them with their own age group.
6. Reconciling moral dilemmas regarding personal and social values.

Some of the moral problems of the elderly include:

- Family problems such as giving and taking advice, living arrangements, need for care and financial needs.
- Legal problems, including assignment of assets, wills, and conservatorships.
- Work or retirement problems, benefits
- Problems related to personal freedom
- Interpersonal problems with family, friends, neighbors.

It is believed that the resident who successfully resolves these developmental tasks will reach a high level of self-awareness and satisfaction with life. Failure to resolve the tasks may inhibit emotional growth and result in emotional instability.

BASIC NEEDS

We all have very basic human needs. Basic needs have been ranked in order of priority by the psychologist Abraham Maslow, who is the author of a classic book in the field of human behavior called *Motivation and Personality*. Maslow identified these basic needs as follows (Fig. 3-3):

- Physical needs
- Security needs
- Social needs

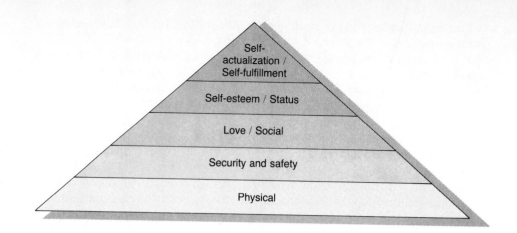

FIGURE 3-3
Five basic human needs.

- Status needs
- Self-fulfillment needs

Physical needs are essential to the survival of each human being. They include the need for food, water, oxygen, rest, exercise, and sex. Even touch is considered necessary for survival. Many studies have been done which show that human beings and animals can become ill or even die when deprived of touch. In your role as a nursing assistant, you will spend a great deal of time assisting residents to meet their physical needs. **Security needs** are concerned with physical safety, feeling protected, having a job and shelter. You help meet the security needs of residents when you:

- Provide a safe, secure environment
- Use side rails or postural supports as necessary
- Help residents feel at home and comfortable in their environment
- Help them develop trust in those who provide their care by keeping your promises and by speaking well about other staff members

Next are the **social needs,** the need for approval and acceptance. You help residents meet their social needs when you:

- Praise the resident for accomplishments
- Encourage the resident to try new things
- Show acceptance of the individual by respecting his or her individuality
- Provide care in a kind, considerate manner
- Provide the essence of human warmth by a gentle touch or a gentle caring voice
- Show interest in the residents and their family and friends

After social needs are met, the status needs, the need for recognition and respect, become most important. You can help residents meet these status needs when you:

- Address the resident by a proper name and title
- Listen to residents' concerns and reminiscences
- Make the resident feel important
- Protect the residents' privacy needs
- Ask their opinion, discuss current issues

The highest level of needs are the self-fulfillment needs. These are the needs to achieve as much as possible and to reach the highest potential of development. You help the resident meet these self-fulfillment needs when you:

- Share health-care goals with the resident and allow the resident to work toward achieving the goal. Nothing succeeds like success.
- Help the resident recognize the purpose and direction in his or her life.
- Help the resident to participate in meaningful activities.
- Help the resident recognize the contribution he or she has made throughout a lifetime.
- Assist the resident to look good! Assist with dressing and grooming as needed.
- Allow the resident to direct and control as much of his or her life as possible. Dependency does not foster self-esteem.
- Allow the resident to participate in and approve the plan of care
- Encourage socialization — the acceptance and approval of friends and family builds self-confidence and self-esteem.

Having control over one's life has been proven to contribute to a positive outlook and good morale. The resident should control as much of his or her daily life as possible. Control is given to the resident by offering choices and following their wishes. Examples of giving choices include:

"Would you like your bath now or after Mrs. Jones?"
"Which dress would you like to wear?"
"Would you like the pink or the white sweater?"
"Would you like to eat your eggs or your cereal first?"

Make offering choices a habit.

PRIVACY

The need for privacy is so important that it requires special mention. Protect privacy of information and privacy of the person as you go about your everyday tasks. Be sure to draw the curtains in the resident's room when performing any kind of personal care. Be aware that the window curtains may also need to be closed. Screen the resident not only from public view but also from view of any roommates who may be present. Never assume that the resident "doesn't mind." Sometimes when you assist a resident to the toilet, she or he may say "leave the door open, so you'll know when I'm finished." Explain that you can't do that but you'll stay within calling distance. Any time a door is closed or curtains are drawn around a resident's unit, ask permission to enter. Avoid giving personal care in public areas or making public comments like, "You've spilled food all over yourself. Let's go clean you up." That is an invasion of the resident's privacy and dignity.

You will be able to identify many more ways in which to meet the basic human needs of residents. Remember, one of the best ways to recognize and meet their needs is to recognize and understand your own needs. If you treat others as you would like to be treated, you will seldom go wrong.

Perhaps one of the greatest challenges you will face in your role as a nursing assistant will be to develop sensitivity to the needs of others (Fig. 3-4). The technical skills are easily taught, but dedication, concern, caring, and wanting to provide the best care possible are traits *you must want to achieve*. A modification of the "Golden Rule" is still the best guide: "Provide care to others as you would have others provide care to you or your loved one."

Aging is inevitable—"unless we can create a world which offers the possibility of aging with grace, honor and meaningfulness, no one can look forward to the future" (Seymour Hallech, *Nursing and the Aged*, McGraw-Hill, 1976).

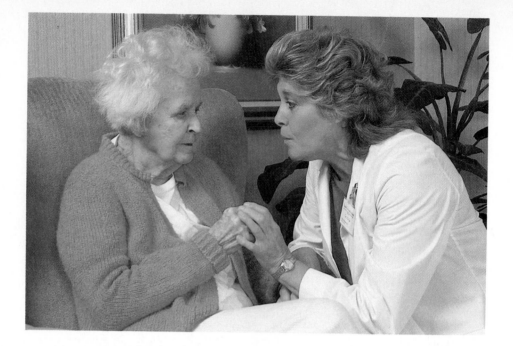

FIGURE 3-4
Developing sensitivity.

SECTION 3 ROLE CHANGES

OBJECTIVES/WHAT YOU WILL LEARN

When you have completed this section, you will be able to:
- Define the term *role*
- List the roles you play
- Differentiate the characteristics of the sick role from those of the well role
- Give three ways the nursing assistant can minimize role changes experienced by the resident

To understand the feelings, attitudes, and behaviors of the resident in an LTC facility, the nursing assistant must understand the concept of roles and role changes.

A **role** is defined as a part one plays in relationship to others (Fig. 3-5). The role we play also affects the way others treat us or respond to us. Roles have specific behavior associated with them. When we are in a particular role, we behave in a particular way.

In a movie or on television, actors are hired to play various roles. Their roles include their lines (the words they speak), their appearance (age, type of clothing), and what they do (behavior). Successful actors are able to perform in many roles during their careers. Even though they personally may be nothing like any of the characters they portray, their skill lies in their ability to convince others that they are.

We, too, play many roles in our everyday lives. Some roles we choose; some are assigned to us. For every role, there are expected behaviors as well as expected ways we are treated. There are roles people associate with age (2-year olds are difficult, teenagers are rebellious; older people are cantankerous); roles associated with sex (men are expected to be strong; women are expected to be weak); roles related to social position (the wealthy are snobbish; the poor are

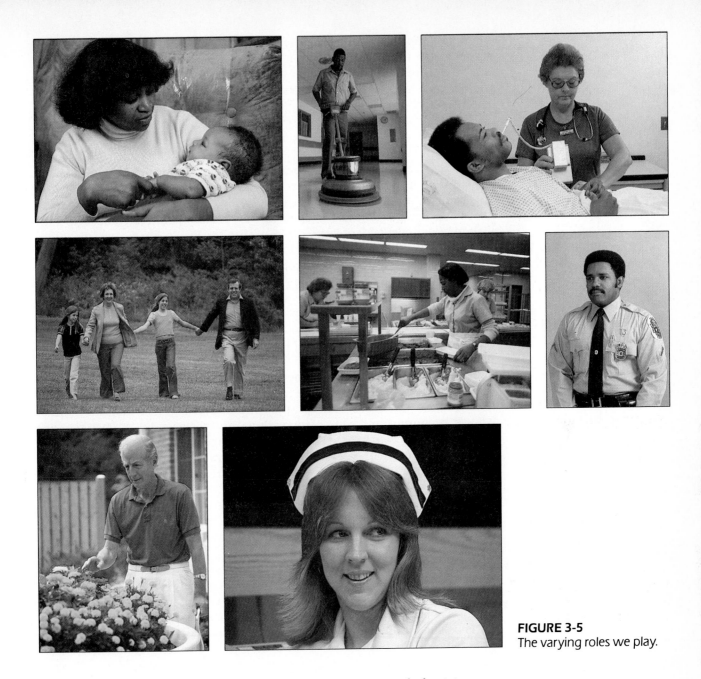

FIGURE 3-5
The varying roles we play.

humble); and roles associated with professions (lawyers and physicians are intelligent, laborers are not).

As you can see from these examples, the expectations that accompany various roles lead to great conflict at times because each of us wishes to be seen as a unique person. We resent being stereotyped or typecast. There are many psychological factors that influence how successful an individual is in meeting role expectations as well as how that person adapts to role changes. Nonetheless, to succeed in a given role, certain behaviors must be adopted. Chapter 1 provided the information you need to assume the role of nursing assistant successfully.

Admission to an LTC facility brings about role changes for the resident, regardless of the facility's effort to minimize these changes. Residents frequently grieve over their lost roles and experience difficulty adopting new ones. The resident may have to give up the role of provider and head of the family. It may no longer be possible to be the grandmother who bakes cookies with the children or the grandfather who takes the children to a ball game. Now it is up to the grandchild to visit or take the grandparents on an outing. The reversal of roles presents a difficult adjustment to many residents.

There are other types of roles that influence residents and their behavior. These are the well role, the sick role, and the disabled role.

The **well role** is characterized by independence, responsibility, usefulness, and decision making. The well person is expected to contribute to the well-being of others and is generally regarded as a valuable member of society.

The **sick role** is characterized by dependence, weakness, control by others, lack of responsibility, and uselessness. While the well person gives, the sick person takes.

The **disabled** person suffers from role confusion, being neither sick nor well. Not only is it difficult to know how to behave, others have difficulty knowing whether to treat the individual as sick or well. Given an opportunity to express their wishes, most disabled people say they prefer to be treated as well. They wish to be as independent as possible, within the limitation of their disability.

Many residents move back and forth between the sick role and the well role. It is important to recognize the role changes that occur and to provide care based on the resident's needs at the time.

Often, people explain a resident's continuing dependency by comparing him or her to a child. An elderly person who may be confused is said to be in his second childhood. This comparison creates a situation where an adult seen as a child is treated like a child and thus continues to behave as a child.

Some residents may behave in childlike ways because of their illness, disability, and dependency. Despite their physical and mental limitations, they are not children and should never be treated like children. Referring to the residents as "kids" or "babies" is never appropriate. By the same token, the manner of dress, grooming, and types of recreational and social activities should be **age appropriate** (appropriate to the chronological age of the person). For example, having adults color in a coloring book with crayons is not age appropriate. Painting a picture or using colored pens to finish a drawing of a farm in the winter would be age appropriate.

Our culture often reinforces or rewards illness by paying special attention to those who are ill. We visit the sick and bring them flowers and gifts. We tell the person that we care for them and show our concern. For some, being sick becomes more desirable than being well.

In order to promote well behavior, the facility and its staff must recognize that sickness does have some attractive features and try to make wellness more desirable than sickness. This is accomplished through praising the resident for all efforts at independence, by spending time with the resident, and by showing concern. The family members also need to be involved so that they work with the facility staff by reinforcing or rewarding well behavior and independence.

Perhaps the most difficult role change occurs when residents have to leave their home or normal surroundings to reside in an LTC facility. This role change can be very difficult for some. You can do a great deal to help the resident change roles successfully by the way you provide care.

SECTION 4 DEVELOPING INTERPERSONAL SKILLS

OBJECTIVES/WHAT YOU WILL LEARN

When you have completed this section, you will be able to:
- List four factors influencing individual behavior
- Identify methods of coping with anger that are acceptable for nursing assistants
- Select the most helpful response by the nursing assistant in sample situations

Performing nursing tasks or skills is quite simple when compared to developing effective interpersonal skills. Although we each have varying abilities to get along with others based on our own personality and life experiences, we can learn to increase our skills in relating to others significantly.

Psychologists and psychiatrists have developed a great body of knowledge about human behavior. Despite many different ideas and philosophies, there are some common principles. Developing skill in interpersonal relations begins with knowing and understanding yourself. Although we are each unique individuals, we are also alike in many ways. We all share the same basic human needs, but we differ in the way we meet those needs.

Our ways of relating to others and our ways of behaving are determined by many factors:

- Heredity — traits we are born with
- Environment — our surroundings, both physical and social
- Culture — habits and customs of our group
- Interests — what we enjoy or care about
- Feelings or emotions — happiness, grief, anger, jealousy, love
- Values — what we consider to be most important
- Standards — what is acceptable and unacceptable to us
- Expectations of others — our behavior tends to conform to what others expect of us
- Learning experiences — we learn which behaviors work in certain situations and discard those that don't work
- Stress (such as illness) — affects our behavior

Because all residents are entitled to equally fine care regardless of their behavior, the nursing assistant must develop patience and tolerance through understanding and acceptance. Recognizing that all behavior has meaning, you must study the behavior in an effort to find that meaning (Fig. 3-6). The more experience you have with a variety of different people, the greater will be your understanding. The principles of behavior management described in Chapter 16 can be very helpful as you deal with the behavior of any resident.

Acceptance of each and every resident requires great effort. The key is to focus on the ways the resident is like you rather than the ways the resident is different from you. Show your interest and caring by listening to the resident, by complying with his or her requests whenever possible, and by giving the resident your full attention whenever you are together.

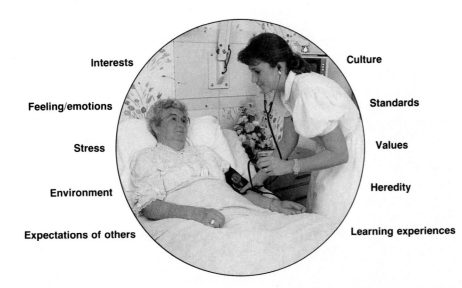

FIGURE 3-6
Factors that determine behavior and ways of relating to others.

Some of the behaviors you will be frequently dealing with are:

- Aggressiveness
- Demanding behavior
- Dissatisfied behavior
- Crying
- Self-centeredness
- Being withdrawn or depressed

In health care, the staff must adapt their own behavior in ways that meet the needs of each resident as best they can. Too often the staff will expect the residents to adapt to staff needs, schedules, and routines. The professional health-care worker learns how to deal with difficult behaviors without losing control or rejecting the resident.

There will be times when you experience anger, frustration, or hurt because of a resident's behavior. Coping with your feelings in an acceptable way is essential. Some acceptable ways of coping include:

- Leaving the room (be sure that it is safe to leave; return when you have "cooled off," or send another staff member in)
- Stating your feelings ("I feel very hurt")
- Discussing or venting your feeling to another staff member in private
- Engaging in physical activity (exercise)

Unacceptable ways of coping include:

- Yelling
- Threatening
- Striking out
- Slamming doors
- Kicking the furniture
- Drinking or eating excessively when off duty

Determining the reason that a person behaves in a certain way helps us know how best to help.

COPING WITH AGGRESSIVE BEHAVIOR

Aggressive behavior can show itself either physically or verbally. As a rule, rational adults do not engage in physical aggression. Usually, the person who strikes out at a staff member is not in control of his or her own behavior due to confusion, mental illness, high fever, or the effects of medication. The individual resident may be frightened by attempts to provide care and can see them as threats of physical harm. This type of behavior can develop if the nursing assistant fails to inform the resident of what he or she is going to do. Imagine a person sleeping soundly at night; the nursing assistant repositions the resident, leaving the light off and saying nothing. Is it any wonder that the resident in the sleeping state might be frightened and fight back? Regardless of the reason for the physical aggression, nursing assistants must protect both the residents and themselves from harm. Usually, it is best simply to back away from the resident rather than try to hold the resident's arms down. If a resident poses a threat to himself or others, seek assistance from your charge nurse immediately. Speak to the resident in a calm, quiet, soothing manner. Give the resident a little time to calm down. Sometimes it is helpful to obtain help from a more experienced staff member or one who knows this particular resident well. Never threaten or attempt to intimidate this resident into cooperating with you. With the right approach, most residents will respond to your requests.

Verbal aggression is a more common event. The key to coping with verbal aggression is to listen without argument or defense and to take action to correct valid complaints. Do not take the attack personally. Your behavior may have nothing to do with the resident's anger.

COPING WITH DEMANDING DISSATISFED BEHAVIOR

Many nurses have the most difficulty dealing with the demanding resident who never seems to be satisfied. This person may ring the signal or call light frequently for what seem like unimportant requests. All efforts to please the resident fail. Each action is met with criticism. You might be asked, for instance, to adjust the pillow. Each time the pillow is moved, it is too much or too little, too high or too low. Chances are great that the pillow will end up back where it started. Part of the frustration is that no matter what you do, it will never be right. It is easy to suffer a loss of confidence and self-esteem if you believe or accept the resident's perception of care provided.

With this type of behavior, the nursing assistant needs to accept the fact that the resident cannot be pleased due to his or her own unique psychological problems. Perhaps because of fears of being alone, excuses are invented to keep the nurse in the room. Sometimes people who suffer from a chronic disease are perceived as demanding because they know more about the condition and their needs than anyone else. After many years of coping with their condition, they develop special ways of doing things that have proved successful. With these residents, it is usually best to do things their way, whenever possible. Imposing your ways and routines on them will only lead to frustration and a poor relationship. Find as many opportunities as you can for the resident to make choices or decisions. Comments like, "Would you like to get out of bed now, or after I finish with Mr. Jones?" or "Would you like to wear the blue pants or the black ones?" are examples of ways you can include the resident in decision making. It is also a good idea to verify with the resident before leaving the room that you have done everything that is needed. Stop by periodically during your shift to see if this individual needs anything. You'll soon find that this person trusts you and will not need to call so often or to invent reasons to keep you in the room.

COPING WITH CRYING AND SELF-CENTEREDNESS

When a resident is crying for any reason, you might feel helpless and uncomfortable. Avoid attempting to stop the resident from crying in order to increase your own comfort. Comments like, "Now, now that isn't necessary" or "Let's put a smile on that face" are not helpful. The role of the nursing assistant is to allow the resident to cry, to convey the fact that crying is helpful, and to listen (Fig. 3-7). Very often, as you listen the resident will express concern and frustration. Sometimes there are actions you can take to resolve some of the frustration, and other times there may be nothing more to do than to convey a feeling to the resident that you are there and you care. Report to your charge nurse any comments or behavior changes that you feel need to be explored further.

Persons who are ill often become very self-centered. Their world seems to become smaller and smaller as they focus attention on their own needs. This person frequently is demanding of your time and attention. Although it may be tempting to scold the resident or to explain that you have other responsibilities or that there are others who are sicker, resist the temptation. This approach not only increases the anxiety of the resident, but it is also not successful in changing the behavior. Attempting to involve this resident in meaningful activities, particularly those that provide him or her with the opportunity to give to others, will do far more to decrease the self-centered behavior.

Some residents may become depressed and withdraw from contact with family, friends, and staff and give the impression of "lingering sadness."

Depression is the most common emotional disorder for all ages in the United States. The older adult who has retired from the work force is often found with feelings of uselessness, loneliness, and boredom. When problems of lost

the word *hospice* referred to a place in the mountains of Switzerland where the monks took care of people as they crossed through the mountains. Gradually, these places for weary travelers also became places for taking care of the sick and dying. In the early 1900s the first British hospice, St. Joseph's, was opened, and Dr. Cicely Saunders, a British physician, became involved. Dr. Saunders was the driving force who not only established other hospice facilities in England, but was also the role model for the first United States hospice in Connecticut. Hospice of Connecticut opened in 1974, and the number of hospice programs in the United States has grown from a handful in the early 1970s to more than 1600 in 1990 according to the National Hospice Association (Fig. 3-10).

Most hospice programs are "home-care"-based, where supportive services are planned and provided by a professional interdisciplinary team. These teams allow patients to die at home surrounded by family and loved ones. However, most home-care programs require the dying person to have someone in the home who is capable of being the "primary caregiver," generally a spouse, child, or sibling. When there is not a primary caregiver or when care becomes too difficult to handle at home, the patient may be transferred to an inpatient hospice unit. The inpatient unit makes every effort to create a homelike atmosphere (Fig. 3-11).

Hospice is a special kind of care uniquely designed to provide sensitive, caring support for both the person who is dying and the dying person's family or loved ones. Hospice philosophy regards death as a normal phase of life and recognizes that the patient and family often need support in order to cope with the difficult transitions and eventual death.

The hospice staff includes highly trained professionals who work exclusively with the terminally ill and their families. The staff includes:

* The patient's personal physician
* The hospice medical director (a physician)
* Licensed nurses
* Nurse assistants
* Home health aide
* Social service workers
* Counselors and pastoral workers
* Therapists
* Volunteers

FIGURE 3-10
The community hospice.

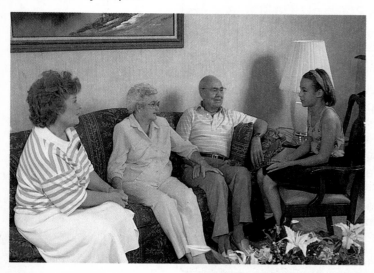

FIGURE 3-11
Hospice unit.

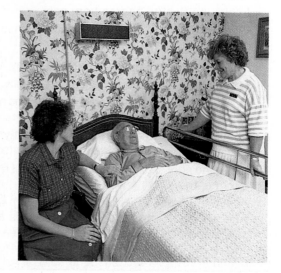

The goals of hospice care are:

- To help the dying person remain as free of pain as possible without sacrificing the person's need to be alert and conscious.
- To allow the dying person and her loved ones as much control as possible over the circumstances of her dying.
- To provide the highest "quality" of life possible when the "quantity" of a person's time for living is limited.
- To assist family and loved ones following the death through bereavement counseling. (**Bereave** means to be left desolate by death.)

As a nursing assistant, you may have the opportunity to work in a hospice inpatient unit, in a hospice home-care program, or in a LTC facility where hospice care is provided for the terminally ill residents. Residents who meet the criteria established by Medicare under the Medicare hospice benefit may receive hospice care in a LTC facility.

The hospice interdisciplinary team works along with facility personnel to plan and provide care to both the terminally ill resident and his or her family. Facility personnel receive special training from the hospice staff.

Regardless of where you provide care to the terminally ill resident, it must be done with knowledge, sensitivity, and concern. The guidelines for care of the dying resident (page 85) must be understood and followed. The long-term relationship that you will develop with residents of your facility provides you with a unique opportunity to assist them to die with dignity in a loving supportive environment.

STAGES OF DYING

Generally, people who are dying react in similar ways. Dr. Elisabeth Kübler-Ross identified the phases or stages that she observed in her work with the dying (Fig. 3-12). Although individuals do not necessarily proceed in an orderly fashion from one stage to another, some people seem to follow a pattern. These stages occur when any major loss is experienced — loss of a job, loss of a husband or wife through divorce, death, or even loss of a treasured possession.

The dying person may remain in any of the various stages or may go back to an earlier stage or go forward to the next (Fig. 3-13). The role of the health-care worker is to accept the person wherever he or she happens to be.

Initially, there is a period of shock and denial. The person simply cannot believe what is happening. They say things like "Oh no, not me. This can't be

FIGURE 3-12
Stages of dying.

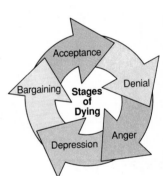

FIGURE 3-13
Losing friends and loved ones is one difficult aspect of growing older.

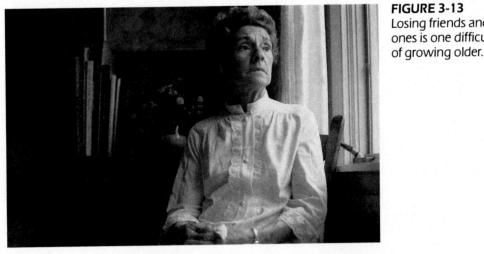

happening to me. There must be a mistake." This is a time when the person prepares to face the truth. While some may deny the truth until the time of death, most people only deny until they are able to believe. Denial protects the person and gives him or her time to adjust. When an individual is in the denial stage, *never* force the truth or try to persuade the person to face the truth. Simply listen and allow the person to express her or his feelings.

When the need for denial is past, the person usually becomes angry, saying, "Why me? What did I do to deserve this?" Blame may be placed on God, the physician, or on family members, or on themselves. The anger may also be directed toward the nursing staff through refusal to cooperate or lashing out verbally. During this time, the nursing staff continues to provide care in a kind, consistent manner, allowing the person to talk. The anger may take the form of constant complaints about the food, the nursing care, or the environment. Those complaints that are legitimate should be taken care of without defensiveness by the staff.

The period of anger is often followed by depression. As the anger passes, the person may feel sad and may withdraw. The resident may refuse to eat, drink, or talk. For many nurses, this is the most difficult part of the grief process. It may seem impossible to get any response from the resident. Never push or pressure the resident to talk. The staff often feels as helpless and hopeless as the resident does. At this point, the staff should continue to show their caring by giving good physical care and by being available to the resident.

Some residents may make efforts to "bargain" for more time or for a pain free death. They may ask God to let them live "until my grandson graduates" or "until spring." In exchange for this time, promises are made. The staff may or may not be aware that the resident is experiencing the stage of bargaining.

For many residents, acceptance comes just before death. Acceptance is best defined as acknowledgement of the fact that death is real and that it is happening. Acceptance does not always mean death is welcomed or desired. The person approaching death with acceptance often prefers to be with only one or two close family members or friends. There is usually very little talking at this point. Nursing actions may be confined to providing physical comfort and quiet loving support.

The dying person should not be left alone for long periods of time. A friend or family member sitting at the bedside holding the resident's hand is often the most important kind of comfort.

PROVIDING CARE FOR THE DYING RESIDENT

Research has shown that most people realize or sense in some way when they are dying. They often will ask the physician to confirm their suspicions, and they may also question you. Information of this nature should only come from the physician. The role of the nursing assistant is one of listening rather than talking. Listening without inserting any of your own experiences or the experiences of others is helpful. It is never appropriate to say, "I understand how you feel" because we really are not able to put ourselves in the place of a person who is dying. It does help to say, "I'm here, I will help in whatever way I can." You don't have to have the answers; just the fact that you are there and listening can be a great source of comfort to the dying resident.

Guidelines for communication with residents who have limited life expectancy and their families or loved ones:

- Remember that dying residents need to be treated like living people; talk to and with them normally.
- Avoid whispering. Speak in your normal voice to the resident as well as to others in the room.

- Don't say things you wouldn't want the resident to hear. The dying person's hearing is usually one of the last senses to fail.
- Continue to talk to and touch the resident. Encourage the family to do the same.
- Respect the need for spiritual support. Learn the policy in your facility concerning religious observances and requirements at the time of death. For example, if a Roman Catholic resident wishes to see a priest and appears to be close to death, a priest should be called. Because the body of an Orthodox Jewish resident should not be touched after death until the rabbi of proper religious authority arrives, it is important to straighten the resident's limbs before death occurs.
- Be sincere and offer support and assistance without assuming control. The dying resident needs to remain in control of his or her own life and the circumstances of their environment as much as possible.
- Allow residents and/or family members to express their grief openly — remember, crying is a natural reaction to loss.
- Create an atmosphere of comfort and let the dying resident set the pace in their communication about dying and related matters.
- Allow each resident to deal with their death according to their own needs and value system. Do not confuse your needs or impose your values on the dying resident.

You may also care for residents who wish to die. They may feel that life has nothing left to offer them or that they are so ill or so debilitated that they do not wish to continue living. They may refuse medications or stop eating. When you observe these behaviors or when they make comments to you about choosing to die, pass on the information to your charge nurse. There are some ethical and legal issues that must be addressed with the resident, the family, the physician, and the facility.

GUIDELINES FOR CARE OF THE DYING RESIDENT

- Keep the room well ventilated and lighted as usual. Because the dying resident's eyesight may be failing, a dark room may be frightening.
- Change the resident's position at least every 2 hours, and more often if necessary, to ensure comfort and to prevent skin breakdown.
- The dying resident may lose control of bowel and bladder and soil the bed often. Keep the resident clean at all times. Take steps necessary to keep the room as odor-free as possible.
- Change the bedding whenever necessary to prevent skin irritation and to increase comfort.
- The resident may be given softer food in smaller amounts than usual or may refuse food. Liquids are given as long as the ability to swallow remains. This helps to keep the mouth moist.
- The resident approaching death needs special mouth care. If the mouth is dry, use an applicator with glycerine (or other lubricant) to swab the mouth and lips or keep the mouth moist with toothettes moistened with water. When there are a lot of secretions in the mouth, tell the charge nurse, who may use suction to remove the material.
- If the resident has dentures, ask your charge nurse if you should leave them in or take them out. If you remove the dentures, place them in a denture cup with the resident's name on the cover.
- A resident's nostrils may also become dry and encrusted. If you notice dryness, clean the nostrils with cotton swabs moistened slightly with glycerine (or other lubricant).

Try to spend as much time with the resident as possible, especially if no family or loved ones are present. Even though there is often very little you can do, just letting the resident know someone is there can be very comforting. Often a gentle touch, the simple gesture of taking the resident's hand, rubbing an arm or shoulder, or touching the cheek will reassure the person that she or he is not alone.

PHYSICAL SIGNS THAT DEATH IS NEAR

Death comes in different ways. It may come quite suddenly after a resident seemed to be recovering, or it may come after a long period during which there has been a steady decline of body functions. Here are some signs showing that death may be near:

- Blood circulation slows down, making the resident's hands and feet cold to the touch. A conscious resident may complain of feeling cold, requiring extra covers for comfort.
- The resident's face may become pale because of decreased circulation, or gray and mottled.
- The eyes may stare blankly into space. There may be no eye movement when you pass your hand across the line of vision.
- The resident may perspire heavily, even though the body is cold.
- The resident loses muscle tone, making the body seem limp. The jaw may drop, and the mouth may stay partly open.
- Respirations may become slower and more difficult.
- Mucus collecting in the resident's throat and bronchial tubes may cause a sound that is sometimes called the "death rattle."
- The pulse is often rapid, but it becomes weak and irregular.
- Just before death, respiration stops and the pulse gets very faint. You may not be able to feel the pulse at all. If you notice any of these signs or any change in resident's condition, report to your charge nurse immediately.

In some states the physician must determine that death has occurred; in others the nurse may do so.

CARE OF THE BODY AFTER DEATH

The body *must* always be treated with dignity and respect after death. Usually any roommates are taken out of the room, or the privacy curtains are drawn. You will be instructed about whether or not the family will be viewing the body before you begin physical preparation of the body.

Although procedures vary with the individual facility, there are some general guidelines:

- There is no laughing or joking while caring for the body after death
- Providing privacy and treating the body with respect is essential
- The body is carefully bathed
- All tubings and dressings are removed
- Clean dressings are applied if indicated
- Dentures are placed in the mouth
- Limbs are straightened

Some facilities have special kits used to prepare the body. Preparations vary from simple to complex. In many facilities, the mortuary arrives promptly and completes some of the preparations, including identification and positioning.

Other residents will ask about the resident who died. The current thinking is that they should be informed of the death openly and honestly. The custom of closing all the doors to the resident's room when the body is removed is questionable since the other residents usually know that this means that someone has died. They also watch how the deaths of others are handled, knowing that their own death will be dealt with in the same way. Most people wish to be remembered and to have their death acknowledged and mourned.

Many LTC and hospice facilities conduct brief memorial services for those who have died or pause for a moment before a meal to remember that person. The terms used in discussing death give some indication of the degree of comfort the person has with death. The correct terms are *died* or *expired*.

THE FAMILY AND GRIEVING

After death, attention is turned toward the family or friends of the resident. They may need someone to listen or perhaps provide coffee and a place to sit and talk. Your support comes not from trying to say "the right thing" but from listening to what the family has to say. A wonderful quote by Doug Manning emphasizes this point: "The ear is the most powerful part of the human body. People are healed by the laying on of ears."

Family and friends will experience the **grief process** in much the same way the dying resident did, even though the death may have been expected (Fig. 3-14). The grief process is characterized by many different emotions experienced by people following a loss.

The way someone dies and the relationship to the person mourning the loss influences the length of time they spend in each phase. People in the "shock phase" can be compared to someone under anesthesia; they are "numb." You can be most helpful to the person in the denial-shock phase by just listening — let the person know you want to listen and that you will take time to listen.

Denial is the part of grieving that deals with, "It can't be true" or "No, he is not really gone" kinds of feelings. Losing a loved one is such a loss that it is natural to deny the truth. In some ways, denial allows people to protect themselves temporarily from the pain and hurt their loss brings until they are better prepared to handle it.

Anger is part of the protest, a reaction most commonly seen once the reality of the death has been faced. Anger may be toward God or toward medical science, other family members, or even directed at the person who died and left them. Sometimes anger is directed toward those who have provided care. If this occurs, never try to argue or defend; allow the person to talk and encourage them to speak to the licensed nurse. Be sure to report any angry behavior to your charge nurse. Anger is a feeling that will not last, and most often people begin to defuse their own anger as they see things more clearly. Sometimes people use their anger constructively to address issues that might have contributed toward the death of their loved ones. A good example of this is MADD (Mothers Against Drunk Drivers), an organization designed to bring about constructive

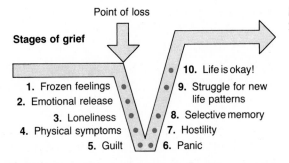

FIGURE 3-14
Stages of grief.

Point of loss

Stages of grief

1. Frozen feelings
2. Emotional release
3. Loneliness
4. Physical symptoms
5. Guilt
6. Panic
7. Hostility
8. Selective memory
9. Struggle for new life patterns
10. Life is okay!

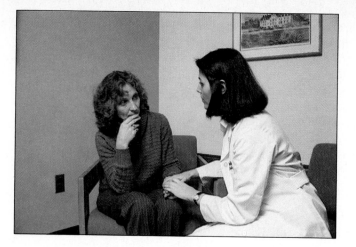

FIGURE 3-15
The grieving family.

changes in laws related to drunk drivers. MADD was founded by a mother whose daughter was killed by a drunk driver.

During the disorganization phase, depression and withdrawal occur as the mourner faces an emptiness that feels like it will never go away (Fig. 3-15). There is a clear realization that the loved one will *never* return. Where anger and pain once were are now feelings of aimlessness and loneliness. Frequently during this phase people may lose or reduce contacts with family and friends. Sometimes it helps to drop a note, letting the person know that someone is thinking of him or to call with, "I just wanted to call and let you know I was thinking of you." Many times during a prolonged illness and death, facility staff can go a long way to helping people through their grieving and back toward a meaningful life in spite of their loss. In the final phase of reorganization, a philosophical acceptance of the death comes, and the individual begins to find new interests, increases socialization, and gradually returns to the mainstream of life and society.

As you provide care to the dying resident and support family members as they grieve, you must be aware of how your own feelings and attitudes toward death will influence how you are in providing care. For this reason, special training as well as selected reading materials are encouraged.

CHAPTER 4

Basic Nursing Care

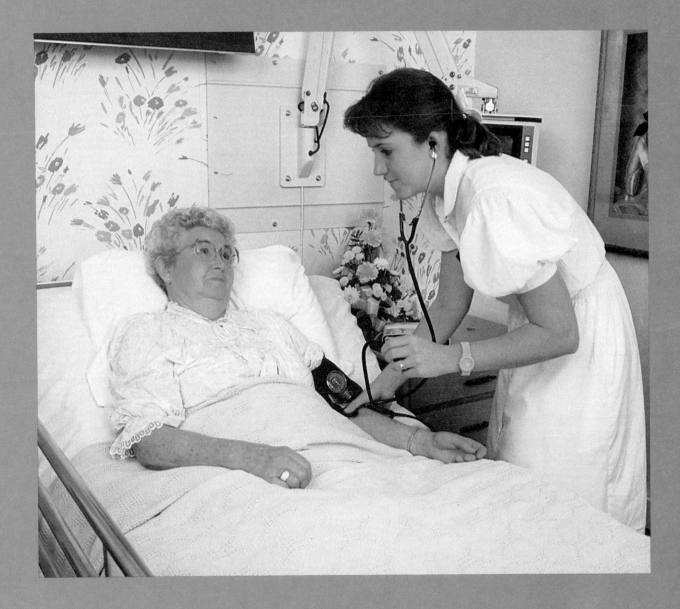

OBJECTIVES/WHAT YOU WILL LEARN

When you have completed this section, you will be able to:

■ Review the health-care plan of ten residents in your facility and list the different health-care disciplines involved

■ Explain how the nursing assistant can contribute to the development of the plan of care

■ List four ways the health-care plan can help you as you provide daily care

CHARACTERISTICS OF THE HEALTH-CARE PLAN

The **health-care plan** is similar to an architect's blueprint — it gives members of the health-care team the written guidelines for providing care. A building is never successfully completed without a plan. Similarly, good resident care cannot be provided without a plan!

An **individualized** health-care plan is a legal requirement for all residents of a health-care facility. Just as we are all different, with our own problems and needs, each resident must be viewed as a unique individual, and a plan of care must be tailored to reflect the individuality of each resident. You can test whether a care plan is individualized by reading the plan and seeing if you can identify the resident without referring to name or room number. Good health-care plans are sketches of the residents and their problems and needs. An individualized care plan is tailor made to reflect the unique needs of a single resident.

To develop an individualized health-care plan, all members of the health-care team must interview the resident, family, or friends as well as gather data from the physician and the health-care record. All needs of each resident must be considered. For this reason, the multidisciplinary health-care team meets regularly to develop, update, and review the residents' health-care plan.

Residents and families are encouraged to participate in the development of the plan and resident's must approve their plan of care. As you review the health-care plans of residents in your facility, identify the entries made by other members of the health-care team.

It is important to include the resident and family members in the development of the health-care plan whenever possible. It's surprising to see how positively residents respond when they are involved in planning their own care. Residents generally are more motivated to achieve goals when they have taken part in the goal-setting process.

As a nursing assistant, you are in the best position to gather important information about the residents' needs and problems. You can contribute to the development of the care plan by:

- Making factual observations
- Reporting and recording those observations accurately

USING THE HEALTH-CARE PLAN

Too often the health-care plan is developed carefully but not used appropriately. It is of no value if the caregivers do not follow the plan! If actions or approaches listed are not effective, they must be changed. When the health-care plan is well

Care Plan

Date No. Problem/Needs	Goals /Objectives	Approach	Discipline
REVIEW DATE: 01/01/00			
LONG TERM GOAL: INCREASED INDEPENDENCE IN ADL'S WITHOUT EPISODES OF ACCIDENT OR INJURY.			
DISCHARGE PLAN: POTENTIAL FOR DISCHARGE LIMITED, DUE TO UNAVAILABILITY OF CAREGIVERS.			
************************************	**************	**	
01 01/01/00 00 AP4 IMPAIRED MOBILITY - POS. REQUIRES EXTENSIVE ASSIST RELATED TO: OSTEOARTHRITIS	01 04/01/00 AP4B RESIDENT WILL BE FREE OF COMPLICATIONS OF INACTIVITY THRU 04/01/00.	01 04/01/00 AP4B1 UTILIZE PRESSURE REDUCING DEVICE - WATER MATTRESS.	LN
		02 04/01/00 AP4B2 USE POSITIONING DEVICE HANDROLL-RIGHT HAND ONLY TO MAINTAIN PROPER BODY ALIGNMENT & POSITIONING.	NL
		03 04/01/00 AP4B3 REPORT CHANGES IN SKIN TEMP, REDDENED OR EXCORIATED AREAS TO SUPERVISOR.	LN
		04 04/01/00 AP4B9 REPOSITION MINIMUM Q 1-2 HOURS.	N
		05 04/01/00 AP4B4 PROVIDE ACTIVE/PASSIVE ROM Q DAY.	N
		06 04/01/00 AP4B6 INSTRUCT RESIDENT REGARDING NEED FOR REPOSITIONING REGIMEN.	L
02 01/01/00 00 CV2 CARDIAC OUTPUT DECREASED RELATED TO: CONGESTIVE HEART FAILURE.	01 04/01/00 CV2A FLUID VOLUME STABILIZED AS EVIDENCED BY NORMAL RESP. FUNCTION/ABSENCE OF EDEMA BY 04/01/00.	01 04/01/00 CV2A1 EVALUATE BREATH SOUNDS AND REPORT CRACKLES, WHEEZING, DYSPNEA, TACHYPNEA, ORTHOPNEA.	L
		02 04/01/00 CV2A2 LIMIT FLUID INTAKE TO 900 CC/7-3, 600 CC/3-11 300 CC/11-7 TO TOTAL 1800 CC/24HR.	LN
		03 04/01/00 CV2A3 REPORT INCREASED FATIGUE TO SUPERVISOR.	LN
		04 04/01/00 CV2A4 WEIGH RESIDENT Q WEEK REPORT WEIGHT GAIN OR LOSS OF 3 LBS. TO PHYSICIAN.	LN
		05 04/01/00 CV2A5 ASSESS/EVALUATE EFFECTIVENESS OF PRESCRIBED DIURETIC MEDICATIONS.	L

ADD-ON #7

Physician: P075 RYAN, J. M.D.	Diagnosis	428.0 CONGESTIVE HEART FAILURE

ADMIT DATE: 01/01/00   AGE: 73   Allergies   PENICILLIN, DAIRY PRODUCTS, DEMEROL M/S HYDRALAZINE, SULFA DRUGS
                        SEX: F
Name   MABEL JOHNSON   88-0101-1   ROOM: 202-0

FIGURE 4-1
Patient care plan.

developed and used appropriately, it is *the single most important tool* in providing high-quality care to residents (Fig. 4-1).

Without a plan, residents generally get the same care. What is right for one resident may not be right for another. When an individualized plan of care is not used, psychosocial needs are almost never met.

There are a number of ways the health-care plan can help you as you provide daily care.

- *It provides specific instructions regarding care to be given:* for example, "keep head of bed elevated at all times; report any complaints of burning, frequency, or pain on urination."
- *It provides necessary information needed prior to giving care:* for example, "hard of hearing — face resident and speak slowly; unsteady when ambulating — ambulate with assistance only."
- *It provides all caregivers with the same guidelines:* **Continuity** means

```
                        ADD ON HEALTH CARE DEVELOPMENT SYSTEM
   07/14/90   16:15        PATIENT MEDICAL RECORDS MAINTENANCE              PAGE   1
   ------------------------------------------------------------------------------
   88-0101-0   JOHNSON, MABEL
   -----CATAGORY----------ASSESSMENT-----------------------------------------------
```

```
    1.      ADL/AMB.    AMBULATION-EXTENSIVE     ASSIST.-ASSIST OF 2
    2.      ADL/BATHING BATH/SHOWER - REQUIRES   LIMITED ASSISTANCE
    3.      ADL/DRESSING DRESSING REQUIRES       EXTENSIVE ASSISTANCE
    4.      ADL/EATING  EATING - REQUIRES        SUPERVISION
    5.      ADL/HYGIENE GROOMING - REQUIRES      EXTENSIVE ASSISTANCE
    6.   ADL/POSITION.  POSITIONING REQUIRES     SUPERVISION
    6.   ADL/POSITION.  POS. DEVICE - PILLOWS    RIGHT HAND ONLY
    7.   ADL/TOILETING  TOILETING - REQUIRES     LIMITED ASSISTANCE
    8.   ADL/TRANSFER   TRANSFER REQ. EXTENSIVE  ASSISTANCE (2 PERSON)
   12.   GENITO/URIN.   BLADDER-OCC. INCONTINENT (2+X/WEEK BUT NOT DAILY)
   13.   INTEGUMENTARY  DERMATITIS/RASH          PERINEAL AREA
   16.   PSYCHOSOCIAL   ORIENTED TO NAMES AND    FACES
   16.   PSYCHOSOCIAL   COMMUNICATES W/O ANY     LIMITATIONS-UNDERSTOOD
   18.    RESPIRATORY   SHORTNESS OF BREATH/     DYSPNEA
   19.        SENSORY   HEARING - SPEAKER MUST   ADJUST & SPEAK DISTINCTLY
   19.        SENSORY   HEARING APPLIANCE (RT/LT) HEARING AIDE BOTH EARS
   19.        SENSORY   VISION - IMPAIRED - SEES LARGE, NOT REGULAR PRINT
   19.        SENSORY   WEARS GLASSES
   20.         SAFETY   REQ. PROTECTIVE DEVICE   VEST IN W/C
   20.         SAFETY   USE OF BEDRAIL           BOTH UP WHILE IN BED
   20.         SAFETY   SMOKES
```

FIGURE 4-2
Nursing assistant
information listing.

doing the same things in the same way — when everyone works together to achieve the same goal, positive results are more likely to occur. Residents feel more secure and comfortable when there is continuity of care.

- *It provides the nursing assistant with essential data or facts necessary for organizing and planning work:* You will be able to determine what special assignments or tasks must be performed, such as Clinitests, I & O, scheduling of special appointments or tests. You will also be better prepared to set your priorities in giving care when you have all the data available.

Remember: The health-care plan is your most important resource in providing care. Each LTC facility will have specific policies and procedures related to the health-care plans. Be sure you understand how to use them in your facility.

Some facilities use a **nursing care Kardex** to make information about the nursing care of the resident more readily available to the nursing assistant (Fig. 4-2). Information from the health-care plan is transferred to a Kardex, or "nursing assistant information" record, which may be handwritten or printed from a computer. The nursing assistant uses the Kardex to complete his or her daily assignment and as a reference for charting.

SECTION 2 ORGANIZE YOUR TIME

OBJECTIVES/WHAT YOU WILL LEARN

When you have completed this section, you will be able to:
- List the four steps involved in organizing time
- Define the term *planning*
- Place four tasks in the sequence in which they should be completed
- Write a sample plan for completing your assignment for one day

When you are doing your job as a nursing assistant, you will soon realize that there is not enough time to do everything you would like to do. In fact, lack of time is a common complaint of most people. Unfortunately, there is only so much time — 60 minutes in a hour, 24 hours in a day. Since you cannot control time, you must learn to control or manage yourself.

ORGANIZING

Organizing or managing yourself in order to complete your assignments is a four-step process that includes:

- Gathering information
- Planning
- Carrying out the plan
- Revising the plan

Your job description provides the foundation of information on which you base your organization. Begin with obtaining your assignment from your charge nurse. You'll be told which residents you'll be caring for and given specific task assignments. These tasks may vary from taking vital signs to cleaning the utility room. Most facilities use a written assignment form. Some are designed to show all the assignments for the unit, while others are individualized to each nursing assistant. You may complete the form yourself or it could be written in advance for you. Review the sample (see Fig. 4-2) to see the kinds of information you would need to plan and organize your work.

Check the health-care plan or nursing care Kardex to find out the specific needs of each resident. Determine if any residents have timed schedules that must be followed, such as testing urine before meals or keeping an appointment inside or outside the facility. You must also find out any planned events that affect the facility as a whole. Check the activity calendar for resident activities. Find out if there are employee classes or meetings scheduled.

Gathering information includes making **rounds** of your assigned residents. Making rounds means going to each resident to determine briefly whether they have any immediate needs.

PLANNING

Once all the information is gathered, it is time to plan (Fig. 4-3). **Planning** is devising a way of getting the job done. It includes thinking about the information you have gathered and writing down your plan. The written plan may

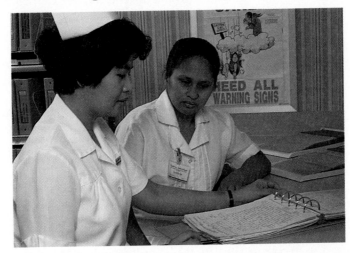

FIGURE 4-3
Planning.

simply be a "things to do" list or notes that list the names of the residents to whom you're assigned and specific tasks to be done. Planning involves:

- What you are going to do
- How you are going to do it
- When you are going to do it

SETTING PRIORITIES

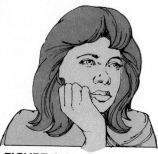

FIGURE 4-4
Setting priorities.

Setting priorities is part of planning. It refers to looking at all things that need to be done and putting them in order of what should be done first, second, and so on. You must decide who needs your attention first as well as which tasks must be done and which can, if necessary, wait until later (Fig. 4-4). Priorities tend to change from moment to moment, so there are no set rules. Your common sense will help you decide which jobs are most important. The charge nurse will help you set priorities.

There are some principles that will guide you in your planning:

- Protecting the welfare and safety of the resident is always a high priority. This includes, for example, staying with the resident in the shower, rescuing a resident who is falling, or carrying out emergency procedures in case of choking.
- Carrying out specific orders from the physician.
- Helping those who are most dependent or ill. Needs of residents always take priority over cleaning duties.

Once your plan is developed, it is time to **implement** or carry out the plan. Learning to think through each task in advance will save you both time and energy. One of the biggest wasters of time is procrastination. **Procrastinating** is putting off doing something until some other time. People most often put off tasks that they find unpleasant. Successful managers of time do not procrastinate. In fact, they usually do unpleasant tasks first so they are free to enjoy more pleasant ones.

Performing a task usually consists of three steps—preparation, action, and completion. Preparation involves gathering needed equipment. This will save you much time and energy. Action is the actual doing of the procedure or task. Remember to follow principles of good body mechanics and infection control. In giving direct care to a resident, you can be more efficient if you describe out loud what you will be doing in a step-by-step manner. Not only will the resident know what to expect, but you will also do a better, more efficient job.

One of the most effective ways you can make your job easier is to allow for and to encourage self-care. At first, it may take more time for residents to feed, dress, or groom themselves. Many of your residents may be very slow. If you find yourself becoming impatient, leave the room briefly or do some other tasks in the room. Don't just stand and watch. Once they have learned, they benefit by feeling better, and you benefit by having less work to do.

To complete a task, there is usually "cleanup" to do. You must return equipment to the proper place and dispose of waste materials properly.

Throughout the day's work, you might have to revise your plan. If you are getting behind or are unable to complete a particular task, ask your charge nurse for help. Be sure to ask as soon as possible so that the job can be completed. Don't wait until the shift is over to say, "By the way, I didn't have time to . . . "

Just as you can ask for help from your co-workers, be ready to help them when they ask. Be particularly sensitive to the needs of new employees. In addition to showing a friendly and welcoming attitude, take time to help. You'll benefit in the long run by having a stronger and more capable co-worker and team member. At the end of your shift of duty, take time to make rounds one last time to be sure that your residents' needs have been taken care of and that your assigned tasks have been done. Then you will be able to leave work with the knowledge and good feelings of a job well done.

SECTION 3 OBSERVATION AND CHARTING

OBJECTIVES/WHAT YOU WILL LEARN

When you have completed this section, you will be able to:
- Define the term *observation* and explain why it is an important responsibility of the nursing assistant
- Differentiate between statements that are fact and those that express an opinion
- List three basic principles of making entries into the resident's health record
- Identify proper charting principles
- Match abbreviations and symbols with their definitions

ELEMENTS OF OBSERVATION

One of the responsibilities of the nursing assistant is to observe, report, and record changes in the resident's condition and her or his response or lack of response to care and treatment provided. Because you, the nursing assistant, provide *more direct care* than anyone else on the health-care team, you are the most valuable resource available for observation of the resident!

Observation is recognizing and noticing a fact or occurrence. It means taking note of or paying attention to what is happening around you. Developing your ability to make accurate observations will take time and practice. You must be alert to obvious visible changes as well as to subtle changes in a resident's physical condition, mental attitude, or behavior patterns. Observation is not merely looking — it is planned, careful, and focused. *Observation involves using all the senses* (Fig. 4-5).

In order to recognize changes, you must have "stored information" as to what is normal for a particular resident. If you make a habit of quickly observing the "head-to-toe" condition of each resident as you provide care, you will be prepared to recognize any changes.

It is very important to learn to make **objective observations.** Objective observations are facts you notice that are not distorted by your personal

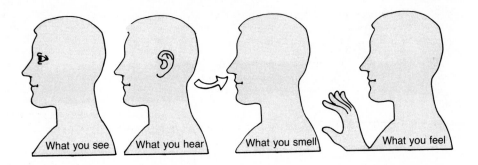

FIGURE 4-5
Observation involves using all the senses.

feelings. In other words, objective means free from bias or judgment. Entries in the health record must be fact, not judgments or impressions.

Subjective observations are individual judgments based on personal feelings. Although it is not appropriate for you to make subjective statements, you may record subjective information when you quote or describe a resident's statement of how he or she feels.

Examples of objective and subjective observations are:

Objective	Subjective
The dress is red.	The dress is pretty.
The resident weighs 80 pounds.	The resident is thin.
The resident wanders from the facility twice a day.	The resident is confused.
The resident refused a shower today.	The resident is uncooperative.
The resident was crying after her daughter visited.	The resident was depressed by the daughter's visit.

CHARTING

In addition to making accurate observations, you must write them in the resident's health record (Fig. 4-6). The amount of charting you will do, as well as the kinds of information you record, will vary from state to state and from one facility to another. *Usually you will record:*

- Care and treatment provided to each resident.
- Their response or lack of response to care and treatment provided
- The safety measures you use in providing care that protect the resident
- What you do with the resident's personal belongings or property
- Any events which occur that involve the resident

FIGURE 4-6
Charting.

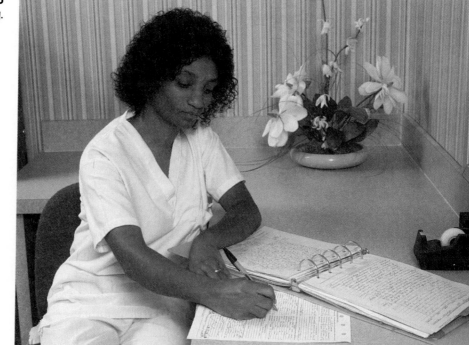

Your charting should reflect the fact that you are carrying out the actions specified on the health-care plan and indicate the resident's progress toward achieving the established goals. Review the care plan as you give care and as you record the care given.

The resident's health record is most commonly called the medical record or chart. The chart is a permanent legal record. The physician uses it to direct the care to be given, to record observations and progress, and to check what care has been given.

The physician will also gather information from entries made by other health team members to use in further diagnosis and treatment. The nursing staff uses the chart as a resource on how to provide care (based on the physician's orders) and also records all observations, progress, or lack of progress. The chart should contain an accurate picture of the resident, the care provided, and the resident's response to the care. The information and observations contained in the chart assist other health team members in planning the care to be given. Although you'll be learning new terminology and abbreviations, remember that clear communication is most important. If you don't know or aren't sure of the medical term, just use simple descriptive words.

PRINCIPLES OF CHARTING

There are certain principles of charting that you should follow:

- All entries must be made in *ink* and should be printed or written so they are *legible.*
- All entries must be *signed* with your first initial and full last name along with your title.
- All entries must be in *chronological order* (in the sequence of occurrence) and must contain *date* and *time* in order to determine when entries are made.
- All entries must be *factual* because the chart is a legal document.
- The chart must be *complete* — it must contain all information regarding the resident.
- All entries should be *brief* and *exact.*
- The chart is a *confidential* record. Each resident is guaranteed the right to confidential treatment of his or her medical records.
- The chart is the *property of the facility* and should not be removed from the premises.
- There should be no empty spaces left on a line when charting. Draw a line through the center of an empty space. This prevents anyone charting in a space signed by someone else.
- When an error is made while charting, no erasures, whiteouts, or any type of obliteration of any entry may be made. If an incorrect entry is made, a single line should be drawn through the entry and a notation made (Fig. 4-7).
- Use the present tense on all entries and use only approved abbreviations. Ditto marks are not acceptable.
- Make sure that any new forms added to the chart are properly identified with the resident's name, room number, and physician's name.

FIGURE 4-7
Correcting an error on the chart.

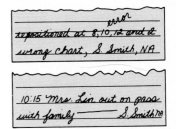

The following charting tips should be helpful as you make entries into the resident's health record.

As you continue to improve your skills in observation, you will find yourself relying on more of your senses to note unusual signs and symptoms. Being a good observer and putting your observations into clear, concise language takes skill and practice.

Describe what you see:

- The activity of the resident, including activities of daily living (dressing, bathing, feeding, personal hygiene, ambulation, continence, etc.)

  Describe what *kind* of assistance is required (total, minimal) and describe what the resident is able to do.

  Describe how the resident tolerates the activities — (fatigued, short of breath, without difficulty, etc.)

  Describe the resident's reaction to performing activities of daily living, by recording the resident's nonverbal reactions (looks of disgust, shaking fist, uninterested look, etc.)

- The resident's appetite or lack of appetite

  Describe what percentage of the food was eaten. If less than 50%, list and report what was eaten.

  On diabetic residents, list any food items not eaten, and report.

  Describe unusual food habits, likes/dislikes (always eats fruit and dessert, never eats meat, is always eating food from other trays, etc.)

- The resident's body position: how the resident appears while in bed, up in chair, ambulating

  Describe contractures or other limitations of movement, posture, gait; special assistive devices (cane, walker, etc.)

- The resident's skin condition: any changes from normal; always refer to the location, size, and special characteristics of any abnormal skin condition

  Describe unusual dryness, discolored areas, breaks in the skin, drainage, scratches, bruises.

- The presence of any abnormal discharge or drainage from any part of the body or present in excretions of the body

  Describe the substance, the amount, the color, the odor, and the consistency.

COMMONLY USED ABBREVIATIONS

If you look at a typical medical dictionary, you will see that the medical profession has developed a language of its own. This section introduces you to common abbreviations used in long-term care facilities so that you can accurately record data in the resident's health record. Study the following abbreviations and definitions until you can use them comfortably.

Related to Time

a.c.	before meals	**a.m.**	morning
p.c.	after meals	**p.m.**	afternoon or evening
q.d.	every day	**h.s.**	hour of sleep (bedtime)
b.i.d.	two times a day	**n.o.c.**	night

Describe what you hear:

• The way the resident talks	Describe any difficulties in speaking, special patterns of speech (repetitive words, mumbling, slurred speech, etc.)
	Describe any differences in how the resident talks to different people (staff, family, friends, etc.)

• What the resident says: ordinary conversations need not be described, but any unusual comments or conversations should be recorded and reported

State exactly what the resident has said that is unusual. Clarify with residents any statements made to obtain additional information and to avoid misunderstandings or "snap" judgments. If the resident complains of pain, ask and record:

- How and when it occurs
- What kind of pain
- Where it is
- How long it lasts

• Unusual sounds or noises made by the resident

Describe any unusual coughing, wheezing, gurgling, sounds in throat, and so on.

Describe what you smell:

• Note changes in the normal odors of the resident's body; poor personal hygiene can lead to disease and infection.

Describe unusual odors (fruity, ammonia-like, foul, sour, etc.)

• Bad mouth odor can indicate an infection in the mouth

• Drainage from wounds is usually foul-smelling when present

Describe what you touch:

• Use your hands to examine the resident; note reactions of the resident to touch

Describe any abnormal areas (smooth, enlarged, swollen, tender, thin, flat, distended, etc.)

Notice and describe changes you feel in skin temperature (cold, clammy, hot, dry, etc.) Describe the resident's reactions to touch (painful, no sensation).

Related to Time *(cont.)*

t.i.d.	three times a day	**stat**	immediately
q.i.d.	four times a day	**P.R.N.**	as necessary
q.o.d.	every other day	**D/C**	discontinue or stop
q.h.	every hour	**c̄**	with
min.	minute	**s̄**	without

Related to Diagnostic Terms and Body Parts

abd.	abdomen	**nephro**	kidney
ax	axilla	**O.D.**	right eye
Ca	cancer or carcinoma	**O.S.**	left eye
CHF	congestive heart failure	**O.U.**	both eyes
CVA	cerebral vascular accident (stroke)	**osteo**	bone

Related to Diagnostic Terms and Body Parts (cont.)

DX	diagnosis	**psych**	related to psychology
Fx	fracture	**pneumo**	lung
gastric	stomach	**resp**	respirations
G.I.	gastro-intestinal	**Rt**	right
G.U.	genito-urinary	**R.B.C.**	red blood cell
H.O.H.	hard of hearing	**staph**	staphylococcus
Lt	left	**S.O.B.**	short of breath
M.I.	myocardial infarction (heart attack)	**W.B.C.**	white blood cell
N/V	nausea/vomiting		

Related to Measurements

amt.	amount	**lb**	pound
approx.	approximately	**L**	liter
C	centigrade or Celsius	**min**	minim
cc	cubic centimeters	**mg**	milligram
dr	dram	**no**	number
F	Fahrenheit	**oz**	ounce
g	gram	**ss**	one-half
gr	grain	**tbsp**	tablespoon
gtt	drop	**tsp**	teaspoon
ht	height	**wt**	weight
kg	kilogram	**I, II, III, IV**	one, two, three, four

Related to Treatments

B/p	blood pressure	**Sub-Q**	subcutaneous (injection just into the superficial layers of skin)
cap	capsule	**PT**	physical therapy
cath	catheter or catheterization	**R**	rectal
C/S	culture and sensitivity (laboratory procedure)	**ROM**	range of motion
drsg.	dressing	**Rx**	prescription
EEG	electroencephalogram (brain wave tracing)	**S/A**	sugar/acetone (test of urine)
EKG or **ECG**	electrocardiogram (tracing of heart function)	**supp**	suppository
Foley	type of urinary catheter	**SSE**	soap suds enema
H₂O	water	**tab**	tablet
H₂O₂	hydrogen peroxide	**TPR**	temperature, pulse, respiration
O₂	oxygen	**TWE**	tap water enema
IM	intramuscular (injection into the muscle)	**U/A**	urinalysis (laboratory procedure)
IV	intravenous (injection within the vein)	**UNG**	ointment
		V/S	vital signs (temperature, pulse, respiration, blood pressure)

Related to Resident Orders/Activity

ADL	activities of daily living	**C/O**	complains of
ad lib	as desired	**Dr.**	doctor
amb	ambulate	**pt**	patient
assist	assistance	**I & O**	intake and output
BM	bowel movement	**NPO**	nothing by mouth
BR	bathroom	**PCP**	patient care plan
BRP	bathroom privileges	**W/C**	wheelchair

Each facility has a particular form or type of charting to be completed by the nurse assistant. The goals, however, are the same: to provide a record of care and treatment given and to record resident response to the care and to record changes in condition, unusual observations and events. In addition to observing and recording changes in the resident's condition, the nursing assistant must report to the charge nurse:

- Accident with or without injury
- Change in:
    appearance
    behavior
    function
    appetite
    elimination
- Presence of unusual odors
- Reddened or broken skin
- Complaints of pain or nausea
- Presence of swelling
- Presence of drainage
- Any bleeding
- Any tubes that are dislodged

SECTION 4 WEIGHT AND VITAL SIGNS

OBJECTIVES/WHAT YOU WILL LEARN

When you have completed this section, you will be able to:
- List the necessary criteria for obtaining accurate weights
- Weigh a resident on a standing scale
- Weigh a resident using a mechanical lift
- Weigh a resident on a bed scale
- Measure a resident's height using a tape measure
- Distinguish between conditions that increase body temperature from those that decrease body temperature
- Identify temperature readings that should be reported to the charge nurse immediately
- Read sample thermometers accurately
- Measure an oral, rectal, and axillary temperature using a glass thermometer
- Measure an oral, rectal, or axillary temperature using a battery-operated electronic thermometer
- Identify four sites on the body where the pulse can be measured
- Distinguish between those conditions that increase the pulse from those that decrease the pulse
- Measure the resident's pulse accurately
- Identify different types of respirations
- Measure a resident's respirations accurately
- Identify which reading represents the systolic blood pressure and the diastolic blood pressure
- Identify those conditions that cause the blood pressure to increase and those that cause it to decrease
- Measure a resident's blood pressure accurately

As part of the admission procedure, and on a periodic basis thereafter, residents are weighed. Many facilities weigh residents monthly or more often according to the physician's orders.

The weight of the resident is important because it is one indicator of both the nutritional status of the resident and a change in her or his medical condition. The weight taken at the time of admission gives the physician a standard to compare with future weights. *Weight measurements must be accurate to be useful!*

There are many types of scales used to weigh residents in long-term care facilities. They include the bathroom scale like the one you have at home, the standing scale, scales attached to hydraulic lifts, wheelchair scales, and bed scales (Fig. 4-8).

You need to learn how to use the scales in your facility safely and correctly. Scales used in your facility might measure the resident's weight according to the U.S. customary scale (pounds and ounces) or the metric scale (kilograms and grams). There are 2.2 pounds in each kilogram. If you wish to change kilograms into pounds, multiply the number of kilograms by 2.2. You may have to

FIGURE 4-8 Types of scales: (a) standing scale, (b) wheel chair scale, (c) bed scale, (d) scale with mechanical lift.

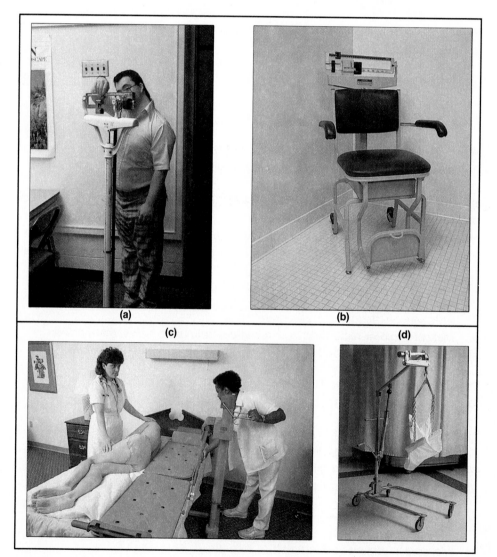

(a)

(b)

(c)

(d)

"read" the numbers on the scale, or it may have a digital readout that prints the numbers.

There are some basic guidelines you should follow when weighing residents.

- Residents should always be weighed each time at the same time of day. (Weight varies during different periods of the day, so when weights are compared, they need to be taken as close as possible to the same time of day.)
- Residents should be weighed each time wearing the *same* type or amount of clothing.
- Residents should be weighed using the *same* scale each time.

As with any procedure, the safety of the resident is most important. Be sure the equipment is in proper working order and that you know how to use it. If you need help or instructions, ask. Never risk injuring the resident!

The most commonly used scales are the standing balance scale, the scale with a hydraulic lift, and the bed scale.

Residents who are unable to stand can be weighed using a chair scale, a modification of the standing balance scale that is operated in the same fashion. Allowance is made for the weight of the chair and platform by subtracting a certain amount from the weight or by having the scale adjusted to allow for the extra weight. Follow the procedures established in your facility for the specific equipment used.

Another method of weighing a resident who is unable to stand is with a mechanical lift with a scale attached. Mechanical lifts operate using a hydraulic pump to raise and lower the resident. There are different types of lifts. Since one of the most commonly used lifts was made by the Hoyer Company, the mechanical lift may be called the Hoyer lift.

Although mechanical lifts are designed to allow one person to lift the resident, it is a good idea to use two people whenever possible. The lift may seem frightening to the resident, so explain the procedure carefully and reassure the resident that the procedure is safe.

PROCEDURE

WEIGHING THE RESIDENT ON A STANDING BALANCE SCALE

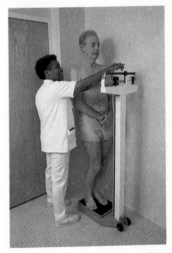

1. Prior to weighing the resident, obtain the previous weight from the chart. If this is an admission, ask the resident what his or her normal weight is. This provides a standard for comparison.
2. Explain to the resident what you are going to do.
3. Take the resident to the scale (scales will remain accurate longer if they are moved as little as possible).
4. Level the scales if necessary. Some have a level bar with a bubble that is centered when the scale is level. Balance the scale. (With both weights at zero, the balance beam should be balanced in the center. If not, use the balance adjustment to bring the scale to balance.)
5. Assist the resident to stand on the scale with hands at the sides. Be sure the resident is balanced and centered on the scale. If the resident is unable to stand alone safely, another type of scale should be used.
6. Adjust the weights until the scale is in balance.
7. Write down the weight immediately.
8. Assist the resident to return to the room.
9. Record the weight in the proper place and report any weight losses or gains to the charge nurse.

WEIGHING THE
RESIDENT WITH A
MECHANICAL LIFT

1. Assemble your equipment at the bedside:
   - Lift
   - Sling
   - Clean sheet
2. Explain to the resident what you are going to do.
3. Provide privacy.
4. Roll the resident on one side and place half the sling between the shoulders and the knees. Roll the resident to the opposite side and pull the other half of the sheet and sling under.
5. Wheel the lift into place over the resident with the base beneath the bed.
6. Attach the sling using the chains and hooks provided.
   Note: The open part of the hook should be *away* from the resident.
7. Using the hand crank or pump handle, raise the resident until the buttocks are clear of the bed. Make sure that the resident is aligned in the sling and is securely suspended.
8. Swing the feet and legs over the edge of the bed. If the bed is low enough and lift goes high enough for the resident to be clear of the bed, weigh the resident while still over the bed.
9. If not, move the lift back from the bed so that no part of the resident's body is in contact with the bed.
10. Adjust the weights until the scale is balanced. Follow the balancing directions for the scale in use. Read and record the weight shown immediately.
11. Return the resident to a position over the bed.
12. Slowly release the knob and lower the resident onto the bed.
13. Remove the sheet and sling from beneath the resident.
14. Position the resident comfortably with call signal within reach.
15. Return equipment to proper place.
16. Report any weight losses or gains to the charge nurse.

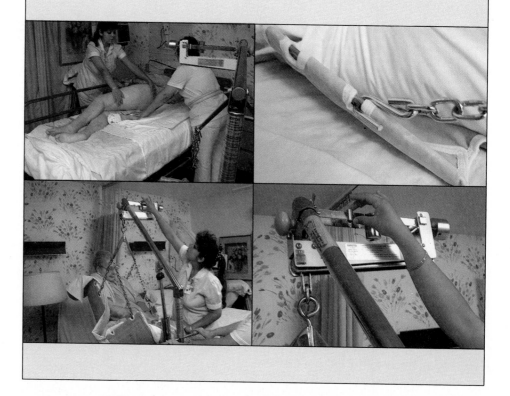

Remember, the resident's weight measurement must be accurate. This information is vital in the diagnosis and treatment prescribed by the physician. If you have any questions as to the accuracy of the weight obtained, ask your charge nurse to verify the weight with you. You can test the accuracy of the scales by weighing yourself and comparing the results to your known weight.

1. Assemble your equipment at the bedside.
   - Scale
   - Clean sheet
2. Explain to the resident what you are going to do.
3. Provide privacy.
4. Roll the resident toward one side and place the clean sheet beneath the resident. (Use a folded sheet to allow you to use it as a lift sheet.) Roll the resident to the opposite side and pull the other half of the sheet under.
5. Place the bed scale next to the bed, or if possible, roll the scale so that the platform is over the bed.
6. Lock the wheels of the scale.
7. Using two people, either
   a. Roll the resident on to the weighing platform, or
   b. Use the lifting sheet to lift the resident on to the platform
8. Release the brake and move the resident and scale away from the bed.
9. When using a digital scale, read and record the weight provided. If weights are used, add until the scale is balanced. Record the weight immediately.
10. Return the resident to the bed by rolling or lifting him or her from the scale onto the bed.
11. Remove the sheet from under the resident.
12. Position the resident comfortably.
13. Place the call signal within reach.
14. Return the equipment to the proper place. Disinfect pads on bed scale unless sheets were used. (Sheets must be changed.)
15. Wash your hands.

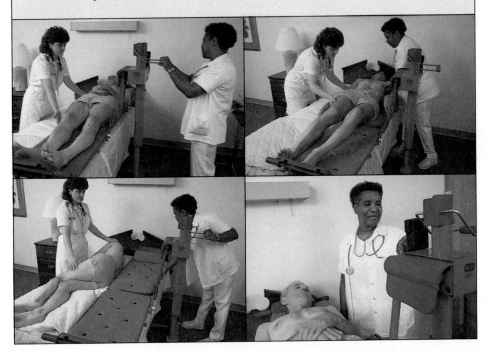

In order to determine the appropriate or ideal weight for an individual resident, it is necessary to know the resident's height. You may be asked to measure height by using either the height measurement device on the standing scale or by using a tape measure.

Height is measured in feet, inches, or centimeters. When using a tape measure, make sure the bed is in a flat position, then position the resident in the supine (back lying) position, with the body extended. Place a mark on the sheet at the top of the head and at the bottom of the feet; then measure the distance between the marks. An alternative for a resident who cannot "straighten out" due to contractures is to extend one arm so that it is **perpendicular** (at a right angle) to the body. Measure from the center of the neck to the tip of the longest finger, multiply the result by 2 and subtract 2 inches. The final number will be the resident's height.

BODY TEMPERATURE

Body temperature is measured by a clinical thermometer, and it represents a balance between the heat produced by the body and the heat lost by the body (Fig. 4-9). The normal adult temperature is measured in degrees **Fahrenheit (F)** or degrees **Celsius** or **centigrade (C).** The normal adult body temperature taken orally is 98.6°F or 37°C.

Factors that *increase* the body temperature include:

- Infection
- Shivering
- Physical activity and exercise
- Warmer external environment (hot weather, warm blankets or clothing, hot bath)
- Dehydration (lack of enough fluid in the body)

Factors that *decrease* the body temperature include:

- Shock (decreased circulation)
- Colder external environment (cold weather, cold shower, alcohol sponge bath)

FIGURE 4-9
Vital signs.

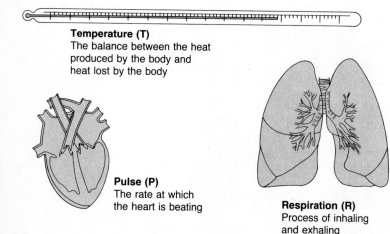

Temperature (T)
The balance between the heat produced by the body and heat lost by the body

Pulse (P)
The rate at which the heart is beating

Respiration (R)
Process of inhaling and exhaling

Blood Pressure (BP)
Force of blood pushing against the walls of the arteries

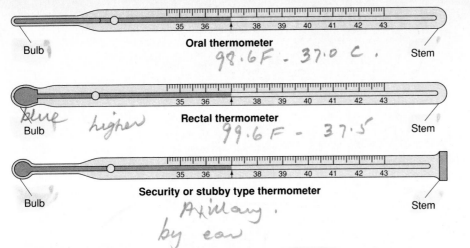

Oral thermometer

Bulb   *Stem*

98.6F - 37.0 C.

Rectal thermometer

blue   higher

Bulb   *Stem*

99.6 F - 37.5

Security or stubby type thermometer

Bulb   *Stem*

Axillary.

by ear

95 - 32 = 63

63 x 5/9

FIGURE 4-10
Types of glass thermometers.

FIGURE 4-11
Temperature conversion.

- Age (older people tend to have a lower "normal" body temperature)
- Drugs such as aspirin or acetaminophen

Regulation of temperature is one of the many ways the body protects itself. The temperature increases to fight infection and decreases to save strength and energy.

TYPES OF THERMOMETERS AND INDICATIONS FOR USE

We measure body temperature with a clinical thermometer. There are glass thermometers (Fig. 4-10), battery-operated electronic thermometers, and chemically treated paper or plastic single-use thermometers.

Glass thermometers are filled with mercury, a silver liquid that expands with heat. The thermometer is **calibrated** (marked) in degrees and fractions of degrees (Fig. 4-11). There are thermometers with Fahrenheit scales and thermometers with centigrade scales (Fig. 4-12).

TYPES OF MEASUREMENT

The Fahrenheit thermometer has been most commonly used in the United States. The numbers start at 94°F and go up to 110°F (Fig. 4-13). The long lines represent 1 degree, the short lines represent two tenths of a degree. There is usually an arrow at 98.6°F, which is the "normal" body temperature reading.

Temperature Conversion		
	43	109.4 / 109.0
Centigrade	42	108.0 / 107.0
To convert Fahrenheit to Centigrade, subtract 32 from degrees F and multiply by 5/9	41	106.0 / 105.0
	40	104.0 / 103.0
	39	102.0 / 101.0
	38	100.0 / 99.0
Fahrenheit	37	98.0
To convert Centigrade to Fahrenheit, multiply degrees C by 9/5 and add 32	36	97.0 / 96.0
	35	95.0 / 94.0
	34	93.0 / 92.0
	33	91.0 / 90.0
	32	89.0
	31	88.0 / 87.0
	30	86.0 / 85.0
	29	84.2

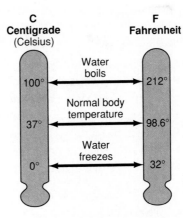

C
Centigrade
(Celsius)

F
Fahrenheit

Water boils

100°   212°

Normal body temperature

37°   98.6°

Water freezes

0°   32°

FIGURE 4-12
The two major scales used for measuring temperature in the United States.

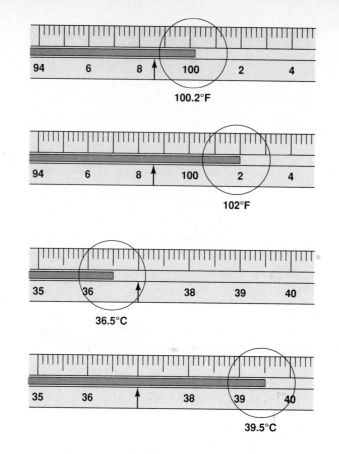

FIGURE 4-13
Fahrenheit thermometer.

FIGURE 4-14
Centigrade thermometer.

The centigrade thermometer begins with 34°C and ends at 43°C (Fig. 4-14). Each long line represents 1 degree; each short line represents one-tenth of a degree.

The parts of a thermometer consist of the **bulb,** which is the portion placed in direct contact with the resident's body, and the **stem,** which is the opposite end of the thermometer.

Temperature is measured orally (by mouth), axillary (under the armpit), or rectally (inserted through the anus into the rectum). These sites are chosen because each has a rich supply of blood close to the surface that will produce an accurate temperature reading.

METHODS OF MEASUREMENT

The decision as to how a temperature should be measured will depend on several factors. In some instances, the physician will specify which method to use. Other factors are related to the condition of the resident. For example, you would never measure an **oral** (in the mouth) temperature on an unconscious or very confused resident who might accidentally bite down on the thermometer. Generally, a **rectal** (in the rectum) temperature is ordered when the resident:

- Has a history of seizures
- Is under 8 years old
- Cannot keep his or her mouth closed around the thermometer
- Is unable to breathe through the nose
- Is restless, unconscious, or confused
- Has coughing or sneezing spells
- Is receiving warm or cold applications to the face or neck

Rectal temperature should *not* be measured under the following conditions:

- When the resident has any sign of hemorrhoids or rectal bleeding

- When the resident is very combative
- When the resident has diarrhea

The **axillary** (in the armpit) method of measurement is the least reliable and should only be used if the oral and rectal methods would be unsafe.

Thermometers vary according to how the temperature is to be measured. One type is used for oral and axillary, another is used for measuring rectal temperature.

The "normal" reading varies with the method of measurement and the type of thermometer used.

	Fahrenheit	Centigrade
3 mis Oral	98.6	37.0
3 mins Rectal	99.6	37.5 *higher by ear → Same as normal*
10 ~ 8 mins Axillary	97.6	36.4 *lower*

Memorize these normal readings so that you can recognize an abnormal reading and report it promptly. There are small variations in body temperature that are considered normal. For example, the body temperature is generally lower in the morning and increases in the afternoon. However, when the temperature reaches any of the following readings, it should be considered out of the normal range and reported immediately.

Oral	100°F or 37.6°C
Rectal	101°F or 38.0°C
Axillary	99°F or 37.2°C

Glass thermometers are quite fragile and must be handled with care. The thermometer should be inspected for cracks and chips before each use. Although mercury rises with heat, it does not constrict with cold. This means that to move the mercury column down after it has risen, the thermometer must be shaken down. To shake the thermometer down, stand away from objects that you might hit with the thermometer. Grasp the stem end securely between your thumb and index finger. Using a snapping motion of your wrist, shake the thermometer three times, then check to see how far the mercury column has gone down. Shake again if necessary. It should be below the 94°F or 34°C mark before the thermometer is ready for use.

Reading the thermometer consists of locating the end of the mercury column and reading or calculating the number of degrees represented (Fig. 4-15). Write the information down immediately. Don't try to remember it.

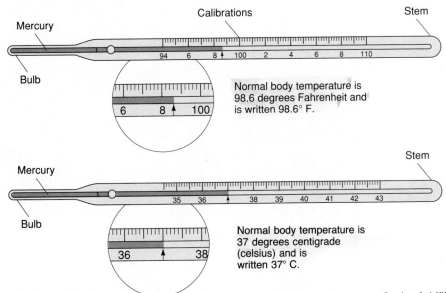

FIGURE 4-15
Using an oral thermometer.

Normal body temperature is 98.6 degrees Fahrenheit and is written 98.6° F.

Normal body temperature is 37 degrees centigrade (celsius) and is written 37° C.

Accuracy is essential! Practice reading as many thermometers as possible and have your charge nurse verify your readings to ensure that you have learned to read a thermometer correctly.

Remember that you will always use a rectal thermometer for taking rectal temperatures. Note that the rectal thermometer has a small round bulb on one end. This bulb prevents the thermometer from injuring the sensitive lining of the resident's rectum.

PROCEDURE

READING A FAHRENHEIT THERMOMETER

1. With your thumb and first two fingers, hold the thermometer at the stem.
2. Hold the thermometer at eye level. Turn the thermometer back and forth between your fingers until you can clearly see the column of mercury.
3. Notice the scale of calibrations. Each long line stands for 1 degree.
4. There are four short lines between each of the long lines. Each short line stands for two tenths (or 0.2) of a degree.
5. Between the long lines that represent 98 and 99, look for a longer line with an arrow directly beneath it. This arrow points to "normal" oral body temperature (98.6).
6. Look at the end of the mercury. Notice the line where the mercury ends. If it is one of the short lines, notice the previously longer line toward the bulb end. The temperature reading is the degree marked by that long line plus two, four, six, or eight tenths of a degree. If the mercury ends on the second short line after 99, the temperature is 99.4°F. If the mercury ends between two lines, use the closer line.
7. Write down the temperature reading right away. The temperature reading may be written 99.4°F or 99⁴. If the temperature is taken rectally, write 99.4 R. If the temperature is taken in the axilla, write 99.4 A. If not marked R or A, the temperature is assumed to be an oral reading.

1. Assemble your equipment:
   - Oral thermometer
   - Pen or pencil and paper
   - Tissue or paper towel
   - Disposable plastic shield
2. Wash your hands.
3. Identify the resident.
4. Tell the resident that you are going to measure the temperature.
5. Ask if the resident has recently had hot or cold fluids, or been smoking. If yes, wait 20 minutes before taking an oral temperature.
6. If the thermometer has been soaking in a solution, rinse it with cool tap water, and dry with paper towel or tissue.
7. Shake the mercury down, if necessary.
8. Gently put the bulb end in the resident's mouth under the tongue. The mouth and the lips should stay closed.
9. For the most accurate reading, leave the thermometer in the resident's mouth for 8 minutes.
10. Take the thermometer out. Hold the stem end and wipe the thermometer with the tissue from the stem toward the bulb.
11. Read the thermometer.
12. Record the temperature. Report any abnormal reading immediately to your charge nurse.
13. Shake the mercury down. Replace the thermometer in its container or return it to the proper area for cleaning.
14. Make the resident comfortable.
15. Wash your hands.

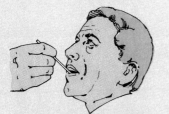

A Insert the thermometer gently into the resident's mouth under the tongue.

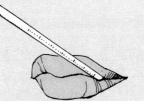

B Position the thermometer to the side of the mouth.

3 mans

C Instruct the resident to keep the thermometer under the tongue by gently closing the lips around the thermometer.

MEASURING RECTAL
TEMPERATURE

3 mins

1. Assemble your equipment:
   - Rectal thermometer
   - Tissue or paper towel
   - Lubricating jelly
   - Disposable gloves
   - Pencil or pen and paper
2. Wash your hands.
3. Identify the resident.
4. Provide privacy.
5. Tell the resident that you are going to measure the temperature by rectum.
6. Place the bed in a flat position, if possible.
7. Inspect the bulb of the thermometer carefully for cracks or chipped places. A broken thermometer could seriously injure the resident. **Never** use a chipped, cracked, or broken thermometer.
8. Shake the thermometer down, if necessary.
9. Put a small amount of lubricating jelly on a piece of tissue. Then lubricate the bulb of the thermometer with the lubricated tissue. This makes insertion easier and also makes it more comfortable for the resident.
10. Assist the resident to turn to one side. Turn back the covers just enough so that you can see the buttocks. Avoid overexposing.
11. Put on your gloves.
12. Raise the upper buttock until you can see the anus (the opening of the rectum) and gently insert the bulb one inch through the anus into the rectum.

PROCEDURE

MEASURING AXILLARY
TEMPERATURE

9 - 10 mins

1. Assemble your equipment:
   - Oral thermometer
   - Tissue or paper towel
   - Pen or pencil and paper
2. Wash your hands.
3. Identify the resident.
4. Tell the resident that you have to measure the temperature.
5. Provide privacy.
6. If the thermometer is kept in a solution, rinse the thermometer with cool tap water and dry it with tissue.
7. Shake the mercury down if necessary.
8. Remove the resident's arm from the sleeve of the gown. If the axillary region is moist with perspiration, dry it with a towel.
9. Place the bulb of the thermometer in the center of the armpit (axilla). The thermometer then should be held upright by the arm.
10. Put the resident's arm across the chest or abdomen.
11. If the resident is unconscious or too weak to help, you will have to hold the thermometer in place.
12. Leave the thermometer in place for 10 minutes. Stay with the resident.
13. Remove the thermometer. Wipe it off with tissue from the stem to the bulb.

13. Hold the thermometer in place for 3 minutes. Never leave a resident with a rectal thermometer in the rectum.

14. Remove the thermometer. Holding the stem, wipe it with a tissue from stem to bulb to remove any particles of feces.

15. Read the thermometer.

16. Remove your gloves.

17. Record the temperature. Note that this is a rectal temperature by writing an R after the figure. Report any abnormal readings immediately to your charge nurse.

18. Return the thermometer to the appropriate area for cleaning.

19. Wash your hands.

20. Make the resident comfortable.

21. Place the call signal within reach.

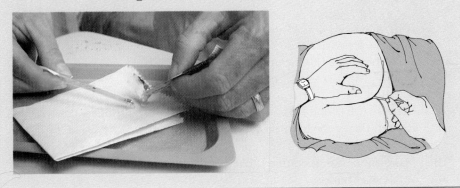

14. Read the thermometer and record the temperature. Note that this is an axillary temperature by writing an A after the figure. Report any abnormal readings immediately to your charge nurse.

15. Replace the thermometer in its container or return it to the proper area for cleaning.

16. Put the resident's arm back in the sleeve of the gown.

17. Make the resident comfortable.

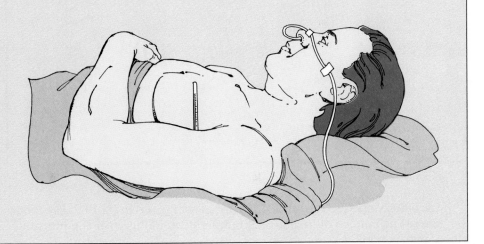

USING A
BATTERY-OPERATED
ELECTRONIC
THERMOMETER

1. Assemble your equipment:
   - Battery-operated electronic thermometer
   - Plastic disposable probe cover
   - Appropriate attachment for type of temperature (oral, rectal, axillary)
   - Pen or pencil and paper
   - Gloves for rectal temperature
2. Wash your hands.
3. Identify the resident.
4. Tell the resident that you are going to measure the temperature.
5. Provide privacy.
6. Remove the probe from its stored position and insert it into the probe cover.
7. Insert the covered probe into the appropriate opening (mouth, rectum, or axilla). If taking the temperature rectally, lubricate the probe cover with a water-soluble lubricant.
8. Hold the probe in place.
9. Wait for the buzzer or beep to signal that the temperature reading is complete.
10. Remove the probe and discard the prove cover without touching it.
11. Return the probe to its stored position.
12. Record the temperature.
13. Make the resident comfortable.
14. Wash your hands.
15. Report any abnormal reading to the charge nurse.

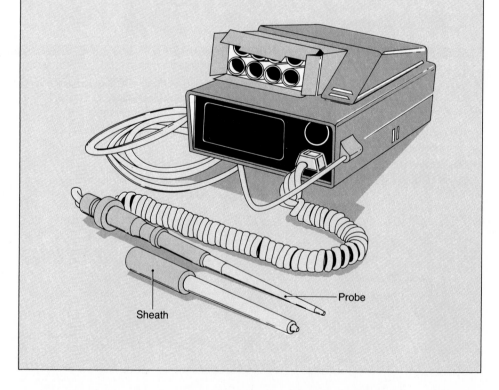

Sheath   Probe

If the battery-operated electronic thermometer is used in your facility, follow the general principles of measuring temperature along with the manufacturer's instructions.

CHARACTERISTICS OF THE PULSE

Each time the heart beats, it pumps a certain amount of blood into the arteries. This causes the arteries to expand (get bigger). Between heartbeats, the arteries contract, returning to their normal size. The heart pumps the blood in a steady rhythm. The rhythmic expansion and contraction of the arteries, which can be measured to show how fast the heart is beating, is called the **pulse** (Fig. 4-16).

Measuring the pulse is a simple method of determining how the circulatory system is functioning. The pulse measures how fast the heart is beating. The pulse can be felt at certain places on the body. The normal pulse can be felt easily by your fingertips. If circulation is decreased, the pulse can be weak or absent.

One of the easiest places to feel the pulse is at the wrist (Fig. 4-17). This is called a **radial pulse** because you are feeling the radial artery. When measuring the pulse, you must accurately note the following.

- **Rate** — the number of pulse beats per minute
- **Rhythm** — the regularity of the pulse beats
- **Force of the beat** — weak or bounding

Each person has a "normal" rate somewhere within the normal range. The nursing assistant must report any significant changes in pulse rate, rhythm, or force. If the resident's rate is below sixty or above ninety beats per mintue, report this to your charge nurse immediately. Remember, the pulse rate will increase with physical activity, stress, emotional disturbances, fever, and some illnesses. Make sure that you measure the routine pulse when the resident is at rest.

Normal Pulse Rates (Per Minute) for Different Age Groups

Childhood Years	80–115
Adult Years	72–80
Later Years	60–70

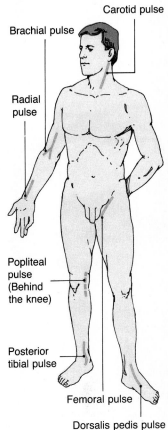

FIGURE 4-16
Places where the pulse may be taken.

Carotid pulse
Brachial pulse
Radial pulse
Popliteal pulse (Behind the knee)
Posterior tibial pulse
Femoral pulse
Dorsalis pedis pulse

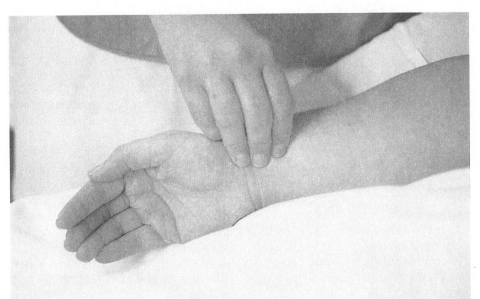

FIGURE 4-17
Radial pulse.

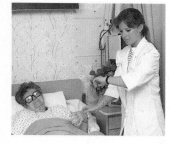

1. Assemble your equipment:
   - Watch with a second hand
   - Pen or pencil and paper
2. Wash your hands.
3. Identify the resident.
4. Tell the resident that you are going to measure the pulse.
5. His hand and arm should be well supported and resting comfortably.
6. Find the pulse by placing the tips of your middle three fingers on the palm side of the resident's wrist, in a line with the thumb, directly next to the bone. Press lightly until you feel the beat. If you press too hard, you may stop the flow of blood and the pulse. Never use your thumb. It has its own pulse and you might count your own pulse instead of the resident's. When you have found the pulse, note the rhythm. Is the beat steady or irregular? Note the force of the beat. Is it strong or weak?
7. Note the position of the second hand on your watch. Count the pulse beats until the second hand comes back to the same position.
   - Method A: Count the pulse beats for 1 full minute and report the full minute count. Always do this if the resident has an irregular beat.
   - Method B: Count for 30 seconds, until the second hand is opposite from the position when you started. Then multiply the number of beats by 2. This is the number you record. For example, if you count 35 for 30 seconds, the count for 1 full minute would be 70.
8. Record the pulse count.
9. Make the resident comfortable.
10. Wash your hands.
11. Report to your charge nurse:
    - If the pulse rate was under 60 or over 90 beats per minute
    - If the rhythm was irregular
    - If the force was weak or bounding
    - If there was a change in rate, rhythm, or force from previous measurements

APICAL PULSE

The pulse rate should be the same as the heart rate. However, in some residents, the heartbeats are not strong enough to be felt along the arteries. This can be due to some forms of heart disease. For these residents, an apical pulse would be taken with a stethoscope (Fig. 4-18).

An **apical pulse** is a measurement of the heartbeats at the apex of the heart, located just under the left breast (Fig. 4-19).

You will be using a stethoscope to listen to the apical pulse. The **stethoscope** is an instrument used to listen to various sounds in the body, such as the heartbeat or breathing sounds. The stethoscope is a tube that picks up sound when it is placed against a part of the body. One end is either bell-shaped (called a bell), or it is round and flat (called a diaphragm) (Fig. 4-20). The other end of the tube is split into two parts. These parts have tips on the ends and fit into the listener's ears.

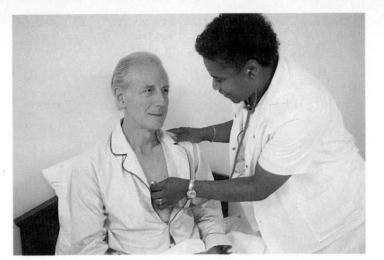

FIGURE 4-18
Taking an apical pulse with a stethoscope.

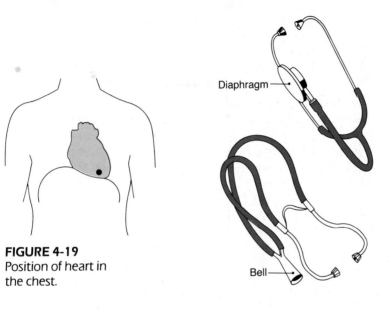

FIGURE 4-19
Position of heart in the chest.

FIGURE 4-20
Stethoscopes.

MEASURING RESPIRATIONS

Respiration is the process of inhaling and exhaling. One respiration includes breathing in once and breathing once. When a person breathes out, the chest contracts (gets smaller). When you count respirations, you watch the resident's chest rise and fall or feel the chest rise and fall with your hand.

When a person knows that respiration is being counted, he or she may not breathe naturally. What you want to count is the natural breathing rate. Normally, adults breathe at a rate of 16 to 20 times a minute. Children breathe more rapidly. The elderly breathe more slowly. Exercise, digestion, emotional stress, disease, drugs, stimulants, heat, and cold can all affect the number of times per minute that a person breathes.

While you are counting the resident's respirations, it is important to observe and make note of anything about the breathing that appears to be abnormal. Different types of abnormal respiration include:

- **Labored** — the resident struggles or works hard to breathe and may make gurgling, rattling, or wheezing sounds.
- **Stertorous** — the resident makes abnormal noises like snoring when breathing.
- **Abdominal** — breathing using mostly the abdominal muscles.

1. Assemble your equipment:
   - Watch with a second hand
   - Pen or pencil and paper
2. Wash your hands.
3. Identify the resident.
4. Provide privacy.
5. Hold the resident's wrist as if you were measuring the pulse. Count the respirations immediately after counting the pulse rate.
6. One rise and one fall of the chest counts as one respiration.
7. If you cannot clearly see the chest rise and fall, hold the resident's arms across the chest and feel the chest rise.
8. Count the respirations for one full minute.
9. Write down the figure.
10. Make the resident comfortable.
11. Wash your hands.
12. Report any unusual observations to your charge nurse immediately.

- **Shallow** — breathing with only the upper part of the lungs.
- **Irregular** — the depth of breathing changes and the rate of the rise and fall of the chest is not steady.
- **Chenye-Stokes** — irregular breathing. At first the breathing is slow and shallow, then respiration becomes faster and deeper until it reaches a kind of peak. It then slows and becomes shallow again. Breathing may stop completely for 10 seconds and begin the same pattern again.

Temperature, pulse, and respiration (TPR) are usually measured at the same time as one procedure. Careful, accurate recording of this information is very important. The procedures for measuring the vital signs must be practiced many times for you to be able to carry them out skillfully and accurately (Fig. 4-21).

BLOOD PRESSURE

Blood pressure is the force of the blood pushing against the walls of the blood vessels. When you measure a resident's blood pressure, you are measuring the force of the blood flowing through the arteries.

FIGURE 4-21
Learning basic skills.

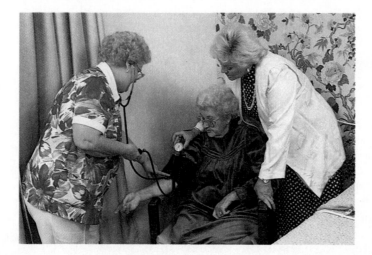

There is always a certain amount of pressure in the arteries. This is because the heart, by pumping, is constantly forcing blood to circulate. The amount of pressure in the arteries depends on two things:

- The rate of the heartbeat
- How easily the blood flows through the blood vessels

The heart contracts as it pumps blood into the arteries. When the heart is contracting, the pressure is highest. This pressure is called **systolic pressure.** As the heart relaxes between each contraction, the pressure goes down. When the heart is most relaxed, the pressure is lowest. This pressure is called the **diastolic pressure.** When you measure a resident's blood pressure, you are measuring the systolic and diastolic pressures.

In healthy adults, the normal systolic blood pressure range is between 100 and 140 millimeters (mm) of mercury (Hg). The normal diastolic pressure is between 60 and 90 millimeters (mm) of mercury (Hg). The way to write these figures is: 120/80. The systolic pressure is always the first or top number.

When a resident's blood pressure is higher than the normal range for his or her age and condition, it is referred to as **hypertension** or high blood pressure. When a resident's blood pressure is lower than the normal range, it is referred to as **hypotension** or low blood pressure.

The elderly tend to have higher blood pressure due to a loss of elasticity of the arteries. There are many residents with hypertension in LTC facilities. The blood pressure will normally increase with physical activity, stress, emotional disturbances, fever, and some illnesses. It will decrease when the resident is sleeping or at rest or if the resident is in shock (a condition related to the circulatory system). Certain medications also increase or decrease blood pressure. All individuals have a "normal" range of blood pressure for their age and physical health. Any significant changes in blood pressure should be reported to the charge nurse immediately.

The position of the resident will also change the measurement. Generally, the blood pressure increases when the resident is lying flat, and it decreases when the resident is in a sitting or standing position. You should try to measure the blood pressure each time with the resident in the same position (usually sitting if tolerated).

INSTRUMENTS FOR MEASURING BLOOD PRESSURE

When you measure blood pressure, you will be using a stethoscope and an instrument called a as sphygmomanometer. **Sphygmomanometer** is a combination of three Greek words:

- *Sphygmo,* meaning pulse
- *Mano,* meaning pressure
- *Meter,* meaning measure

This instrument, however, is usually called a *blood pressure cuff.* The four main parts of this instrument are the manometer, valve, cuff, and bulb.

Two kinds of manometers are used for taking blood pressure. One is called the mercury type (Fig. 4-22). The other is called the aneroid (dial) type (Fig. 4-23). Both have an inflatable cloth-covered rubber bag or cuff. The cuff is wrapped around the resident's arm. Both kinds also have a rubber bulb for pumping air into the cuff. The procedure for measuring blood pressure is the same, except for reading the measurement. When you use the mercury type, you will be watching the level of a column of mercury on a measuring scale. When you use the dial or aneroid type, you will be watching a pointer on a dial.

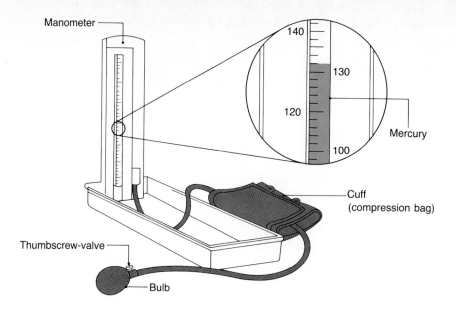

FIGURE 4-22
Mercury
sphygmomanometer.

When you measure a resident's blood pressure, you are doing two things at the same time. You are listening to the brachial pulse as it sounds in the brachial artery in the resident's arm. You also are watching an indicator (either a column of mercury or a dial) in order to take a reading.

Accurately measuring blood pressure requires a lot of practice. Blood pressure can vary each time it is taken and in each arm. If you need to repeat the measurement, allow the resident several minutes to rest. Do not inflate and deflate the cuff several times in a row because the results will be inaccurate. The cuff that wraps around the resident's arm must fit properly in order to obtain an accurate result. For this reason, there are cuffs made in small (pediatric) sizes as well as extra-large sizes. For residents who are so thin that the cuff slides up and down on the arm, request a small cuff. If the resident is so heavy that the cuff just barely meets, ask for a large cuff.

Usually, blood pressure is measured in the left arm in order to have consistent readings. Do not measure blood pressure in an arm with an IV, an A-V shunt (dialysis patient), a cast, or any kind of wound or sore.

FIGURE 4-23
Aneroid
sphygmomanometer.

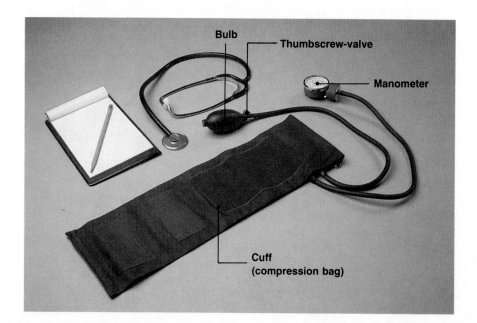

1. Assemble your equipment:
   - Sphygmomanometer
   - Stethoscope
   - Antiseptic pad
   - Pen or pencil and paper
2. Wash your hands.
3. Identify the resident.
4. Tell the resident that you are going to measure the blood pressure.
5. Wipe the earplugs of the stethoscope with antiseptic pads.
6. Have the resident resting quietly, either lying down or sitting in a chair.
7. If you are using the mercury type, the measuring scale should be at eye level.
8. The resident's arm should be bare up to the shoulder.
9. The resident's arm from the elbow down should be resting fully extended on the bed or on the arm of a chair.
10. Unroll the cuff and loosen the valve on the bulb. Then squeeze the compression bag to deflate it completely.
11. Wrap the cuff snugly and smoothly around the resident's arm about 1 inch above the elbow with the arrows on the cuff pointing toward the brachial pulse. Do not wrap it so tightly that the resident is uncomfortable from the pressure.
12. Be sure the manometer is in position so that you can read the numbers easily.
13. Put the earplugs of the stethoscope into your ears.
14. With your fingertips, find the brachial pulse at the inner side of the arm above the elbow. Place the diaphragm or bell of the stethoscope there. It should be held firmly against the skin, but should not touch the cuff.
15. Tighten the thumbscrew of the valve to close it. Turn it clockwise. Be careful not to turn it too tightly or you will have trouble opening it.
16. Hold the stethoscope in place. Inflate the cuff so that the dial points to 170 (200 on an older person), and you no longer hear the pulse.
17. Open the valve counterclockwise. This allows the air to escape. Let it out *slowly* until the sound of the pulse comes back. A few seconds must go by without any pulse sounds. If you do hear pulse

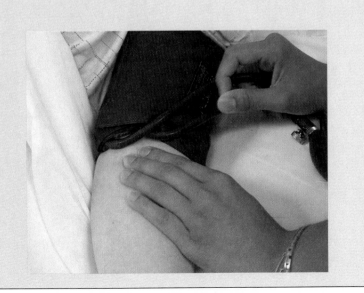

SECTION 1 INTRODUCTION TO ANATOMY AND PHYSIOLOGY

OBJECTIVES/WHAT YOU WILL LEARN

When you have completed this section, you will be able to:

- Explain why it is helpful for the nursing assistant to understand basic principles of anatomy and physiology
- Define the terms *anatomy* and *physiology*
- Explain the concept of homeostasis
- List five basic physical needs
- Match the parts of a cell with their function
- Identify the four components in the organization of the body
- Identify the various organs of the body

BASIC PHYSICAL NEEDS

All people have basic human needs that must be met to survive. These needs are divided into two categories:

- Basic psychosocial needs (mind)
- Basic physiological needs (body)

The psychosocial needs have been studied in Chapter 3. In the chapters dealing with the body systems, you will study the physiological needs. In addition to the sections on basic human physiology, systems, and the senses in this and following chapters, also study the color illustrations of these topics presented in each chapter.

- Need for air (oxygen)
- Need for food and fluids
- Need for activity and rest
- Need for protection (shelter)
- Need for elimination of body wastes

During your study of normal body structure and function, you will see how chronic illness, disease, injury, and age-related problems interfere with the resident's ability to meet these basic physical needs.

ANATOMY AND PHYSIOLOGY

As you provide residents with care, you will need to understand the *anatomy* (basic structure) and *physiology* (function) of the body. This knowledge will help you understand why certain kinds of nursing care are necessary.

- **Anatomy** is the study of body parts, how the body is made, and what it is made of.
- **Physiology** is the study of how the body functions and how all the body parts work independently and together.

In the study of anatomy, all terms of reference are made in relation to the **anatomical position** (Fig. 5-1). When in the anatomical position, the person is standing straight facing you, with palms out and feet together. When you look

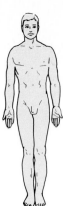

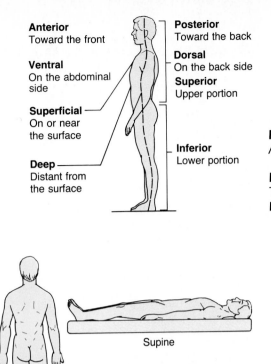

Anterior
Toward the front

Ventral
On the abdominal
side

Superficial
On or near
the surface

Deep
Distant from
the surface

Posterior
Toward the back

Dorsal
On the back side

Superior
Upper portion

Inferior
Lower portion

FIGURE 5-1
Anatomical position.

FIGURE 5-2
Terms that describe where
body parts are located.

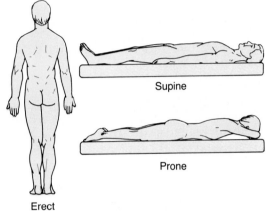

Supine

Prone

Erect

FIGURE 5-3
Terms that describe
anatomical postures.

at a person in the anatomical position, the left side is always on your right side—like looking into a mirror.

Many of the terms used to describe body parts and their relationships are familiar words, but they assume different meanings when used in anatomical description (Figs. 5-2 and 5-3). For example, **superior** means toward the head and **inferior** means toward the feet. These terms may also be used to describe the position of an organ in the body. For example, the shoulder is superior to the elbow.

HOMEOSTASIS

The human body is a complex structure. This section provides you with only a basic introduction to the study of anatomy and physiology. A very important concept in the field of physiology is homeostasis. **Homeostasis** is the body's attempt to keep its internal environment stable or in balance.

Examples of the body's ability to maintain homeostasis are:

- The body temperature stays very constant
- The blood pressure stays within specific limits
- The chemistry of the blood stays within certain normal limits

Only when illness, disease, injury, or emotional disturbances occur does this balance of our inner environment change. The body then has a great ability to adapt to overcome these problems.

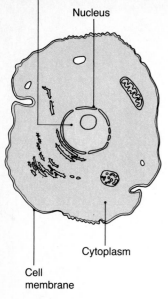

Nucleoplasm

Nucleus

Cytoplasm

Cell
membrane

FIGURE 5-4
Structure of the cell.

THE CELL

The **cell** is the fundamental "building block" of all living organisms (Fig. 5-4). Cells are so small they can be seen only through a microscope. The human body is made of about 100 trillion cells. There are many different kinds of cells and each kind has a special function. Living cells have many things in common. Cells:

- Come from preexisting cells
- Use food for energy
- Use oxygen to break down the food
- Use water to transport various substances
- Grow and repair themselves
- Reproduce themselves
- Die

Cells are made of **protoplasm,** the basic substance of life. The cell consists of three main parts:

- **Nucleus**—directs the activities of the cell, like a command center. The nucleus directs the growth of the cell and cell division. Cells also contain **chromosomes,** threadlike structures that carry the genetic material.
- **Cytoplasm**—the protoplasm *outside* the nucleus. It contains structures that have specialized functions in performing the work of the cell (work center of the cell).
- **Cell membrane**—the rim or edge of the cell. It keeps the protoplasm in but allows certain other materials to pass in and out of the cell.

All living cells carry out complex processes that use oxygen and give off carbon dioxide. These processes are called **metabolism,** or the work of the cell.

Cells are constantly dying; therefore, they must reproduce themselves. Cells reproduce by dividing. Cell division simply means that the cell splits into two parts, each exactly like the other. Then these two parts divide again and again.

Currently, there is a great deal of research involving the cell and its environment. Because the cell is considered the building block of all living matter, scientists are constantly searching for new knowledge that can lead to cures for diseases such as cancer, muscular dystrophy, and leukemia.

TISSUE

Cells usually do not work alone but are organized together into tissue. **Tissue** is a group of the same type of cells functioning in the same way. The types of body tissue are grouped into five distinct categories (Fig. 5-5):

- Epitheleal
- Connective
- Nervous
- Blood and lymph
- Muscular

Tissues do not work alone, they combine to form organs (Fig. 5-6). An organ is a body part where two or more tissues work together to perform a particular function. Examples of important organs and their location within the body are shown on page 128 (Figs. 5-7 and 5-8).

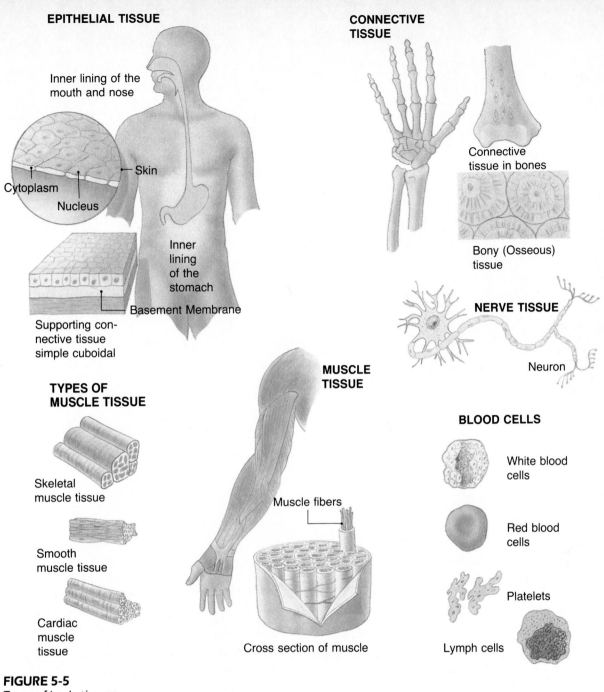

EPITHELIAL TISSUE

Inner lining of the mouth and nose

Cytoplasm

Nucleus

Skin

Inner lining of the stomach

Basement Membrane

Supporting connective tissue simple cuboidal

CONNECTIVE TISSUE

Connective tissue in bones

Bony (Osseous) tissue

NERVE TISSUE

Neuron

TYPES OF MUSCLE TISSUE

Skeletal muscle tissue

Smooth muscle tissue

Cardiac muscle tissue

MUSCLE TISSUE

Muscle fibers

Cross section of muscle

BLOOD CELLS

White blood cells

Red blood cells

Platelets

Lymph cells

FIGURE 5-5
Types of body tissues.

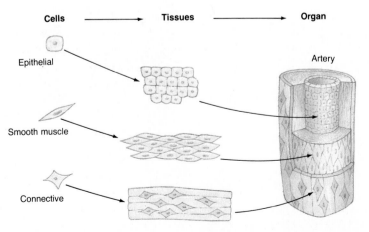

Cells → Tissues → Organ

Epithelial

Smooth muscle

Connective

Artery

FIGURE 5-6
Cells combine to form tissues, and tissues combine to form organs.

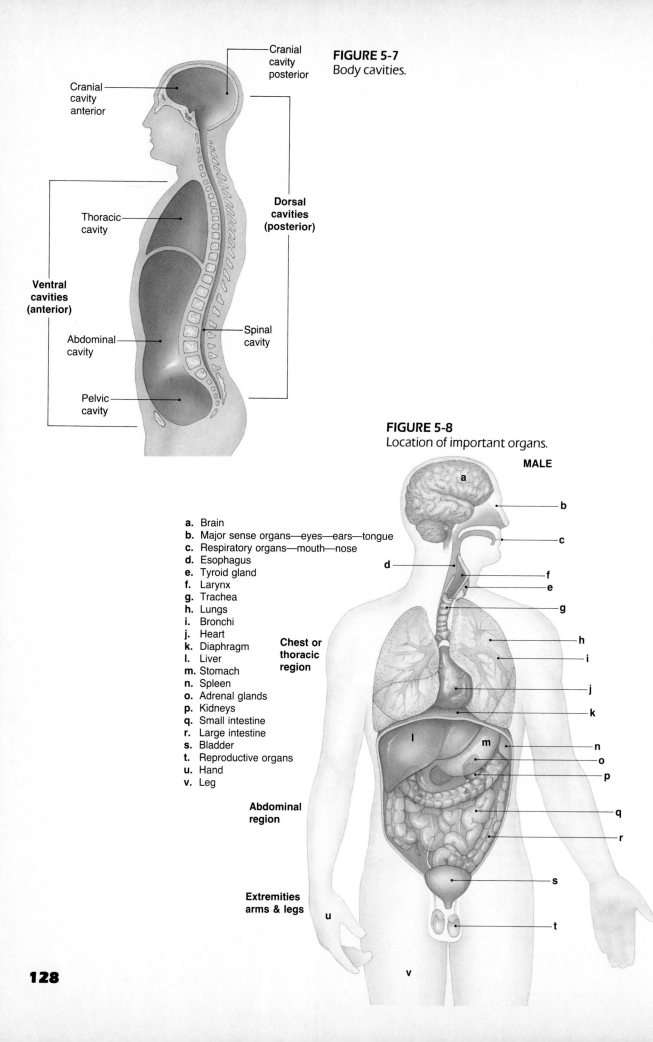

FIGURE 5-7
Body cavities.

Cranial
cavity
posterior

Cranial
cavity
anterior

Dorsal
cavities
(posterior)

Thoracic
cavity

Ventral
cavities
(anterior)

Spinal
cavity

Abdominal
cavity

Pelvic
cavity

FIGURE 5-8
Location of important organs.

MALE

a. Brain
b. Major sense organs—eyes—ears—tongue
c. Respiratory organs—mouth—nose
d. Esophagus
e. Tyroid gland
f. Larynx
g. Trachea
h. Lungs
i. Bronchi
j. Heart
k. Diaphragm
l. Liver
m. Stomach
n. Spleen
o. Adrenal glands
p. Kidneys
q. Small intestine
r. Large intestine
s. Bladder
t. Reproductive organs
u. Hand
v. Leg

**Chest or
thoracic
region**

**Abdominal
region**

**Extremities
arms & legs**

128

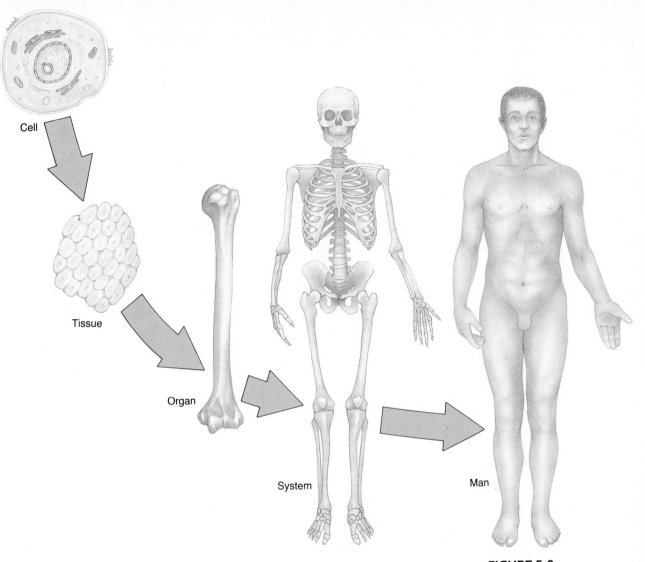

Cell

Tissue

Organ

System

Man

FIGURE 5-9
From cell to man.

SYSTEMS

Organs do not function independently either. They work together with other organs to perform a specific function, thereby creating a body system. A system consists of a group of organs that perform the same function (Fig. 5-9). The systems of the body are:

- Integumentary
- Digestive
- Skeletal
- Respiratory

- Muscular
- Circulatory
- Nervous

- Endocrine
- Urinary
- Reproductive

When all the body systems are working normally, a person is "physically well." As you review each body system, you will study:

- The normal anatomy and physiology of each system
- The common abnormalities associated with each system
- Age- and disuse-related changes associated with each system
- The related nursing measures and skills associated with each body system

SECTION 2 CANCER

OBJECTIVES/WHAT YOU WILL LEARN

When you have completed this section, you will be able to:
- Describe the basic mechanisms of cancer
- List cancer's seven warning signals
- Describe the three most common types of cancer treatment

Cancer is often considered a disease of modern humanity caused by chemical irritants, pollution, and radiation. However, some of the earliest writings refer to the Greek work *kapklvoo*, which means "crab," spreading its pincers throughout the body to choke off life.

Cancer is a form of cellular disorder in which the normal mechanisms of the cell that control the rate of growth, cell division, and movement are disturbed. If you think of the cell as a tiny computer, when cancer invades the cell's normal mechanisms that control rate of growth, cell division and movement are destroyed (Fig. 5-10). The American Cancer Society describes cancer as "a group of diseases caused by the runaway growth of useless cells that crowd out tissues needed for essential body functions . . . such as digestion, circulation, motion, excretion, etc."

Research has identified approximately 100 viruses and over 1000 substances capable of producing cancer in animals when concentrations of these substances are high. There continue to be many advances made in the prevention, diagnosis, treatment, and rehabilitation of cancer victim, yet no "miracle cure" has been discovered.

Cancer cells can originate in any body tissue and grow to invade other tissues, or cancer can **metastasize** (spread) to other parts of the body through blood and lymphatic vessels, where the cancer cells continue to grow. There are over 250 different kinds of cancer that can occur in different sites in the body (Fig. 5-11). The two main types of cancer are:

- **Carcinoma**—found most often in skin and the lining of hollow organs and passageways
- **Sarcoma**—found most often in bone, muscle, cartilage, and lymph systems

FIGURE 5-10
Cancer cell surrounded by killer T cells. Unregulated cells that avoid detection by T cells cause cancer.

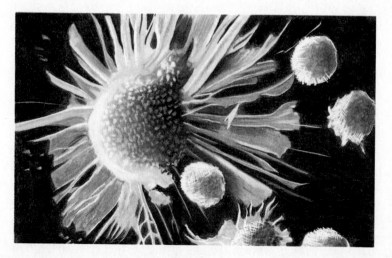

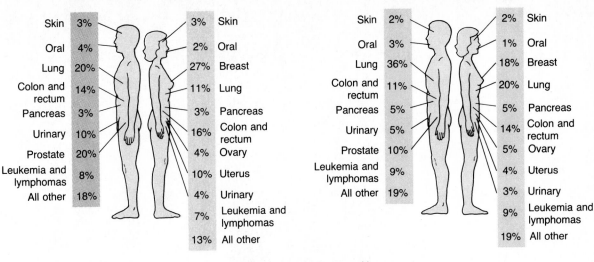

Cancer incidence by site and sex †

Skin	3%		3%	Skin
Oral	4%		2%	Oral
Lung	20%		27%	Breast
Colon and rectum	14%		11%	Lung
Pancreas	3%		3%	Pancreas
Urinary	10%		16%	Colon and rectum
Prostate	20%		4%	Ovary
Leukemia and lymphomas	8%		10%	Uterus
All other	18%		4%	Urinary
			7%	Leukemia and lymphomas
			13%	All other

Cancer deaths by site and sex

Skin	2%		2%	Skin
Oral	3%		1%	Oral
Lung	36%		18%	Breast
Colon and rectum	11%		20%	Lung
Pancreas	5%		5%	Pancreas
Urinary	5%		14%	Colon and rectum
Prostate	10%		5%	Ovary
Leukemia and lymphomas	9%		4%	Uterus
All other	19%		3%	Urinary
			9%	Leukemia and lymphomas
			19%	All other

† Excluding non-melanoma skin cancer and carcinoma in situ.

FIGURE 5-11
Cancer incidence and death by site and sex—1987 estimates.

Cancer is the second leading cause of death behind heart disease in the United States. Of the 250 million Americans now living, approximately 75 million will develop cancer. Cancer will strike about three of four families.

In 1937 when the National Cancer Institute was founded, only 20 percent of those diagnosed were cured. By 1950 the cure rate had increased to 33 percent. Currently, the cure rate exceeds 42 percent. One of every three diagnosed will be saved—a more positive outlook than ever before. Of the approximately 965,000 new cases of cancer diagnosed in the United States each year, 375,000 will be alive with no evidence of recurrence in five years. Still 483,000 people will die of cancer in the United States—about one person every 65 seconds. It is estimated that 160,000 to 170,000 of these cancer patients could have been cured if treated earlier. Early detection and prompt treatment increase the possibility of both control and cure. Annual check-ups which include examination of the mouth, breast, rectum, cervix, prostate, and skin are very important in detecting cancer early. When people neglect regular physical examinations and wait until symptoms occur, valuable treatment time is lost.

Research has helped to identify **carcinogens** (substances known to cause cancer) (Fig. 5-12). Education and control are directed toward either removing carcinogens from the environment or minimizing the exposure to them. For example, it is well known that cigarette smoking increases the risk of lung cancer and that overexposure to the sun increases the risk of skin cancer.

Cancer is frequently referred to as a disease of old age—*50 percent of all cancer cases occur after the age of 65.* It is the second leading cause of death in the elderly. Because cancer is so common among the elderly, it is very important for all members of the health-care team to be aware of cancer's seven warning signals. Being alert and recognizing a problem can make the difference between life and death.

Cancer's Seven Warning Signals

- Change in bowel or bladder habits
- A sore that does not heal
- Unusual bleeding or discharge
- Thickening or lump in breast or elsewhere
- Indigestion or difficulty swallowing
- Obvious changes in a wart or a mole
- Nagging cough or hoarseness

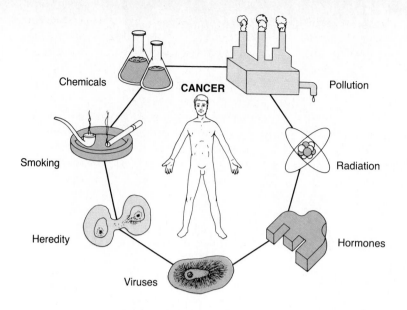

FIGURE 5-12
Possible causes of cancer.

Report any observations of the above to your charge nurse immediately.

Diet is now considered a *suspected* risk factor. Studies suggest that diets high in fat as well as obesity increase the risk of developing cancer.

The American Institute for Cancer Research lists the following dietary guidelines to lower cancer risk:

- Reduce the intake of dietary fat—saturated and unsaturated—from the current average of approximately 40 percent to a level of 30 percent of total calories.
- Increase the consumption of fruits, vegetables, and whole-grain cereals.
- Consume salt-cured, smoked, and charcoal-broiled foods in moderation only.
- Drink alcoholic beverages in moderation only.

The diagnosis of cancer evokes many negative emotions, including shock, denial, anxiety, and fear. Fear of the unknown, fear of pain, and fear of dying are some of the most commonly expressed concerns. The diagnosis of cancer has a tremendous impact on all aspects of a resident's life as well as on those family members and friends who are in regular contact. There are many agencies that can provide support to residents and families during this difficult period.

The Cancer Information Service (CIS) is a toll-free telephone inquiry network funded by the National Cancer Institute, Bethedsda, Maryland 20205. It is affiliated with state divisions of the American Cancer Society. It is an important resource available to everyone. Specially trained volunteers and professionals are available to answer questions. Call (800) 638-6694. Each state has local numbers that can be obtained from the national center.

Once cancer is diagnosed, treatment is generally directed toward:

Goal of treatment →

- **Cure**—to correct or remove a problem
- **Control**—to stop or limit growth
- **Palliation**—to relieve symptoms
- **Rehabilitation**—to restore or return function

Cure is most often achieved by **surgery** that removes the cancerous tissue by means of an operation. The use of radiation and chemotherapy are the second and third most commonly used forms of treatment.

In the LTC facility, you will see residents who have already experienced one or more of the above treatments and, in some cases, are currently receiving either radiation therapy or chemotherapy on an outpatient basis through an acute care hospital or oncology center (treatment center for cancer patients).

Radiation therapy is the use of high-energy rays to stop cancer cells from growing and multiplying. Radiation destroys the ability of *all* cells, both cancerous and normal, to grow and reproduce. Radiation therapy may be either external or internal. In external therapy, the most common type of treatment, a machine beams high-energy rays toward the cancer site. The treatment itself is painless, but unpleasant side effects frequently result. With internal radiation therapy, a very small amount of radioactive material is placed inside the body and left for a short time period. This type of therapy is carried out in the acute care hospital.

Radiation is sometimes used alone to destroy cancer and sometimes used with chemotherapy and surgery. Radiation is an aggressive form of cancer treatment and will often affect normal tissues, causing side effects. The side effects vary according to the extent of the cancer, the amount of radiation given, the part of the body being treated, and the individual resident's response. There are a number of nursing measures to help the resident receiving radiation therapy to tolerate the treatments better. Review these nursing measures carefully in the next section.

Chemotherapy refers to the use of drugs or medications to treat disease. It comes from combining the two words *chemical* and *treatment*. Chemotherapy may be given:

- **Orally** (taken by mouth)
- **Intramuscularly** (injection into muscle)
- **Intravenously** (injection into the vein)

These medications enter the bloodstream and are distributed to all parts of the body. The medication acts to interfere with the duplication and growth of the rapidly multiplying cancer cells. Unfortunately, anticancer drugs also affect normal cells, especially those that normally divide rapidly, like those of the bone marrow and gastrointestinal tract. However, these normal cells have the ability to regenerate and usually repair themselves.

Anticancer drugs produce side effects in some but not all people. Each drug may react differently in different people. Generally, chemotherapy drugs affect:

- Gastrointestinal tract
- Mouth
- Bone marrow
- Hair
- Skin
- Reproductive system (ovaries and testes)
- Urinary tract
- Emotional state

There are a number of nursing measures to help reduce the side effects of chemotherapy, which will be explained in the next section. After finishing a treatment program of either surgery, radiation, chemotherapy, or some combination of these, the patient waits and hopes for control or cure. Many are optimistic and are able to move positively toward any necessary rehabilitation and a return to normal life. Others face recurrence of the disease accompanied by emotional trauma and disappointment. Even those who have experienced cure or control live with the fear that the disease will recur. One patient stated, "It's like living on top of a powder keg, a time bomb. You don't know when it's going to go off and destroy you!"

For those residents or patients whose cancer has reached an uncontrollable state, the goals of treatment change from cure and control to palliative. Palliative measures are used to reduce pain and discomfort. Pain control and symptom management are the primary focus of care.

Treatment must not only be directed toward destroying cancerous cells, it must also take into consideration the emotional and psychosocial needs of each resident. Family members and friends must be assisted and given support to help them deal with the shock, fear, anxiety, frustration, and role changes they face when a loved one has cancer. The trauma to a family can be tremendous, and the responsibilities overwhelming.

SECTION 3 CARE OF THE RESIDENT WITH CANCER

OBJECTIVES/WHAT YOU WILL LEARN

When you have completed this section, you will be able to:
- List four common side effects associated with radiation and chemotherapy
- List two specific nursing measures that can help reduce side effects or complications
- Describe ways you would like others to provide you with emotional support if you were a cancer victim

CANCER TREATMENT

Because cancer treatment is almost always aggressive, it can extend over weeks and months. The side effects are not easy to deal with, and frequently the resident feels more illness and discomfort from the side effects of treatment than from the disease itself. The following guidelines will help you provide better nursing care to the resident receiving radiation or chemotherapy.

- *Fatigue*—Residents easily become tired because the body uses a good deal of its energy to fight the cancer and to rebuild injured cells. Allow residents time for rest and recognize their limitations. Help them understand why they feel so tired.

- *Loss of appetite leading to malnutrition*—Nausea and vomiting are frequently associated with chemotherapy. Loss of appetite is common. It is especially important for residents to maintain good nutrition because the body needs wholesome food to restore its strength and to rebuild and repair injured cells.
  The following tips can help the resident maintain good nutrition:
  — Provide food whenever they feel hungry, even if it is not mealtime.
  — Encourage smaller meals more frequently, offering fluids 1 hour before meals rather than with meals.
  — Have nutritious snacks available, cottage cheese, juice, milk. Discourage sweets and fatty foods.
  — Create a pleasant mealtime atmosphere to make it a positive experience.
  — If the odor of hot foods increases nausea, provide cold substitutions.
  Encourage the resident to chew food well so that it is easily digested. Instruct the resident not to lie down flat for 2 hours after eating. Food is digested easier if the resident is not supine and if activities are limited. Notify the charge nurse so that medications prescribed to reduce nausea and vomiting can be given promptly.

- *Skin effects*—Sometimes the skin may begin to look reddened or irritated or even burned during radiation therapy. A variety of rashes and itching can develop during chemotherapy:

— Keep skin clean.

— Avoid any type of irritation, pressure, or injury to the skin.

— Report rashes, irritation, or broken areas to the charge nurse immediately.

- *Mouth effects*—Some anticancer drugs can cause the mouth and throat to be dry and sore. Radiation therapy to the head and neck can cause difficulty swallowing and chewing. The following tips should increase the patient's comfort:

  — Cut food into small pieces or if necessary mechanically alter the diet so that it is tolerated by the resident.

  — Discourage rough or coarse foods.

  — Encourage plenty of fluids.

  — Keep the mouth very clean, using a soft brush.

  — Avoid use of commercial mouth washes that contain alcohol and are drying to the mucous membranes of the mouth.

- *Hair effects*—The hair follicles of the scalp, beard, eyebrows, eyelashes, armpits, and pubic areas are very sensitive to some of the anticancer drugs and radiation therapy, resulting in loss of scalp and body hair. This side effect is called **alopecia.**

  This is a particularly disturbing side effect, as it changes the body image drastically. Once treatments are finished, the hair generally grows back, but in the meantime help the resident to select some form of head covering, such as a wig, scarf, turban, or hat.

- *Emotional effects*—Having cancer and receiving treatments is a very stressful experience. The side effects of therapy can be very distressing, and many residents have difficulty accepting them. They find it hard to believe they are "getting better" when they feel so ill. Some emotional changes are directly related to the drug therapy—feelings of depression, fear, anger, and even apathy (not caring) are common.

There are other side effects that should be observed for and reported at once:

- Fever
- Sudden weight loss or gain
- Bleeding or hemorrhage
- Changes in vital signs
- Intense or severe pain
- Changes in behavior
- Severe constipation or diarrhea

One of the most important aspects of providing care is to be sensitive to the emotional needs of the cancer resident and the family and friends (Fig. 5-13).

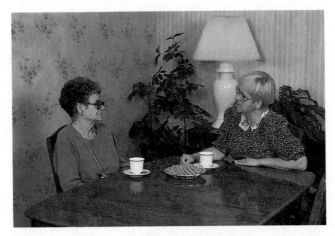

FIGURE 5-13
Being sensitive to the emotional needs of the cancer resident.

You must allow them to express their feelings and fears. It is not appropriate to give false cheer and try to lift the resident's spirits; this merely keeps the residents from being able to express what they really feel. Listening, sharing, being yourself is the best you can offer. There is no "right thing" to say or do in most cases. Just being there and conveying to the resident "I care" may be enough.

There are always ways to find hope during difficult times. Even if the future is uncertain, there may be remissions or periods of control. There can still be good days, special times, and shared experiences.

The cancer resident needs to stay as involved as possible with responsibilities, diversions, and activities. It seems that cancer patients who have things to do live longer. Help your residents engage in useful and meaningful activities.

Caring for the resident who has cancer requires an understanding of the nature of the disease and its side effects and, most important, an understanding of the unique individual who is experiencing the disease. There are a number of excellent references and resource groups that will assist you in expanding your knowledge and understanding.

SECTION 4 THE SENSES

OBJECTIVES/WHAT YOU WILL LEARN

When you have completed this section, you will be able to:
- Match three types of visual disturbance with their descriptions
- Identify age-related changes in the sense of taste
- Describe how loss of sensation of temperature and pain can pose a hazard to the safety of the resident

SENSORY SYSTEM

The sensory system (Fig. 5-14) consists of:

- Eyes
- Ears
- Nose
- Tongue
- Skin

FIGURE 5-14
The sensory system.

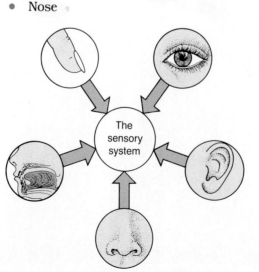

The functions of the sensory system are:

- Vision
- Hearing
- Balance
- Smell
- Taste
- Touch

Through the actions of specialized cells called **sensory neurons,** a person is made aware of changes in the outside environment. These changes are referred to as **stimuli** (an action or agent that causes a response in an organ or organism).

- Eyes respond to visual stimuli (what you see)
- Ears respond to sound stimuli (what you hear)
- Membranes lining the nose respond to smells
- Taste buds located chiefly on the tongue respond to bitter, sweet, sour, and salty tastes
- Skin responds to touch, pressure, heat, cold, and pain

THE EYE

The eye is similar to a camera. It has a lens, a shutter, and an adjustable opening, as well as light-sensitive film (Fig. 5-15).

The parts of the eye:

- *Sclera*—white of the eye

The body has the sense of vision, hearing, balance and equilibrium, touch, pain, heat, cold, pressure, taste, and smell.

The eye can receive and focus light and then convert this energy into nerve impulses to be sent to the brain. The nerve impulses originate from the retina. Visual receptors in the retina called rods can work in low intensity light. They have no color function. The visual receptors called cones operate in high intensity light and do receive colors.

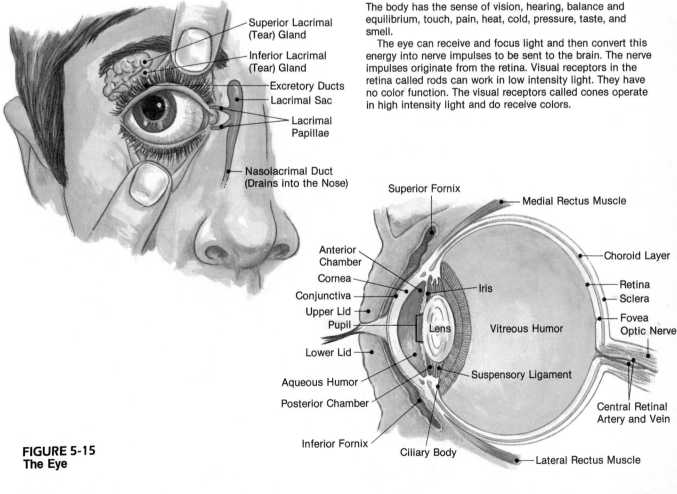

FIGURE 5-15
The Eye

- *Vitreous humor*—transparent liquid that fills the eyeball
- *Aqueous humor*—fluid produced in the eye. Fills space between cornea and lens
- *Cornea*—clear plasticlike covering
- *Iris*—circle of color
- *Pupil*—the opening in the center of the iris through which light enters
- *Lens*—directly behind the pupil, focuses the image upon the retina
- *Retina*—back part of the eye, receives image and sends impulses to the optic nerve
- *Optic nerve*—receives impulses from the rods and cones in the retina and transmits them to the brain

AGE-RELATED CHANGES AND ABNORMALITIES OF THE EYE

As a person ages, various changes occur and diseases of the eye are common. Generally, there is a decrease in peripheral (side) vision and vision at night. The eye also adjusts more slowly to changes in both light and distance.

Some conditions of the eye include:

- **Presbyopia**—lens of the eye loses its ability to focus clearly due to loss of elasticity of the lens. The individual with presbyopia must hold small print at arm's length in order to read. Frequently, eyeglasses will improve vision. If an individual has difficulty seeing at a distance, bifocals (glasses with two different lenses) might be needed.
- **Cataract**—the lens undergoes changes that decreases its transparency. The lens becomes more and more opaque (cloudy) to the point of complete blindness. The only cure for a cataract is surgery. Many recent advances in surgical technique make this a relatively safe and simple procedure. A person with cataracts may describe his or her vision "like looking through glasses covered with Vaseline." The individual usually experiences sensitivity to bright light and glare.
- **Glaucoma**—occurs when pressure within the eye increases. This pressure can increase to dangerous levels leading to blindness from pressure on the optic nerve. The resident may complain of pain over the eye at night, indicating the pressure is increasing. Glaucoma is usually treated with eye drops. If this therapy fails, a small hole is made surgically to reduce pressure. Glaucoma may be acute, with sudden severe symptoms, or chronic, with slowly developing symptoms. The person may describe "halos" around lights and decreased peripheral and central vision. Such things as physical strain and emotional stress tend to increase the pressure within the eye and to increase the damage done by the pressure.

THE EAR

The ear is a special sense organ associated with hearing and equilibrium (balance). The ear has three main parts (Fig. 5-16).

- *Outer ear*—leads to the small sound opening of the middle ear. The small membrane that separates the outer and middle ear is the eardrum.
- *Middle ear*—contains three small bones that serve as a bridge to the inner ear. The middle ear also contains the eustachian tube arising from an area of the throat.
- *Inner ear*—contains canals that hold fluid necessary for maintaining equilibrium or balance. Also within the inner ear are tiny hairlike nerve cells that receive sound and send signals to the brain.

Good nursing care
(Fig. 5-18). Some exar

- *Sight*—television,
  above the bed, bull
  newspapers, outdc
- *Hearing*—radio, te
  activities, pets
- *Smell*—flowers in
  personal cleanline
  popcorn
- *Taste*—offering a
  temperature, offer
- *Touch*—gentle tou
  pats on the should
  animals, or childr

Even the **uncons**
environment, must b
know what is unders
treated as if he could
   When giving care
what you are going to
chatting with one an
in the presence of the

VISUAL IMPAIR

Visual problems are
in a LTC facility. Ab
problem. These appr

- Identify yourself
  assistant."
- Describe what yo
  now."
- Keep the residen
- Relocate possess
  where you are pl
- Describe events
  word picture.
- Watch for safety

   All staff member
dent from withdrav
feed oneself is an in
not change this. Wh
ious items on the tr
use a clock as a refer
5-19). You may also
be served separately
feeding themselves
success.
   If the blind resid
well as the content
too. Determine if t

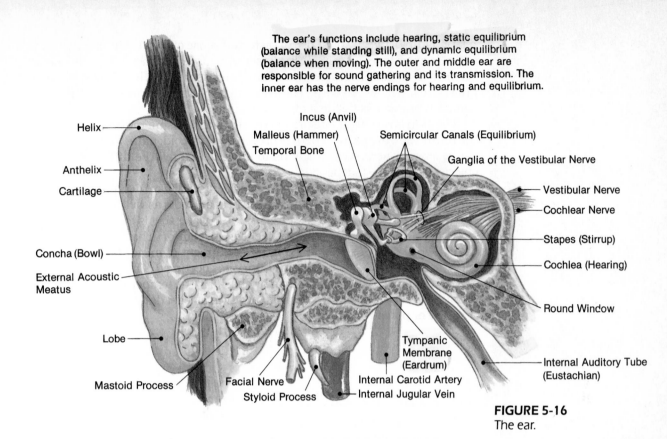

The ear's functions include hearing, static equilibrium (balance while standing still), and dynamic equilibrium (balance when moving). The outer and middle ear are responsible for sound gathering and its transmission. The inner ear has the nerve endings for hearing and equilibrium.

Helix
Anthelix
Cartilage
Concha (Bowl)
External Acoustic Meatus
Lobe
Mastoid Process
Facial Nerve
Styloid Process

Incus (Anvil)
Malleus (Hammer)
Temporal Bone

Semicircular Canals (Equilibrium)
Ganglia of the Vestibular Nerve
Vestibular Nerve
Cochlear Nerve
Stapes (Stirrup)
Cochlea (Hearing)
Round Window
Internal Auditory Tube (Eustachian)

Tympanic Membrane (Eardrum)
Internal Carotid Artery
Internal Jugular Vein

FIGURE 5-16
The ear.

Sound waves enter the outer ear and strike the tympanic membrane (eardrum), causing it to vibrate. The vibration of the membrane causes the tiny bones of the middle ear to move, carrying the sound to the inner ear. Through a complex process, sound stimuli are transmitted to nerves that transport the signal to the brain.

AGE-RELATED CHANGES AND ABNORMALITIES

Disturbances of any part of the hearing mechanism can lead to partial or complete deafness. Most elderly people experience some hearing loss as a result of the aging process. Ninety percent of the elderly have some hearing loss. A progressive hearing loss of high pitched sounds is most common. The hearing loss may be compared to a radio that is not quite tuned correctly. There is distortion of sound that is not improved by turning up the volume. Severe loss of hearing can seriously interfere with a person's ability to interact and communicate with others. This loss of socialization can contribute to increased confusion, disruptive behavior, and withdrawal. You have an important nursing responsibility to assist hard-of-hearing residents in all aspects of communication.

FIGURE 5-17
The tongue.

SMELL, TASTE, TOUCH

Olfaction or the sense of smell is associated with the special lining of the upper part of the nose. Of all the senses, the sense of smell is the least understood. You can detect, by smell, various substances and can even tell the difference between substances. How this occurs is not known. The sense of smell is often affected when infection of the nasal sinuses occurs. The sense of smell decreases during the aging processes.
   Generally, the sense of taste is associated with the tongue. The tongue allows us to tell the difference between sweet, sour, bitter, and salty tastes (Fig. 5-17). The taste buds are special sensory nerve cells. There is an important

Bitter
Sour
Sweet and salt

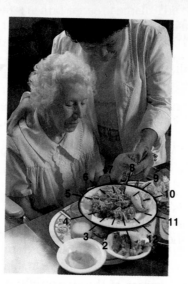

FIGURE 5-19
Use the clock as a reference.

another or a bite or two of each food. Allow the resident to make as many choices as possible to help him or her feel less dependent, more in control.

When assisting blind residents to ambulate, have them take your arm rather than you taking their arm. Describe where you are going, mentioning obstacles along the way. Most facilities have rooms and bathrooms marked with raised numbers or symbols. Show the resident how to locate these numbers. When staff consistently explain locations of items inside and outside of the room, most residents will be able to function more independently.

Be sure to assist the blind resident with grooming and hygiene. The loss of vision need not make the resident less attractive in appearance. It is up to you to be the eyes of the resident and be sure that her or his appearance is neat, clean, and appropriate.

In a fire or disaster, the blind resident will require your assistance to leave the building. A list of the blind residents is kept at the nursing station, and some type of sign is placed at the bedside. You should be aware of those residents who have visual impairments; but remember, even though many can have the same disability, each is a unique individual with different ways of coping.

HEARING LOSS

Communicating with the hard-of-hearing or deaf resident will be more effective if you follow these guidelines:

- Always face the person when speaking (this provides visual cues and increases understanding).
- Do not cover your mouth with your hand.
- Touch the person to gain his or her attention.
- Speak slowly and clearly, but do not pronounce words unnaturally (avoid overarticulating or mumbling).
- If you are not understood, find new words to say the same thing rather than repeating the same words at a higher volume.
- Use gestures and body movements to help to get your point across.
- Avoid talking while chewing gum or smoking.
- Do not shout. Since the resident hears distorted sounds, making them louder does not make them easier to understand.
- Speak slowly.
- Write hard-to-understand messages on paper or a "magic slate."

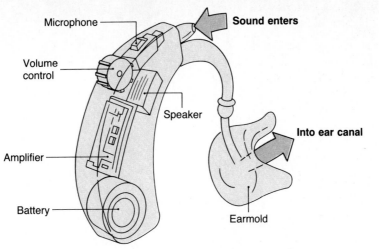

Microphone

Volume
control

Speaker

Amplifier

Battery

Sound enters

Into ear canal

Earmold

FIGURE 5-20
Hearing aid.

There is a tendency to avoid contact with residents who have communication problems because of the difficulty and frustration in communicating. It is very important to make every effort to establish contact. It may take patience, time, and understanding on your part to accomplish good communication with the resident who has a hearing loss, but it is necessary to prevent isolation, withdrawal, and deprivation.

Some types of hearing loss can be improved through use of a **hearing aid** (Fig. 5-20). Only an **otologist,** a specialist in hearing, makes this determination. Hearing aids are mechanical devices used to make certain sounds louder. They do not make sounds clearer.

When a resident has a hearing aid, you will be responsible to help care for and properly use this expensive device. There are many different devices. Some are quite small and are contained entirely within the ear, while others may be part of a pair of eyeglasses. Regardless of the type, remember to:

- Protect the hearing aid from damage. Keep it in a safe place when not in use. Do not drop it or expose it to water.
- Turn off the aid when not in use. Report the need for batteries to the charge nurse.
- Observe for wax buildup and sores in the ears, and report any you see to the charge nurse.
- Keep the earmold clean.
- When talking with the resident, keep background noise to a minimum. It may be helpful to turn off the radio or television or close windows and doors.
- Follow the same principles or guidelines for communicating as you do in communicating with the hard-of-hearing resident.

Residents with hearing aids experience a great deal of distortion of sound in large, noisy groups, and they may avoid such situations or turn off the aid during those times. The resident with a hearing loss must be identified, just as the blind person is. In the event of fire or disaster, the deaf resident will need special assistance to leave the building safely. There is usually a list of hard-of-hearing residents at the nursing station. The resident's room or bed may also be identified with a sign or symbol.

CHAPTER 6

The Integumentary System

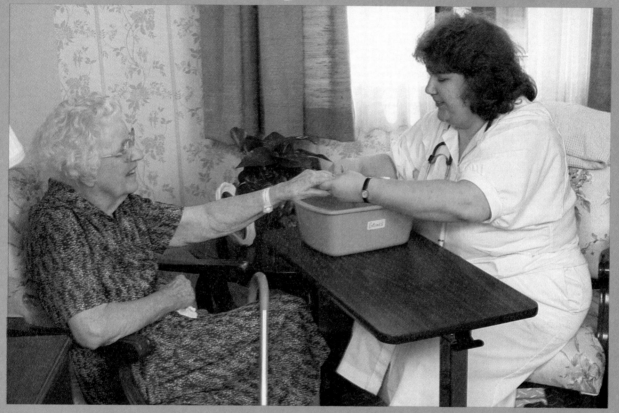

SECTION 1 ANATOMY AND PHYSIOLOGY

OBJECTIVES/WHAT YOU WILL LEARN

When you complete this section, you will be able to:
- List four functions of the integumentary system
- Relate changes in skin condition to possible causes
- Explain how the skin helps to regulate body temperature

THE SKIN

The integumentary system is composed of:

- Skin
- Hair
- Nails
- Sweat and oil glands

The functions of the integumentary system are to:

- Protect the body
- Improve one's appearance
- Eliminate wastes through the sweat glands
- Regulate body temperature
- Produce vitamin D when exposed to sunlight

The skin, which is the largest organ, covers the entire body and has two layers (Fig. 6-1):

- **Epidermis**—the outer layer of skin (the skin you see)
- **Dermis**—the second layer of skin, which is made up of new cells that replace discarded cells from the epidermis

The epidermis or outer layer of skin is quite thin on most parts of the body, with the exception of the palms of the hands and the soles of the feet. Because these areas get the most "wear and tear," the cells there die and rub off constantly, producing dead flaking skin. Within the dermis or second layer of skin, new cells grow to replace the dead ones.

Under the dermis is a fatty tissue. When more food is taken in than is needed, fat is manufactured. Fat is the way the body stores energy until it is needed. Because there are few blood vessels in fatty tissue, the fat acts as insulation for the body, keeping warmth in and cold out. Fat also adds protection or padding to the body.

Because of the skin's protective function, it must be kept clean, dry, and properly lubricated. Moisture on the skin picks up dust and particles from the air, which creates an environment where bacteria can grow. Moisture also causes chafing, excoriation, rashes, and lesions, leading to skin breakdown and infection. Injuries to the skin destroy its protective nature and provide openings for disease-producing organisms to enter the body.

Oil glands in the skin keep it lubricated, soft, and flexible, and they also supply the hair **follicles** (roots) with oil. The skin has a role in the production of vitamin D when exposed to sunlight. Vitamin D produces calcium and plays a role in potassium metabolism.

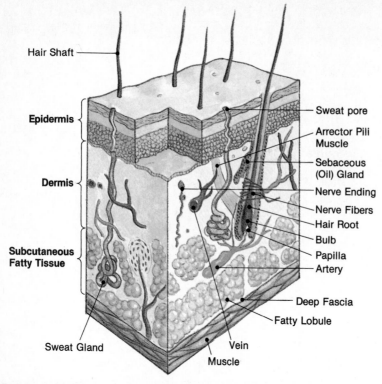

Hair Shaft

Epidermis

Dermis

Subcutaneous
Fatty Tissue

Sweat Gland

Sweat pore

Arrector Pili
Muscle

Sebaceous
(Oil) Gland

Nerve Ending

Nerve Fibers

Hair Root

Bulb

Papilla

Artery

Deep Fascia

Fatty Lobule

Vein

Muscle

The skin is the largest organ of the body. In the adult the skin covers about 3000 square inches (1.75 square meters) and weighs about 6 pounds. It is involved with protection, insulation, thermal regulation, excretion, and the production of vitamin D.

FIGURE 6-1
The skin.

Membranes

Membranes cover or line body structures to provide protection from injury and infection. There are four major classes of membranes. Mucous membranes line those structures that open to the outside world (for example, the mouth, the airway, digestive tract, urinary tract, and vagina). Serous membranes line the closed body cavities and cover the outsides of organs. The cutaneous membrane is the skin. Synovial membranes line joints to reduce friction during movement.

A serous membrane that covers an organ is called a visceral layer. The term parietal layer is used for the part of the serous membrane that lines a cavity. The serous membrane in the thoracic cavity is called pleura (for example, the parietal pleura lines the chest cavity). In the abdominal cavity, it is called peritoneum (for example, the parietal peritoneum). A double layer of peritoneum is called mesentery. The membrane that lines the sac surrounding the heart is pericardium.

The skin helps to eliminate certain body wastes. Perspiration is released from the body through sweat glands, which are distributed over the entire skin surface. Water and salts are excreted through the sweat glands.

Body temperature is controlled by the skin. The skin helps reduce body temperature when blood vessels near the surface of the skin dilate (become larger). This brings more body heat to the skin surface. There the heat is lost through exposure to the cooler air. Even more important, the evaporation of perspiration carries heat away from the skin.

When the body needs to increase its temperature in order to stay warm, perspiration stops. Blood vessels near the surface contract (become smaller). This decreases the heat brought to the surface of the skin, and the skin temperature falls. When we feel too cold, we begin to shiver. This creates warmth due to muscle activity.

The "homeostatic" or balance mechanism is important in keeping body temperature the same most of the time. Only when illness or injury occurs does the body temperature exceed its normal limits.

The hair and nails are **appendages** or attachments of the skin. Fingernails and toenails grow from nailbeds. Some illnesses, diseases, drugs, and injuries affect the growth and condition of hair and nails.

AGE-RELATED CHANGES

Age-related changes in the integumentary system can be seen easily. The skin loses elasticity and becomes dry, wrinkled, thin, and easily damaged. The skin becomes so thin that it almost feels like tissue paper. This fragile skin tears and scrapes easily, which can lead to infection. Because of this the nursing assistant must be very gentle when lifting, moving, positioning, and bathing elderly residents. Remember to use a transfer belt in order to decrease the risk of injury.

There may be brown spots on the skin, particularly on the hands and arms. The hair usually becomes sparse and gray or white. Fingernails and toenails thicken and become abnormally shaped. It is frequently necessary to have a **podiatrist** (foot specialist) care for the toenails of the elderly. Just as you observe the skin for changes, it is also important to observe and report changes in the fingernails and toenails that may indicate a problem (complaints of pain, redness, drainage, or swelling).

Some women experience growth of hair on the face, especially around the mouth and chin. These residents may require special personal care for the removal of facial hair.

Most elderly residents experience loss of the fat under the skin. They lose the comfort from the padding provided by the fat and may become uncomfortable sitting or lying on hard surfaces. Because of the loss of insulation, they often complain of feeling cold even when the room temperature seems fine or even warm to others. For this reason, you must take special care to keep elderly residents warmly dressed or well-covered when giving nursing care.

The protective function of the skin is *very important* in the prevention of disease and infection. Therefore, some of your responsibilities as a nursing assistant are to:

- Keep the resident's skin clean and dry.
- Protect the residents from injury to the skin.
- Report *any* changes in skin condition or color to your charge nurse immediately:
  — Redness of the skin (**erythema**) can mean increased body temperature, prolonged pressure, infection, or injury.
  — A blue or gray color (**cyanosis**) can mean decreased circulation, a life-threatening problem.
  — A black or "scablike" skin area can mean **eschar,** disguising a more serious skin problem underneath. A scab does not necessarily mean a wound is healing well.
  — A very pale or white color can mean circulatory problems related to shock.

Accurate observation and reporting of the resident's skin color and condition is of life and death importance!

SECTION 2 PRESSURE SORES

OBJECTIVES/WHAT YOU WILL LEARN

When you have completed this section, you will be able to:
- List the three causes of pressure sores
- Identify the sites on the body where pressure sores are most likely to occur
- Select those conditions that increase the risk of developing a pressure sore
- List five ways the nursing assistant can prevent pressure sores from occurring
- Describe correct usage of two pressure sore prevention devices

EFFECTS OF IMMOBILITY ON THE SKIN

Immobility can cause serious changes in the skin. The most important is development of **pressure sores,** often called decubitus ulcers or "bed sores." Pressure on an area of skin prevents the flow of blood, resulting in tissue that dies from lack of oxygen and other necessary nutrients. The dead tissue comes off, leaving an open painful sore that provides a way for microorganisms to enter the body, causing infection.

The areas most likely to break down are those parts of the body where little fat exists between the skin and the bone. Examples are the back of the head, rim of the ears, shoulder blades, spine (especially the coccyx or tailbone), shoulders, elbows, hips, knees, ankles, heels, and toes (Fig. 6-2).

The residents most likely to develop pressure sores are those who are unable or unwilling to move.

Residents may be unable to move because of:

- *Paralysis*—due to stroke, spinal injury, or disease
- *Weakness*—may be very frail, ill, or anemic
- *Coma*—illness or injury resulting in unconsciousness

Residents may be unwilling to move because of:

- *Pain*—it hurts to move, as with arthritis
- *Depression*—may have "given up"
- *Disorientation*—not aware of the consequences of remaining in one position

Residents who spend a lot of time sitting may also experience skin breakdown in the center of the buttocks due to pressure from the ischial bones and sacrum (Fig. 6-3). Those who remain on their abdomen (prone) for long periods of time often develop pressure sores on their cheeks, ears, ribs, collar bones, breasts, genitalia, knees, and toes.

Although *intense* pressure can cause death of tissue after only 90 minutes, it usually takes 6 to 8 hours to occur.

Skin breakdown can also be caused by a force called **shearing.** Shearing takes place when the skin moves one way while the bone and tissue under the skin move another way (Fig. 6-4). This pinches the tiny blood vessels and cuts off the supply of oxygen and other nutrients, leading to tissue death. An example of shearing force can be seen when a resident slides down in bed or a wheelchair. The nursing assistant can cause shearing by pulling a sheet from under the resident. If the sheet is wet, the damage increases. This is why the resident should be *rolled* from side to side to remove linens from underneath or assisted to stand if in a wheelchair. The fragile skin of the elderly is highly susceptible to shearing.

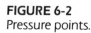
FIGURE 6-2
Pressure points.

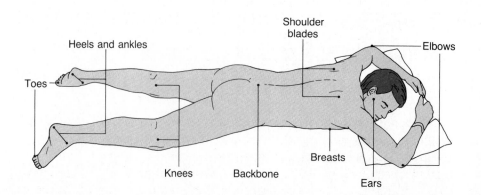

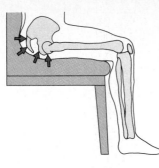

FIGURE 6-3
Pressure from the ischial bones and sacrum with the resident in the sitting position.

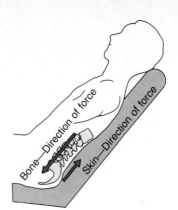

FIGURE 6-4
Shearing of blood vessels due to opposing forces.

In addition to pressure and shearing, moisture is the greatest contributor to skin breakdown. Moisture on the skin from saliva, perspiration, urine, or feces reacts chemically with the skin, leading to redness, irritation, and damage.

RISK FACTORS FOR SKIN BREAKDOWN

Some residents have a higher risk of developing a pressure sore than others. In addition to those unable or unwilling to move, high-risk residents include those who are underweight or overweight, those with **anemia** (usually not enough red blood cells), diabetes, or poor circulation. Also at risk are residents in casts, braces, or splints. It is important for you to be able to recognize which residents are most likely to experience skin breakdown. Then you can take extra precautions to prevent breakdown.

Now that you know why a pressure sore develops, let's examine what happens if nothing is done to prevent or treat it. You've probably heard the expression "an ounce of prevention is worth a pound of cure." In no case is this saying more true than with pressure sores. Once a sore is allowed to develop, it is very difficult to heal. It is also painful to the resident and requires a great deal of nursing time and energy to heal.

STAGES OF DEVELOPMENT FOR PRESSURE SORES

Pressure sores develop in stages or steps (Fig. 6-5). First the skin becomes reddened (or in the case of the dark skinned resident becomes darker). This redness does not immediately disappear when pressure is relieved. To understand the first-stage development of a pressure sore, hold a clear drinking glass tightly in your hand. Notice that your fingers become pale, showing that the supply of blood has been cut off. Let go and note how quickly the blood returns to the area. This is the redness seen when there has been pressure on a particular area. You can see another example simply by crossing your knees for a few minutes and then uncrossing them. Observe the skin. You'll see that it is red from the pressure. In both examples, the skin quickly returns to normal. When a resident is developing a pressure sore, the area remains red even after pressure is relieved.

The reddened area is tender and warm to touch. If nothing is done at this point, the next stage will be development of a blister. The blister then breaks open, leaving a sore that may grow in width and depth. Some might even progress through the tissue and muscle to the bone!

Infection is often recognized when foul-smelling drainage is present and the area is reddened and warm. In its most advanced stages, the sore can be

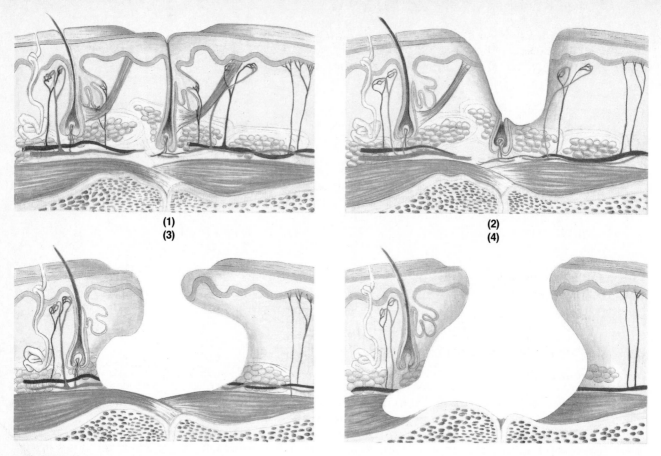

(1)
(3)
(2)
(4)

FIGURE 6-5
Stages of pressure sore
development.

covered with eschar. Eschar prevents healing and must be removed with surgical instruments or medication. This process is called **debridement.**

Remember, regardless of the special preventive devices used, *there is no substitute for position changes and avoidance of prolonged pressure!*

PREVENTING PRESSURE SORES

Other measures to prevent development of pressure sores include keeping the skin clean and dry, providing lotion, and gentle massage, and protecting the skin from scratching, rubbing, or other trauma. Gentle massage helps to increase circulation to the area and is an important preventive measure. The bed should be free of wrinkles or objects that could cause irritation. Clothing, shoes, braces, and splints must fit properly so there is no injury or pressure. The resident's nails should also be kept short and smooth to prevent scratching. Carrying out these measures, together with being sure that the resident is adequately nourished and **hydrated** (receives enough liquids), is necessary to prevent the development of pressure sores.

Frequent changes of position as well as the use of proper positioning techniques are essential! A dependent resident's position should be changed at least every 2 hours. Residents who are very frail or seriously ill may need to be positioned even more often.

You will use certain devices to help decrease pressure and reduce friction or rubbing. Review the chart that follows and study the various devices available as well as the purpose of each. Regardless of the devices used, the resident continues to require frequent position changes. Never assume that because special beds or mattresses are in use that you need not reposition the resident.

All measures used to prevent pressure sores must be documented or recorded in the resident's health record. There is a saying in health care that "if it isn't documented, it wasn't done." Take credit for your efforts by recording them.

PRESSURE SORE PREVENTION DEVICES

Device	Purpose	Precautions for Use
Eggcrate-type mattress Eggcrate-type wheelchair cushion	Provides cushioning and a light redistribution of pressure as well as some circulation of air beneath resident.	Not as effective for incontinent patients unless a very thin plastic sleeve covering is used to protect the mattress. The mattress will retain a urine odor unless protected. It is most effective when used with *only one* loosely applied sheet between the resident and the mattress.
Water mattress	Redistributes the body weight during any movement. Conforms to body shape and weight.	Do not puncture. Must not be over- or under-filled.
Air mattress	Redistributes pressure on a timed automatic basis.	Be careful not to puncture. Be sure that motor and mattress are working correctly. Use only one loosely applied sheet between the resident and the mattress.
Sheepskin pad	Reduces friction or rubbing against sheets.	*Does not* eliminate pressure.
Heel protector Elbow protector	Cushions against trauma. Decreases friction on rubbing against bedclothes.	Must be removed for daily washing of feet/elbows and inspection of skin. Creates warm moist environment favoring growth of bacteria.

Device	Purpose	Precautions for Use
Foot elevator 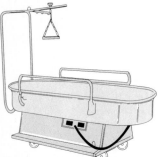	Reduces pressure on heels.	Must be properly applied. Check skin for rubbing.
Wheelchair cushion (solid)	Conforms to body when sitting. Provides comfort.	Place properly in chair. Cover with cloth.
Foot cradle (tent-like device attached to the lower third of the bed)	Keeps bed coverings off legs and feet.	Be sure the bed covering is off legs. Residents may feel cold, requiring pajamas, etc., to provide additional warmth.
Air-fluidized therapy	Relieves pressure through continuous motion. Resident "floats."	Produces heat in the room; resident needs additional fluids to prevent dehydration. Must use wedges to elevate head.

SECTION 3 CARE OF THE SKIN

OBJECTIVES/WHAT YOU WILL LEARN

When you have completed this section, you will be able to:
- List three goals of good skin care
- Give four reasons for bathing residents
- Recognize appropriate guidelines for bathing residents
- Give a complete bed bath
- Give a back rub
- Give perineal care
- Give a tub bath
- Give a shower

GOALS OF SKIN CARE

Nursing care of the skin is designed to:

- Provide cleanliness
- Promote circulation
- Prevent injury

Cleanliness is maintained by bathing. There are several important reasons for bathing the resident. Bathing removes dirt from the resident's body. It also eliminates body odors and cools and refreshes the resident. A bath stimulates circulation and helps prevent pressure sores. Bathing requires movement of certain parts of the body: the resident's legs and arms are lifted, and the head and torso are turned. This activity exercises muscles that might otherwise remain unused. At bath time, the nursing assistant has the opportunity to observe the resident for any unusual body changes, such as skin rashes, pressure sores, or reddened areas. Bath time is also an excellent time to communicate with the resident.

A resident may be bathed in one of four ways, depending on his condition. He may be given a complete bed bath, a partial bath, a tub bath, or a shower. Some areas of the body require daily bathing to remain clean. These areas include the face, hands, underarms, groin, and areas where body folds and creases exist. When a resident perspires greatly (due to fever) or has lost control of bowel and bladder function, bathing is required more often. This type of bathing is called a **partial bath.**

The frequency for giving a total bath will vary with the individual resident. The elderly resident usually receives a complete bath at least twice a week. More frequent bathing is likely to cause further drying of the skin. Younger and more active residents may be bathed more often.

GUIDELINES FOR BATHING A RESIDENT

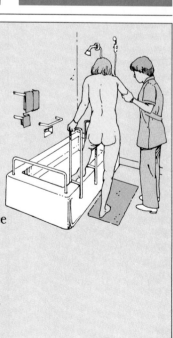

- Always protect the welfare and safety of the resident. Take all safety precautions to prevent slips and falls. *Never* leave a resident unattended in the bath tub or shower!
- Use good body mechanics to protect yourself as well as the resident.
- Rinse the resident carefully. Soap has a drying effect and can cause itching and skin rashes if not rinsed off completely.
- Make bath time a pleasant experience for the resident by:
  — Protecting the privacy of the resident
  — Avoiding exposure or chilling
  — Using comfortably warm water and changing it whenever it becomes soapy, dirty, or cold
  — Talking with the resident so that bath time becomes a social experience
- Always encourage the resident to do as much of the bath as possible.
- Be alert and carefully observe the condition of the resident's skin as you are giving a bath. Report any redness, rashes, broken skin, tender places, or complaints of pain to your charge nurse immediately.
- If you must transport the resident through the halls for a bath or shower, be sure that she is adequately covered to protect her privacy and to keep her warm. It is a good idea to dress and undress the resident in the shower room.

PROCEDURE

GIVING A COMPLETE BED BATH

1. Assemble your equipment on the overbed table:
   - Soap and soap dish
   - Washcloth
   - Wash basin
   - Towels
   - Gloves, if indicated
   - Talcum powder or cornstarch (optional)
   - Clean gown or clothing
   - Bath blanket, if available
   - Orange stick for nail care, if used by your facility
   - Lotion
   - Comb or hairbrush
   - Clean bed linen, stacked on the chair in order of use, if the bed is to be made following the bed bath
2. Wash your hands.
3. Identify the resident.
4. Tell the resident what you are going to do.
5. Provide privacy.
6. Offer the bedpan or urinal (see Chapter 10).
7. Take the bedspread and regular blanket off the bed.
8. Fold them loosely over the back of the chair, leaving the resident covered with the top sheet or bath blanket, if available.
9. Lower the headrest and kneerest of the bed, if permitted. The resident should be as flat as is comfortable for him and as is permitted.
10. Raise the bed to a comfortable working height with the side rail up on the side opposite from where you are working.
11. Assist the resident to move closer to you so you can work easily without straining your back.
12. Remove the gown, but keep the resident covered to avoid chilling.
13. Fill the wash basin two-thirds full of water at 105°F (40.5°C).
14. Put a towel across the resident's chest and make a mitt with the washcloth. This prevents flopping edges from dropping across the skin. Wash the eyes from the nose to the outside of the face. Ask if the resident wants soap used on his or her face. Wash the face. Be careful not to get soap in the eyes. Rinse, and dry by patting gently with the bath towel.
15. Place the towel lengthwise under the arm farthest from you. Support the arm with the palm of your hand under the elbow. Then

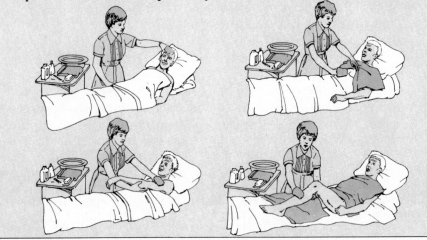

wash the shoulder, axilla (armpit) and arm. Use long, firm, circular strokes. Rinse and dry the area well.

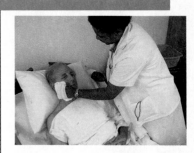

16. Place the basin of water on the towel on the bed. Put the resident's hand into the water. Wash, rinse, and dry the hand well. Place it under the sheet.

17. Wash, rinse, and dry the arm, hand, axilla, and shoulder closest to you in the same way.

18. Clean the fingernails with an orange stick, if used by your facility.

19. Fold the sheet down to the resident's abdomen. Wash and rinse the resident's ears, neck, and chest. Take note of the condition of the skin under the female resident's breasts. Dry the area thoroughly.

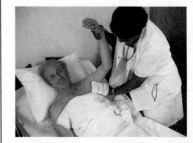

20. Cover the entire chest with the towel. Fold the sheet down to the pubic area.

21. Wash the resident's abdomen. Be sure to wash the umbilicus (navel) and any creases of the skin. Dry the abdomen. Then pull the sheet up over the abdomen and chest and remove the towel.

22. Empty the dirty water. Rinse the basin and fill it with clean water at 105°F (40.5°C).

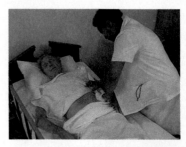

23. Fold the sheet back from the resident's leg farthest from you.

24. Bend the knee, and wash, rinse, and dry the leg and foot. Hold the heel for more support when flexing the knee. If the resident can easily bend the knee, put the wash basin on the towel. Then put the foot directly into the basin to wash it.

25. Observe the toenails and the skin between the toes for general appearance and condition. Look especially for redness and cracking. Remove the basin. Dry the leg and foot and between the toes. Cover the leg and foot with the sheet and remove the towel.

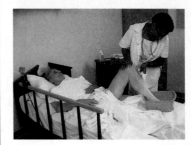

26. Repeat the entire procedure for the leg and foot closest to you. Empty the basin, rinse and refill it with clean water at 105°F (40.5°C).

27. Assist the resident to turn to one side with his or her back toward you.

28. Put the towel lengthwise on the bottom sheet near the resident's back. Wash, rinse, and dry the back, buttocks, and back of the neck behind the ears with long, firm, circular strokes.

29. Look for reddened areas, dry the resident's back, remove the towel, and assist the resident to turn over.

30. Offer the resident a soapy washcloth to wash the genital area. Offer a clean wet washcloth to rinse with, and a dry towel for drying. If the resident is unable to do this, you must wash the resident's genital area. Allow for privacy at all times. Put on your gloves when washing the genital area.

31. Give the resident a back rub.

32. Follow the procedures for dressing the resident (see Chapter 6) and transferring to a wheelchair (see Chapter 8) if indicated. If the resident is to remain in bed, put a clean gown on the resident.

33. Comb the hair if the resident is unable.

34. Change the linens and make the bed.

35. Clean your equipment and put it in its proper place. Discard disposable equipment.

36. Wipe off the overbed table. Discard soiled linen in the dirty linen container.

37. Make the resident comfortable.

38. Place the signal cord within reach.

39. Wash your hands.

40. Report and record your observation of anything unusual.

Rubbing a resident's back is refreshing; it relaxes muscles and stimulates circulation. Because of pressure caused by the bedclothes and the lack of movement to stimulate circulation, the skin of a bedridden resident needs special care.

Back rubs are usually given right after the bath. They are also given:
— as part of bedtime care
— when changing the position of a dependent resident
— for restless residents who need relaxing
— on doctor's orders

Proceed to rub the back as follows:
— Warm the lotion by placing it in a basin of warm water or by pouring a small amount into your hand and using friction to warm it.
— Apply the lotion to the entire back with the palms of your hands. Use long, firm strokes from the buttocks to the shoulders and back of the neck.
— Exert firm pressure as you stroke upward from the buttocks toward the shoulders. Use gentle pressure as you stroke downward from shoulders to buttocks.
— Use a circular motion on each bony area.
— Continue rubbing for 1 1/2 to 3 minutes.

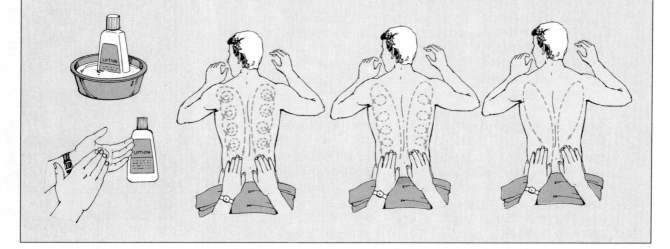

When the term *partial bath* is used in an LTC facility, it refers to bathing only part of the body. A partial bath usually includes face, underarms, hands, and perineal area. The **perineal** area in the female is the area between the vagina and the anus. In the male the perineal area is between the scrotum and the anus. Partial baths are usually given on the days between showers or tub baths and if a resident is very ill or incontinent. When the resident is incontinent, you will always give perineal care.

PROCEDURE

GIVING PERINEAL CARE

1. Assemble your equipment:
   - Disposable bed protector
   - Bedpan
   - Basin of warm water (or special perineal washing solution)
   - Soap
   - Washcloth
   - Towels
   - Gloves

2. Wash your hands.
3. Provide privacy.
4. Explain to the resident what you are going to do.
5. Obtain a basin of warm water, or special peri-wash solution used in the facility.
6. Place the disposable bed protector under the buttocks.
7. Assist the resident onto the bedpan.
8. Put on your gloves.
9. Using a disposable paper cup or peri-wash squeeze bottle, pour warm solution over the perineal area. Spread the labia in the female and wash from front to back. In the uncircumcised male, retract the foreskin and clean thoroughly, rinse thoroughly and dry.
10. If the resident is soiled with urine and feces, use soap and warm water to wash thoroughly. Change water in basin as necessary. Rinse and dry thoroughly. Remember, bacteria normally found in the bowel will cause urinary tract infections—take every precaution to ensure that residents are properly cleaned.
11. Remove the bedpan and disposable bed protector.
12. Cover the resident.
13. Empty, rinse, and clean equipment and return to appropriate storage area.
14. Discard disposable equipment.
15. Remove your gloves.
16. Wash your hands.
17. Assist the resident with handwashing.
18. Reposition and make the resident comfortable, and replace the call signal cord.
19. Wash your hands.
20. Report and record care given and any unusual observations.

1. Assemble your equipment on a chair near the bathtub:
   - Towels
   - Washcloth
   - Soap
   - Bath thermometer, if available
   - Chair (place this near the bathtub)
   - Clean clothing
   - Disinfectant solution
2. Wash your hands.
3. Identify the resident.
4. Tell the resident what you are going to do.
5. Take the resident to the tub room, being sure that he or she is covered to avoid chilling.
6. Wash the tub with disinfectant solution.
7. Fill the tub half full of water at 105°F (40.5°C). Test the temperature with a bath thermometer.

PROCEDURE

(CONTINUED)

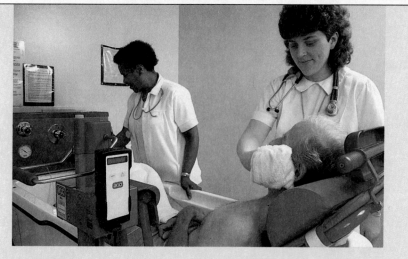

8. Place one towel on the floor where the resident will step out of the tub to prevent slipping.
9. Assist the resident to undress and get into the tub. Get additional assistance if necessary.
10. Let the resident stay in the tub according to your instructions (usually about 15 minutes).
11. Assist the resident with washing as needed.
12. *Never* leave the resident alone in the tub.
13. Put a towel across the chair.
14. Assist the resident out of the tub and onto the towel-covered chair.
15. Dry the resident well by patting gently with a towel.
16. Assist with dressing.
17. Take the resident back to his or her room.
18. Make the resident comfortable.
19. Return to the tub room. Clean the tub with disinfectant solution.
20. Remove all used linen and put it in the dirty linen container.
21. Wash your hands.
22. Record in the chart:
    • That you have given the resident a tub bath
    • Your observations of anything unusual

PROCEDURE

GIVING A SHOWER

1. Assemble your equipment on a chair near the shower:
   • Towels
   • Soap
   • Washcloth
   • Clean clothing
2. Wash your hands.
3. Identify the resident.
4. Tell the resident what you are going to do.
5. Provide privacy.
6. Be sure the resident is properly covered.
7. Turn on the shower and adjust the water temperature.
8. Assist the resident into the shower.

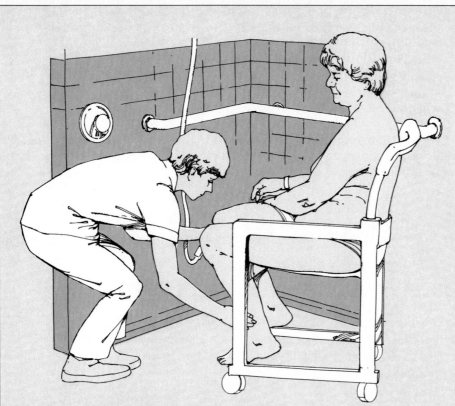

9. Give the resident soap and washcloth so he or she can wash as much as possible. Assist as necessary.
10. Turn off the water and assist the resident out of the shower.
11. Dry the resident well by patting gently with the towel.
12. Assist with dressing.
13. Take the resident back to his or her room.
14. Return to the shower room. Remove all used linen and put it in the dirty linen container.
15. Put your equipment back in its proper place.
16. Wash your hands.
17. Record in the chart:
   • That you have helped the resident with a shower
   • Your observations of anything unusual

Record in the chart the type of bath, shower, or skin care given. Include the response of the resident, degree of independence, and any observations you have made.

Although you have learned many tasks that make up care of the resident's skin, it is important not to treat the person as an object and perform these tasks in a mechanical, routine way. Each resident is unique, and the performance of nursing care activities provides an opportunity to establish meaningful contact with the residents. Such care also allows you to experience the rewards that come from helping others.

It is very important to prevent injuries to the resident's skin when you provide care. The smallest bump or scrape may result in severe bruising or skin tears because the skin of the elderly resident is often very fragile. Ways to prevent injuries to the skin include:

- Taking time to protect limbs when transferring and repositioning
- Padding side rails or wheelchair parts
- Transporting carefully in wheelchair to avoid dragging feet and/or bumping arms against door frames, etc.
- Using long-sleeved clothes
- Keeping shoes and socks on
- Using assistance or mechanical lifts to avoid dragging across bed or wheelchair

When skin tears occur, they are often difficult to heal and frequently become a site for infection. Any bruising or skin tear should be reported to the charge nurse immediately.

SECTION 4 PERSONAL CARE AND GROOMING

OBJECTIVES/WHAT YOU WILL LEARN

When you have completed this section, you will be able to:
- List the procedures included in personal grooming
- List three conditions that increase the need for oral hygiene
- Brush the teeth of a dependent resident
- Care for dentures
- Indicate which residents should not be given nail care by the nursing assistant
- Trim fingernails or toenails
- Care for the hair
- Shave a resident's beard
- Dress a resident in bed
- Dress a resident who is paralyzed on one side
- Explain the terms *AM care* and *PM care*

PERSONAL GROOMING

Personal grooming includes oral hygiene, care of nails, care of hair, shaving, makeup, and dressing. Personal grooming is particularly important to the resident's feelings of self-worth and well-being. The dignity of all human beings is directly related to their grooming. No matter what the personal grooming activity, encourage as much resident involvement as possible. Even if the participation is limited simply to making decisions, the resident must be included in the process.

Residents should be encouraged to use deodorant, perfume, and cosmetics just as they did prior to admission. If you need to apply makeup for the resident, make every effort to obtain a pleasing result. Some residents with poor vision might apply too much makeup and will need your help to determine the right amount.

ASSISTIVE DEVICES

Greater independence can sometimes be achieved through use of assistive devices. Assistive devices are tools designed to help the resident perform tasks that would otherwise be impossible. Use of any assistive devices requires

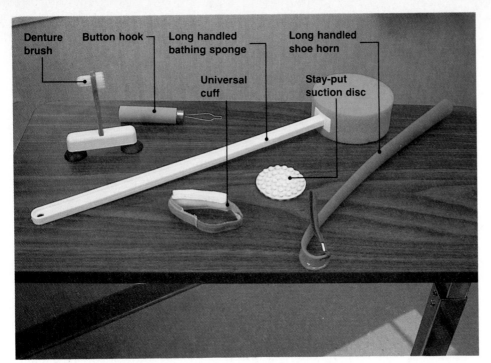

Denture brush   Button hook   Long handled bathing sponge   Long handled shoe horn

Universal cuff   Stay-put suction disc

FIGURE 6-6
Some grooming and dressing devices.

training the resident along with consistent encouragement from the staff. At first, it may take the resident more time to use the device than if you performed the task, but remember the independence and self-esteem that come with it are very important to the resident. A good nursing assistant will not perform tasks for residents that they are capable of doing for themselves. A good nursing assistant will be patient and assist each resident toward independent functioning. Some of the devices available for grooming and dressing are shown in Fig. 6-6.

As you give care to residents, remember that there are many assistive devices available. Do not hesitate to suggest to the charge nurse that they be used when appropriate. The services of an occupational therapist may be indicated to recommend special devices and to train the resident in their use.

ORAL HYGIENE

Oral hygiene is part of the daily care of every resident and includes care of the mouth, teeth, gums, and tongue. The purpose of oral hygiene is to keep the mouth, teeth, gums, and tongue healthy. A mouth in poor condition can be uncomfortable and can cause loss of appetite as well as decreased fluid intake. Poor nutrition and dehydration contribute to lowered resistance of the mouth, tongue, teeth, and gums to infection. When mouth care is poor, tartar, plaque, and food collect around the teeth, leading to irritation, tooth decay, gum disease, and loss of teeth. Other parts of the body are often affected by infection and disease of the mouth.

Residents who are disabled or elderly may be unable to provide their own mouth care (Fig. 6-7). They can fail to recognize the importance of oral hygiene, forget to perform it, or be physically unable to do so. Having a clean, fresh mouth is part of the dignity to which each resident is entitled.

Some nursing assistants find giving mouth and denture care an unpleasant task. It is so important that you must learn to overcome your own feelings and put the needs of the resident first. The more you practice this skill, the less unpleasant it will become.

FIGURE 6-7
Assisting the resident with oral hygiene.

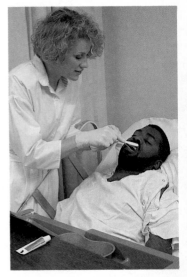

In addition to performing mouth and denture care, the nursing assistant should observe and report signs of disease or injury of the mouth, tongue, teeth, and gums. Report such things as:

- Sores in the mouth
- Bleeding
- Dry, coated tongue
- Loose or broken teeth
- Bad mouth odor

These problems must be reported immediately and recorded in the health record.

Every resident should receive oral hygiene twice daily. Certain residents require more frequent care. They are residents who are:

- Unconscious
- Receiving oxygen
- Unable to take fluids by mouth
- Breathing through the mouth
- Feverish

Brushing the teeth is the most important aspect of mouth care! Although you also may refresh and lubricate the mouth with mouthwash, swabs, and sponge-type devices, there is no adequate substitute for brushing the teeth and gums.

Ideally, a soft-bristle, junior-size brush is used for the resident. This allows you to do a good job without injuring the mouth and gums.

Dental hygienists have recommended that the teeth of long-term residents be brushed using the following principles:

- Wear gloves.
- Use a *dry* brush first to stimulate gums.
- Hold the brush at a 45-degree angle to the teeth.
- Use a circular motion.
- Massage the area where the teeth and gums meet.
- Brush the upper teeth first since brushing the lower teeth produces excessive saliva.
- Brush outer surface, inner surface, then chewing surface.
- After about 1 1/2 minutes, repeat this process using toothpaste.

PROCEDURE

CLEANING DENTURES (FALSE TEETH)

1. Assemble your equipment on the bedside table:
   - Tissues
   - Mouthwash
   - Denture cup
   - Toothbrush or denture brush
   - Towel
   - Denture toothpaste or baking soda
   - Gloves
2. Wash your hands.
3. Identify the resident.
4. Tell the resident what you are going to do.
5. Provide privacy.
6. Spread the towel across the resident's chest to protect the gown and the top sheets.
7. Put on your gloves.

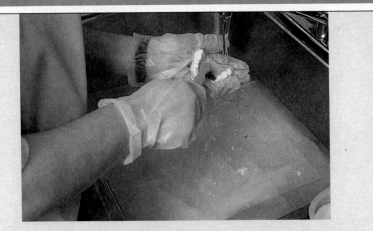

8. Ask the resident to remove the dentures. Assist residents who cannot remove their own dentures by pushing gently to break the suction.

9. Take the dentures to the sink in the denture cup. Hold the dentures securely in the basin.

10. Line the sink with a paper towel or fill the sink with water to guard against breaking the dentures if you drop them.

11. Apply toothpaste or denture cleanser. With the dentures in the palm of your hand, brush them until they are clean.

12. Rinse them thoroughly under cool running water.

13. Fill the clean denture cup with cool water and place the dentures in the cup.

14. Help the resident rinse with the mouthwash and water solution.

15. Have the resident replace the dentures.

16. Leave the labeled denture cup with the clean solution where the resident can reach it easily.

17. Clean all equipment and put it in the proper place. Discard disposable equipment in the proper container.

18. Remove and discard your gloves.

19. Wash your hands.

20. Record and report any unusual observations.

PROCEDURE

GIVING SPECIAL MOUTH CARE TO THE UNCONSCIOUS RESIDENT

1. Assemble your equipment:
   • Towel
   • Emesis basin
   • Mouth care kit of commercially prepared swabs. Or if such kit is not available:
     — Tongue depressor
     — Applicators or gauze sponges
     — Lubricant such as glycerine, or a substance used by your facility, or a solution of lemon juice and glycerine
   • Gloves
2. Wash your hands.
3. Identify the resident.
4. Tell the resident what you are going to do. Even though a resident seems to be unconscious, he or she still may be able to hear you.

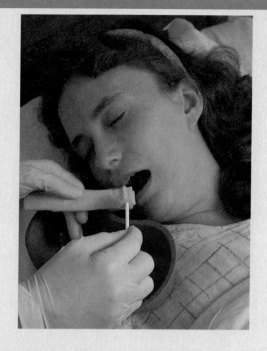

5. Provide privacy.
6. Stand at the side of the bed with the resident facing you.
7. Put a towel on the pillow under the resident's head and partly under the face.
8. Put the emesis basin on the towel under the resident's chin.
9. Put on your gloves.
10. Press on the cheeks and hold the tongue in place with a tongue depressor.
11. Open the commercial package of swabs and wipe the resident's entire mouth, roof, tongue, and inside the cheeks and lips.
12. If a disposable swab is not available, use applicators moistened with diluted mouthwash.
13. Clean your equipment and put it back in the proper place. Discard disposable equipment in the proper container.
14. Remove your gloves.
15. Make the resident comfortable.
16. Wash your hands.
17. Report and record any unusual observations.

If a resident is able to brush his own teeth, he should be encouraged to do so. Your role would be to provide the necessary equipment and supplies and to assist as needed. Use the following procedure when assisting a resident with oral hygiene.

PROCEDURE

ASSISTING THE RESIDENT WITH ORAL HYGIENE

1. Assemble your equipment on the overbed table:
   * Mouthwash
   * Fresh water
   * Disposable cup
   * Straw
   * Toothbrush
   * Toothpaste
   * Emesis basin
   * Face towel

2. Wash your hands.
3. Identify the resident.
4. Tell the resident what you are going to do.
5. Provide privacy.
6. Spread the towel across the resident's chest to protect the gown and top sheet. (If possible, assist the resident into the bathroom.)
7. Dilute the mouthwash with four parts of water to one part of mouthwash. (Full-strength mouthwash may be harmful to delicate gums.)
8. Let the resident take a mouthful of the mixture and rinse the mouth.
9. Hold the emesis basin under the chin so that the resident can spit out the mouthwash solution.
10. Put toothpaste on the wet toothbrush. Encourage the resident to brush his or her own teeth if possible. Assist as necessary.
11. Help the resident rinse out the toothpaste using the fresh water.
12. Make the resident comfortable.
13. Clean and put your equipment in its proper place. Discard disposable equipment.
14. Wash your hands.
15. Record that you have assisted the resident with oral hygiene.

CARE OF NAILS AND HAIR *study*

As a nursing assistant in a LTC facility, you will assist residents with nail care and care of the hair (Fig. 6-8). As with the skin, cleanliness is very important. The hair and fingernails are a critical part of personal grooming and will have an effect on how the residents feel about themselves. Cleanliness and good grooming contribute to the dignity and self-esteem of every resident.

The fingernails and toenails must be kept short, clean, and free of rough edges. This prevents damage to the skin and provides a pleasant appearance. With the inactive or elderly resident, the nails may become thick, brittle, and difficult to trim. For this reason, you will find it easier if the nails are trimmed after soaking in warm water. Trimming the nails weekly also makes the job easier. If the nails are long, they are more likely to split when being trimmed. Usually, clippers are used rather than scissors. Take care not to injure the skin while trimming.

Certain residents will have their nails trimmed only by the licensed nurse or podiatrist. These are residents who have diabetes or poor circulation and heal slowly if injured. Follow the policies and procedures established in your facility regarding trimming the resident's nails. If you are to trim nails, follow this procedure:

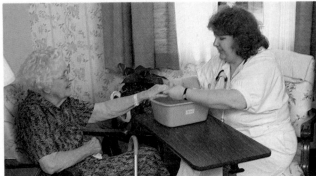

FIGURE 6-8
Assisting resident with nail care.

1. Assemble your equipment:
   - Nail clippers
   - Emery board or file
   - Orange stick, if available
   - Basin of warm water
   - Towel
   - Lotion
2. Wash your hands.
3. Explain to the resident what you are going to do.
4. Protect the bed with a towel.
5. Place the hands or feet in warm water and wash.
6. Clean the nails using the orangewood stick.
7. Dry the hands or feet.
8. Trim the nails using the clippers.
9. File rough edges using an emery board or nail file.
10. Apply lotion and gently massage the hands or feet.
11. Repeat steps 6–10 on the feet or hands.
12. Return the equipment to its proper place.
13. Wash your hands.
14. Record and report your actions and any unusual observations in the chart.
15. Report any injury immediately.

Daily care of the resident's hair consists of combing, brushing, and arranging. Any resident who is able to should be encouraged and assisted to care for her own hair. Your role may be simply to take the resident with the proper equipment to the bathroom to perform her own hair care. Some residents, due to blindness, paralysis, weakness, or disorientation, may need to have their hair care done entirely by you.

The goals for choosing a particular style should include simplicity and neatness, but most important are the preference and dignity of the individual. Most facilities have a professional hairdresser who visits on a regular basis. When an age-appropriate or dignified hairstyle cannot be achieved, the resident may need an appointment with the hairdresser. It is always necessary to obtain permission of the family and the resident before making the appointment.

GUIDELINES FOR SHAMPOOING THE RESIDENT'S HAIR

Shampooing hair is part of the routine care of the resident. Some residents will have a regular appointment with a hairdresser or may even go out to a beauty salon for shampooing. Do not shampoo the hair as part of the shower if the resident has a regularly scheduled beauty salon appointment.

Most often you will shampoo the hair as part of the shower. Younger residents may be shampooed daily, while the elderly may receive a shampoo once a week. Check with your facility for the policy on frequency of shampoos.

Regardless of the method used the procedure should be done in such a way that the:
- Hair is thoroughly cleansed
- Resident is not chilled
- Soap is rinsed completely
- Eyes are not irritated by the shampoo

Residents who are unable to sit in a shower or shampoo chair may have their hair shampooed by placing them on a wheeled stretcher set over the sink, shower, or tub.

SHAVING THE RESIDENT

A regular morning activity for most men is shaving. This is a *daily* activity, not every other day. If the resident is able to shave himself, encourage him and only provide help if necessary.

Shaving can be done with an electric razor or a safety razor. If the resident has his own electric razor, it should be used to shave him. Electric razors are *never* used if the resident is receiving oxygen or if oxygen is being given to any other person in the room because this presents a fire hazard.

PROCEDURE

SHAVING THE
RESIDENT'S BEARD
WITH A SAFETY RAZOR

1. Assemble your equipment on the bedside table:
   - Basin of water at 115°F (46.1°C)
   - Shaving cream
   - Safety razor
   - Face towel
   - Mirror
   - Tissues
   - Aftershave lotion, if available
   - Washcloth
2. Wash your hands.
3. Identify the resident.
4. Tell the resident that you are going to shave his beard.
5. Adjust the light so that it shines on the resident's face.
6. Raise the head of the bed, if allowed.
7. Spread the face towel under the resident's chin. If he has dentures, be sure they are in his mouth.
8. Pat some warm water or use a damp washcloth on the resident's face to soften his beard.
9. Apply shaving soap generously to the face.
10. With the fingers of one hand, hold the skin taut (tight) as you shave in the direction that the hair grows. Start under the sideburns and work downward over the cheeks. Continue carefully over the chin. Work upward on the neck under the chin. Use short firm strokes.
11. Rinse the razor often.
12. Areas under the nose and around the lips are sensitive. Take special care in these areas.
13. If you nick the resident's skin, report this to your charge nurse.
14. Wash off the remaining soap when you have finished.
15. Apply aftershave lotion if the resident prefers.
16. Clean your equipment and put it in its proper place. Discard disposable equipment.
17. Make the resident comfortable.
18. Wash your hands.

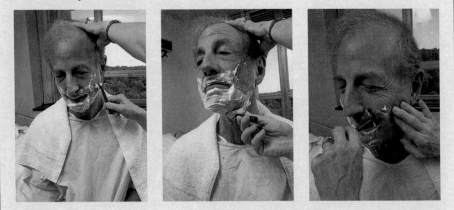

DRESSING THE RESIDENT

In most LTC facilities, residents are encouraged to wear street clothing rather than hospital gowns or pajamas, robes, and slippers. As a nursing assistant you will not only help the resident to dress but also to select clothing that is neat, clean, in good repair, and appropriate for the environment and weather.

Types of clothing that are particularly useful are jogging suits (they are warm and loose fitting, without buttons, snaps, or zippers), brunch coats (loose-fitting dresses that snap down the front), or specially made clothing for those who spend time in wheelchairs or in bed. Most of this type of clothing uses Velcro fasteners and opens in the back. These items can be obtained from some of the major department stores as well as specialty companies.

Offering the resident the opportunity to choose his or her own clothing is one way of encouraging the resident to participate in his or her own care and to make decisions. It also allows the resident a measure of control that is important to most individuals. Elderly residents tend to require warmer clothing due to decreased circulation. Take this need into consideration as you assist with dressing.

For residents who have a problem that results in their constantly disrobing (taking their clothes off), jump suits can be very helpful as a deterrent. For those who don't remain covered when in bed or who are exposed when up in a chair, try pants or pajama bottoms to protect privacy and dignity.

The dressing procedure varies with the abilities and limitations of each resident. You may need to combine parts of the following procedures on dressing, depending on the needs of the residents. Remember to allow residents to do as much for themselves as possible.

PROCEDURE

DRESSING AND UNDRESSING THE TOTALLY DEPENDENT RESIDENT

Note: It is usually easier to dress the dependent resident completely in bed before transferring the resident to a chair. Generally, the resident sleeps in a hospital gown at night.

1. Wash your hands.
2. Identify the resident.
3. Explain what you are going to do.
4. Assist the resident to select clothing.
5. Provide privacy.
6. Fold back the bed covers.
7. Turn the resident to the supine (face up) position.
8. Untie the gown.
9. Remove the gown by pulling the sleeves down and over the arms.
10. Lay the gown across the resident to provide covering.
11. With all the buttons, fasteners, or zippers open, apply the clothing as follows:

    To apply pants or slacks: Gather the pant leg for the leg farthest from you. Reach through the leg to grasp the resident's ankle. Pull the pant leg over your hand and the resident's leg. Repeat for the leg nearest you. Pull the pants up as high as possible. If the resident is able, have him or her raise the buttocks as you pull the pants up to the waist. If the resident is unable to raise the buttocks, roll the

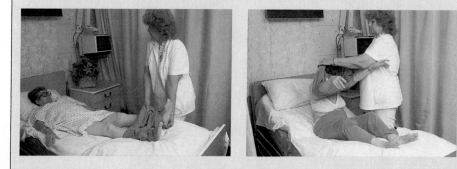

resident on the side away from you as you pull up the other side. Fasten as indicated.

Shirt or dress that opens down the front: Reach inside the sleeve farthest from you and grasp the resident's wrist. Slide the sleeve over your hand and the resident's arm. Roll the resident toward you and tuck the remainder of the item under the resident. Roll the resident away from you and pull the item free. Reach through the sleeve and grasp the resident's wrist. Pull the sleeve over your hand and the resident's wrist. Secure the fasteners.

Pullover-type shirt or dress: Place both the resident's hands, one at a time in the sleeves. Pull the item as high on the arms as possible. Grasp the neck opening and slide over the head. Either assist the resident to sit and pull the item down, or roll the resident from side to side, pulling the clothing down as you go.

12. Apply socks or stockings and shoes.

You may have times when you are dressing residents who have either tubes (feeding tubes or catheters) or intravenous (in the veins) catheters. Use caution so that you do not place any tension on the tube that might dislodge or displace it. Treat the IV and the tubing as a part of the person. Some facilities will provide gowns that snap on over the arm and shoulder to make it easier to dress the resident. If you have no special clothing, be careful in both clothing selection and application. If there is an IV in an arm, use short-sleeved clothing. The nurse needs to be able to observe the site where the needle or catheter enters the vein. Loose-fitting clothing will be easier to apply than tight-fitting clothing. You will be learning more about the purposes and types of tubes and catheters in Chapter 9 and Chapter 10.

1. Wash your hands.
2. Identify the resident.
3. Explain what you are going to do.
4. Assist the resident to select clothing if appropriate.
5. Provide privacy.
6. Remove the gown or shirt from the arm without the IV.
7. Move the gown carefully down the arm containing the IV carefully sliding it over the site and off the hand. Bring the gown over the tubing.
8. Remove the IV bottle or bag from the pole and slide the gown over it. *Do not lower the bag below the level of the resident's arm.*
9. Replace the bag or bottle on the pole.
   Note: If a pump or a rate-control device is attached to the IV, ask the charge nurse to assist you. The nurse will have to disconnect the tubing from the pump and reconnect when you have finished changing the gown.
10. Put on the new gown or shirt by beginning with the arm containing the IV. Remove the bag from the pole and slide the gown over the bag and tubing, being careful not to lower the bag below the level of the arm.
11. Put the other arm through the sleeve.
12. Tie or button as indicated.
13. Make the resident comfortable or proceed with the remainder of the dressing procedure.

Undressing a helpless resident is simply the reverse of the dressing procedure.

Dressing a resident with one paralyzed side, a cast, an IV, or other impairment requires that you remember one thing. *Always dress the affected side first and undress it last.* It is also important that residents be dressed with proper underclothing in keeping with their personal preferences.

Most of the basic skills you have learned in this section are carried out on a daily basis and make up some of the facility routines or daily procedures performed for each resident.

These activities are often referred to as AM care or PM care because of the time of day they are carried out.

AM care includes:

* Providing an opportunity to go to the bathroom (see Chapter 10)
* Washing the resident's face and hands
* Providing oral hygiene
* Preparing the resident for breakfast (see Chapter 9)

PM or **HS** (hour of sleep) **care** includes:

* Providing an opportunity to go to the bathroom
* Washing face and hands
* Providing a bedtime snack or nourishment
* Providing oral hygiene
* Dressing in sleeping attire
* Giving a back rub

Most facilities have specific procedures for both AM and PM care that can include other activities.

SECTION 5 APPLICATION OF WARM AND COLD

OBJECTIVES/WHAT YOU WILL LEARN

When you have completed this section, you will be able to:
■ Describe the effect of heat and cold on blood vessels
■ List appropriate temperatures for different types of heat application
■ List four safety precautions to be followed when using heat or cold

APPLYING HEAT AND COLD

You may be given the job of applying heat or cold to a resident's body. To carry out this task safely requires an understanding of how both heat and cold work (Fig. 6-9) and the safety precautions that must be followed. Each facility has policies that include the kinds of applications used and the personnel who may apply them. Some facilities permit only licensed nurses to apply heat and cold.

Heat is used to speed up the healing process, to decrease swelling, or to relieve pain. When heat is applied to the skin, the blood vessels dilate (open). This causes more blood with oxygen and nutrients to reach the injured area.

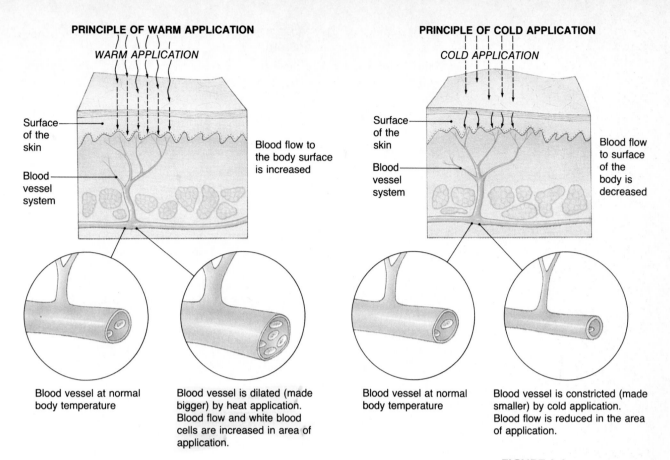

PRINCIPLE OF WARM APPLICATION

WARM APPLICATION

Surface of the skin

Blood vessel system

Blood flow to the body surface is increased

Blood vessel at normal body temperature

Blood vessel is dilated (made bigger) by heat application. Blood flow and white blood cells are increased in area of application.

PRINCIPLE OF COLD APPLICATION

COLD APPLICATION

Surface of the skin

Blood vessel system

Blood flow to surface of the body is decreased

Blood vessel at normal body temperature

Blood vessel is constricted (made smaller) by cold application. Blood flow is reduced in the area of application.

FIGURE 6-9
Principles of warm and cold application.

Fluids that may be causing swelling and pain are absorbed and carried away as the blood circulates. The warmth also relaxes the muscles, decreasing pain due to tension.

Cold is used to prevent swelling, control bleeding, relieve pain, or lower body temperature. When cold is applied, the blood vessels contract (narrow), reducing the flow of blood to the area. The physician will order the kind of heat or cold to be applied, the frequency of application, and the length of treatment. Moist or dry applications may be ordered.

Moist applications include:

- Soak (warm or cold)
- Compress (warm or cold)
- Tub
- Alcohol sponge bath
- Sitz bath
- Cool wet packs

Dry applications include:

- Ice pack and ice collar
- Warm water bottle
- Heat lamp
- Aquamatic K-pad

A **moist application** is one in which water touches the skin. A **dry application** is one in which no water touches the skin. Compresses and soaks are both moist applications. They can be either warm or cold. A compress is a localized application. A soak can be either localized or generalized. In applying a compress, a cloth is dipped into water, wrung out, and applied to a specific area. To apply a soak, you immerse the body or body part completely in water. Warm water bottles, ice caps, and Aquamatic K-pads are considered dry applications because they have a dry surface. Water is used only *inside* the equipment and never touches the skin. Dry applications are sometimes used to keep moist applications at the correct temperature.

Although some facilities still use warm water bottles to apply dry heat, most have discontinued the practice for several reasons:

- The elderly and chronically ill often have decreased perception of the temperature and pain, increasing the risk of burns.
- The weight of the bottle can create additional pressure on an already injured or damaged area.
- It is difficult to keep the bottle in position.
- It is difficult to control the temperature of the water.

Electric heating pads are equally dangerous to older residents. Sometimes families bring in heating pads in an attempt to be helpful. Refer them to the charge nurse, who can explain the dangers to the resident. Most facilities have policies excluding the use of electric heating pads.

Use of a heat lamp also contains great risk of burning the resident. This procedure is being used much less frequently than in the past. A heat lamp can provide soothing and drying to skin irritated from moisture as a result of perspiration or urine. Current knowledge of pressure sore treatment indicates that use of a heat lamp slows down the healing process if the skin is actually broken. In other words, heat lamps are not indicated for any pressure sores except perhaps stage 1.

PROCEDURE

APPLYING THE AQUAMATIC K-PAD

1. Assemble your equipment:
   - Aquamatic K-pad and control unit
   - Cover for pad
2. Inspect the K-pad for leaks, and make sure the cord and plug are in good condition.
3. Wash your hands.
4. Identify the resident.
5. Explain to the resident what you are going to do.
6. Provide privacy.
7. Plug the cord into an electrical outlet.
8. Place the pad in the cover. *Do not use pins!*
9. Place the pump on the bedside table. Arrange the tubing at the level of the pad. Do not allow the tubing to hang below the level of the bed.
10. Gently apply the covered pad to the proper body area.
11. Check the skin under the pad every hour.
12. When the treatment is finished, return the equipment to its proper place.
13. Make the resident comfortable.
14. Wash your hands.
15. Record in the chart:
    - The time the K-pad was applied
    - The length of treatment
    - The area of application
    - Your observations of anything unusual

THE ALCOHOL SPONGE BATH

You can probably remember the experience of perspiring on a warm summer day. You often feel cooler as the moisture evaporates from your skin. As perspiration evaporates into the air, it carries heat away with it and this cools the body. An alcohol sponge bath cools in the same way. Alcohol is applied to the resident's body because it will evaporate from the skin much faster than water. The purpose of the alcohol sponge bath is to lower the body temperature.

Either heat or cold applications can damage the skin if not observed frequently and carefully. Since the elderly and chronically ill residents have fragile skin and a decreased ability to feel pain and temperature, they are at risk for burns.

GUIDELINES FOR GIVING THE ALCOHOL SPONGE BATH

- Alcohol sponge baths are *never* given without doctor's orders.
- Never apply alcohol to the resident's face.
- If the resident starts to shiver, stop the treatment. Call the charge nurse. If the shivering cannot be controlled, the alcohol sponge bath will do no good because the shivering causes increased cell and muscle activity. This produces more heat and causes the body temperature to rise.
- Follow your facility's step-by-step procedures for giving the bath.

GUIDELINES FOR APPLICATION OF WARM AND COLD

- Follow the instructions of the charge nurse.
- Check the application often to keep it at the right temperature throughout the treatment. Suggested times for checking different kinds of applications are:
  — Soaks and intermittent compresses: every 5 minutes
  — Heat lamps: every 5 minutes
  — Continuous compresses: every 30 minutes
  — Ice bags: at least every hour
- Keep the resident comfortable. Make sure that the resident is comfortably positioned during the application of heat or cold.
- If the resident begins to shiver during cold applications, stop the treatment, cover the resident with a blanket, and report to your charge nurse for further instructions.
- For a warm application, always use a bath thermometer to test the temperature of the water. Temperatures for different kinds of heat application are:
  — Warm soak 100°F (37.8°C)
  — Warm compress 115° (46.1°C)
  — Tub bath 105°F (40.5°C)
- For cold applications, use cubed ice if available. Crushed ice will melt too quickly. Also, it may stick to the cloth and be too cold for the resident's skin. Keep the application cold by adding ice as necessary.
- Always dry the bags after checking for leaks.
- Always apply the ice cap with the metal or plastic stopper away from the resident's body. The stopper should never touch the resident's skin. It will burn the resident. Remember, ice can also burn the skin.

- Never put an ice cap directly on the skin. Always cover it with a cloth.
- Never put an ice bag on top of the painful area. The weight will probably increase the pain.
- Check the resident's skin. Watch for too much redness. Look for darker discolorations that might mean the resident is being burned. Listen to any complaints. If you think a resident is being burned, remove the heat application immediately and report to your charge nurse at once!
- Check the resident's skin where cold is being applied. If the area appears to be blanched or bluish, tell the charge nurse at once!
- When you have finished the moist application, dry the resident's skin thoroughly and gently, using a patting motion. Do not rub the resident's skin.

CHAPTER 7

The Skeletal System

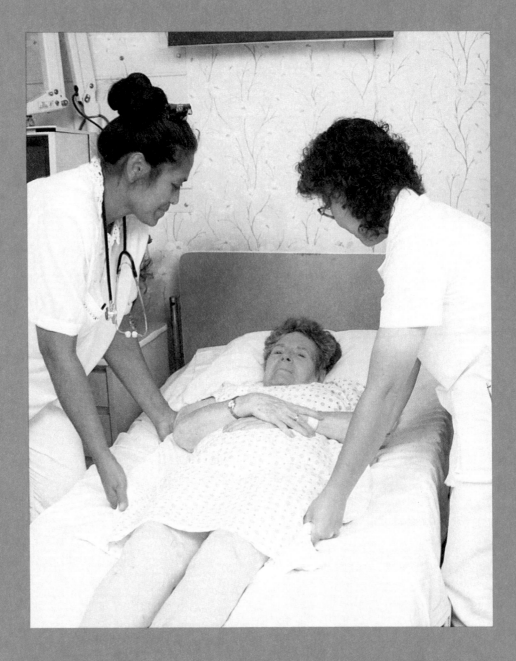

OBJECTIVES/WHAT YOU WILL LEARN

When you have completed this section, you will be able to:

- List four functions of the skeletal system
- Identify examples of the different types of bones
- Define the terms *ligament, tendon, bursa,* and *cartilage*
- Identify two age-related changes that affect the skeletal system

FIGURE 7-1
The skeletal system.

The skeleton is a living framework made by the joining of bones. It serves to provide support, body movement powered by muscular contractions, protection for the vital organs and other soft structures, blood cell production, and storage for essential minerals. There are 206 bones in the adult body, forming the two divisions of the skeletal system. The axial skeleton is comprised of skull, vertebrae, rib cage, and sternum. The upper and lower extremities and the shoulder and pelvic girdles form the appendicular skeleton.

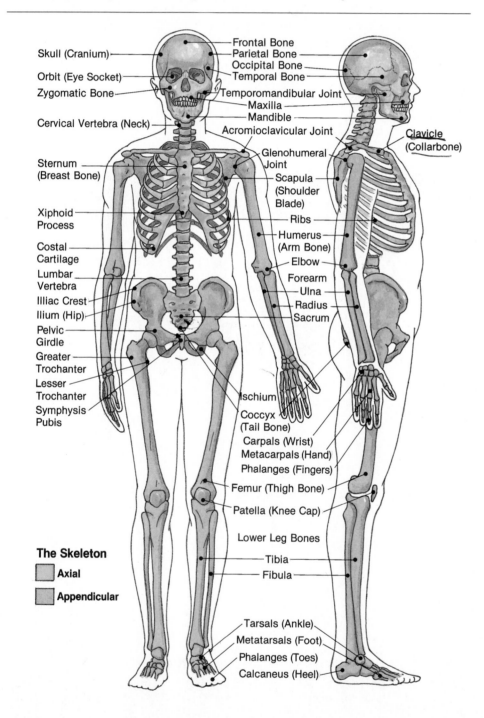

Skull (Cranium)
Orbit (Eye Socket)
Zygomatic Bone
Cervical Vertebra (Neck)
Sternum (Breast Bone)
Xiphoid Process
Costal Cartilage
Lumbar Vertebra
Illiac Crest
Ilium (Hip)
Pelvic Girdle
Greater Trochanter
Lesser Trochanter
Symphysis Pubis

Frontal Bone
Parietal Bone
Occipital Bone
Temporal Bone
Temporomandibular Joint
Maxilla
Mandible
Acromioclavicular Joint
Glenohumeral Joint
Scapula (Shoulder Blade)
Ribs
Humerus (Arm Bone)
Elbow
Forearm
Ulna
Radius
Sacrum

Clavicle (Collarbone)

Ischium
Coccyx (Tail Bone)
Carpals (Wrist)
Metacarpals (Hand)
Phalanges (Fingers)
Femur (Thigh Bone)
Patella (Knee Cap)
Lower Leg Bones
Tibia
Fibula

Tarsals (Ankle)
Metatarsals (Foot)
Phalanges (Toes)
Calcaneus (Heel)

The Skeleton

■ Axial

■ Appendicular

THE SKELETAL SYSTEM

The skeletal system (Fig. 7-1) is composed of:

- Bones
- Joints

The skeletal system functions are to:

- Protect
- Support
- Provide leverage
- Store vital minerals
- Produce blood cells

The human skeleton is made up of 206 bones. The bones act as a framework for the body, giving it structure and support. The bones are passive organs of motion—they do not move by themselves. They must be moved by the muscles of the body, which are stimulated to move by nerve impulses. Most muscles attach to bones, providing the leverage necessary for body movement.

BONES

The bones surround our vital organs and provide protection:

- **Cranium** (bones of the head)—protect the brain (Fig. 7-2)
- **Vertebrae** (bones of the spine)—protect the spinal cord (Fig. 7-3)
- **Bones** of the rib cage—protect the heart and lungs

Bones are composed of living cells called **osteocytes,** which store vital minerals like calcium, phosphorous, magnesium, and sodium that are essential for other body functions. Bones are not dead, they are the site of many body activities. Red blood cells are produced in the marrow of certain bones.

FIGURE 7-2
The skull.

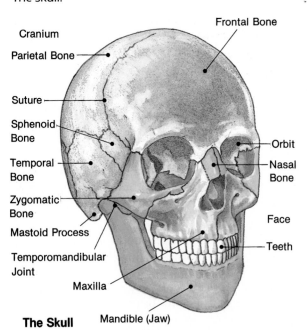

Cranium
Parietal Bone
Suture
Sphenoid Bone
Temporal Bone
Zygomatic Bone
Mastoid Process
Temporomandibular Joint
Maxilla
Frontal Bone
Orbit
Nasal Bone
Face
Teeth
Mandible (Jaw)

The Skull

FIGURE 7-3
The vertebral column (spine).

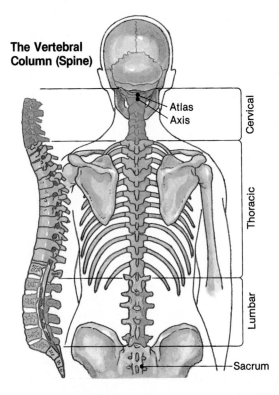

The Vertebral Column (Spine)

Atlas
Axis
Cervical
Thoracic
Lumbar
Sacrum

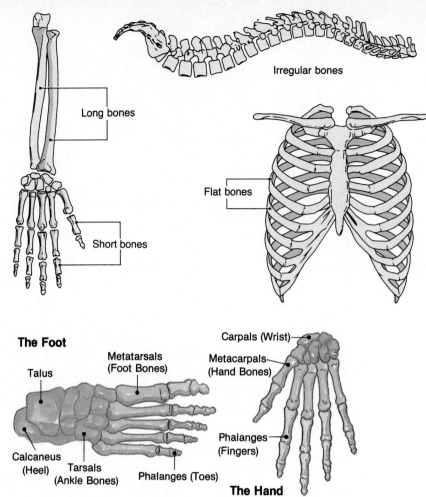

Irregular bones

Long bones

Flat bones

Short bones

FIGURE 7-4
Types of bones.

FIGURE 7-5
Bones of the hand and foot.

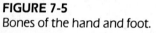

The Foot

Talus

Metatarsals
(Foot Bones)

Calcaneus
(Heel)

Tarsals
(Ankle Bones)

Phalanges (Toes)

Carpals (Wrist)

Metacarpals
(Hand Bones)

Phalanges
(Fingers)

The Hand

There are several types of bones (Fig. 7-4), each of which has a different function. The skeletal system interacts with the muscular system, the nervous system, and the circulatory system to achieve movement of the body. Movement occurs at the joints. Bones of the hands and feet are shown in Fig. 7-5.

JOINTS

Joints are areas where one bone connects with one or more other bones. Joints are necessary as levers in all motion. Joints are classified by their type of motion (Fig. 7-6). Joints are made up of different structures (Fig. 7-7):

- **Ligament**—tough, white, fibrous cord that connects bone to bone.
- **Tendon**—an elastic cordlike structure that connects muscle to bone.
- **Bursa**—small fluid-filled sac that allows one bone to move easily over another. The fluid prevents friction so that the ends of the bones do not wear out. Bursas are located throughout the body, but the most important are in the shoulder, elbow, knee, and hip.
- **Cartilage**—a tough gristlelike substance that forms a pad at the end of or between bones, which acts as a cushion. Cartilage looks like white elastic.

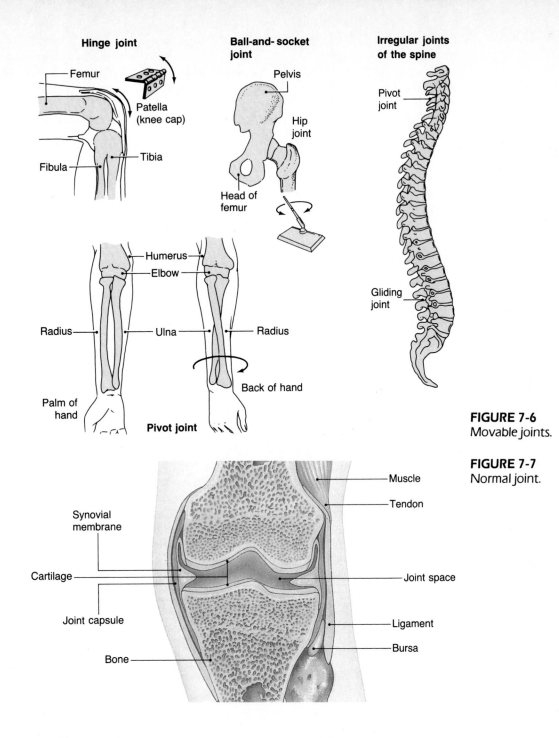

Hinge joint

Femur

Patella (knee cap)

Tibia

Fibula

Ball-and-socket joint

Pelvis

Hip joint

Head of femur

Irregular joints of the spine

Pivot joint

Gliding joint

Humerus

Elbow

Radius

Ulna

Radius

Back of hand

Palm of hand

Pivot joint

FIGURE 7-6
Movable joints.

FIGURE 7-7
Normal joint.

Muscle

Tendon

Synovial membrane

Cartilage

Joint capsule

Bone

Joint space

Ligament

Bursa

ABNORMALITIES OF THE SKELETAL SYSTEM

Abnormalities of the skeletal system include skeletal or postural deformities. Due to aging or chronic illness, scoliosis and kyphosis can occur. **Scoliosis** refers to an S-shaped curving of the spine. **Kyphosis** is a hunchback or forward curving of the spine. Both of these conditions affect the body's balance and distribution of weight. Ambulation is usually affected, resulting in the resident's need to compensate or adjust his gait.

Osteoarthritis is the deterioration and abrasion of joint cartilage, with formation of new bone at the joint surfaces. Osteoarthritis affects many joints but usually the weight-bearing ones—knee, hips, vertebrae, and fingers.

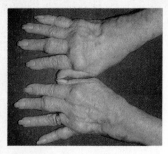

FIGURE 7-8
Crippling effect of
rheumatoid arthritis.

Symptoms include aching, stiffness, and limited motion. Osteoarthritis does not cause inflammation, deformity, or crippling as does **rheumatoid arthritis.**

Rheumatoid arthritis affects people of all ages. The joints become extremely painful, stiff, swollen, red, and warm to the touch. The joints become gradually more deformed and often function is completely lost (Fig. 7-8). The pain experienced is severe, even at rest. Application of heat and gentle massage and medications may provide some relief.

Common injuries of the skeletal system include:

- **Fracture**—breaking or cracking a bone (injury, cancer of the bone, and osteoporosis are common causes).
- **Dislocation**—disruption of the normal alignment of bones where they form a joint.
- **Sprain**—stretched or torn ligaments or tendons that support a joint.
- **Bursitis**—inflammation of the fluid-filled sac causing pain on movement.

Broken bones mend solidly, but the process is gradual. Bone cells grow and reproduce slowly. The blood supply to bone tissue is poor compared to other tissues of the body. This decreased circulation makes bone more susceptible to infection. Once infection is present in bone, it is very difficult to clear up.

AGE AND DISUSE-RELATED CHANGES

Both aging and disuse have profound effects on the skeletal system. There is a loss of bone mass and a shortening of the vertebral column. Some people lose as much as 2 inches in height. If an individual is unable to bear weight (stand), the long bones of the body lose calcium, which is eliminated by the kidneys. This same loss of calcium has been reported when astronauts are in a weightless or "zero gravity" state. With the loss of calcium, the bones become porous and chalklike. The resulting condition is known as **osteoporosis.** The bone is weakened and breaks easily. Sometimes a slight fall or stumble can result in a fracture. Fractures of the hip (the neck of the femur) are life-threatening to the elderly. Confinement to bed while the fracture heals means the resident has a greater risk of developing other complications related to immobility.

SECTION 2 THE RESIDENT WITH A FRACTURE

FIGURE 7-9
Fractures of the femur.

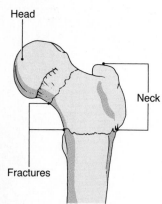

Head

Neck

Fractures

OBJECTIVES/WHAT YOU WILL LEARN

When you have completed this section, you will be able to:
- Define the term *fracture*
- List the three goals of fracture treatment
- Match common problems of the resident with a cast to their related causes

FRACTURES

The term **fracture** refers to a break in a bone (Fig. 7-9). A fracture usually results from some type of trauma, but in the elderly or residents with certain types of disease, it can occur spontaneously. Frequently, hip fractures in the

THE

The r
tions
condi
prom

A.

B.

C.

D.

E.

F.

G.

H

I.

elderly are spontaneous. Instead of falling and fracturing the hip, the spontaneous fracture of the hip causes the person to fall. Regardless of the cause of the fracture, the symptoms are similar.

- Loss of strength and movement
- Bruising and swelling
- Pain and tenderness over the fracture site
- Deformity or misalignment

If any of these symptoms are observed, report and document them immediately.

Any time a resident in your facility sustains a fall or other trauma, the resident should be evaluated by a licensed nurse *before being moved.* The licensed nurse will observe for the signs and symptoms mentioned above. One sign of a fractured hip is misalignment—usually external rotation of the hip (Fig. 7-10).

FRACTURE TREATMENT: REDUCTION, IMMOBILIZATION, REHABILITATION

Whatever the cause of the fracture, the goals of treatment are the same:

- Reduction
- Immobilization
- Rehabilitation

Reduction means setting the bone in a proper position so that it heals correctly. The reduction may be closed (by movement or traction) or open (surgical procedure). Reduction is done by a physician.

Once the fracture is reduced, it must be **immobilized** (unable to move) to allow healing to take place. Immobilization is also done by the physician in several basic ways (Fig. 7-11):

- External (casts, splints, traction)
- Internal (pin and plaster; nails, plates, screws)

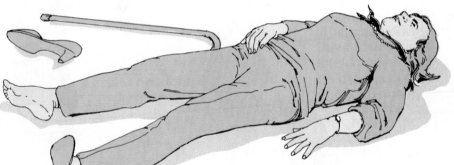

FIGURE 7-10
External rotation of the hip.

FIGURE 7-11
Ways to immobilize.

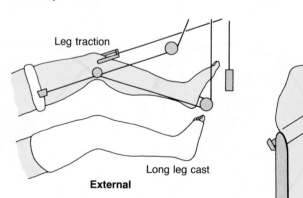

Leg traction

Long leg cast

External

Internal

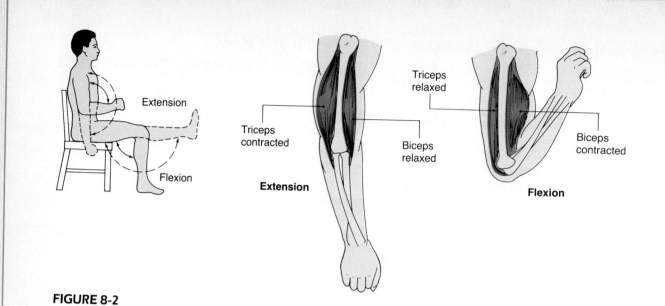

FIGURE 8-2
Coordination of muscles.

FIGURE
Hip frac

Muscles seldom move independently. Most movement is a result of the coordinated action of several muscles (Fig. 8-2). Flex your arm by bringing it toward you. The large muscle, the biceps, on the anterior portion of your upper arm contracts (tightens) while the large muscle on the posterior portion of your upper arm, the triceps, relaxes. When you extend or straighten your arm, the opposite occurs—the triceps contracts and the biceps relaxes.

There is a complex system of chemical reactions that allows muscles to contract and relax, producing movement. The end result of this process is the production of energy (heat). The muscles not only move the body, but they also produce heat. This heat production is increased during physical activity or exercise.

Muscles have an abundant blood supply that delivers oxygen and nutrients to the muscle cells. This rich blood supply makes the muscle tissue more resistant to infection than all other body tissues. The muscles provide support to the bones of the skeleton and give posture to the body.

MUSCULAR SYSTEM ABNORMALITIES

Paralysis means loss of voluntary movement. Paralysis of a body part can occur as a result of injury or illness. Damage to the brain or spinal cord makes it impossible to transmit the necessary signals that tell the muscles to act or react, so voluntary movement is lost.

Muscular dystrophy is a group of related muscle diseases that are progressively crippling due to weakness and atrophy of muscles. It affects the muscles themselves. This disease is different from multiple sclerosis, where the muscles become useless due to damage to the nerves that control them. Muscular dystrophy affects almost a quarter of a million Americans. These people frequently require ongoing nursing care in LTC facilities. At this time, all the causes of muscular dystrophy are not known, and there is no specific cure.

EFFECTS OF AGING AND DISUSE ON THE MUSCULAR SYSTEM

Older persons usually lose some muscle strength and muscle bulk. When people remain physically active, these changes do not occur, or they occur more slowly. Since the body is designed to function most efficiently when movement is present, immobility (the limitation of movement) through disuse results in many changes. Most of these changes are serious and tend to be permanent.

Atrophy—Muscle mass decreases in size (also called wasting of muscle). When muscles are not used for any reason (paralysis, limb in a cast or brace, pain, lack of motivation to move, etc.), atrophy occurs.

Contracture—A permanent shortening of the muscle. When a muscle is not used, it becomes "fixed" or very resistant to stretching. Contractures occur most often in well-developed muscles, usually the muscles that allow flexion or bending of the joints. They commonly occur in the hands, fingers, elbows, hips, and knees. Contractures can lead to permanent disability or loss of function. If untreated, the joints themselves become **ankylosed** or "frozen."

Contractures are painful and unsightly. Even though a resident may never ambulate or perform activities of daily living independently, you should not allow contractures to develop. The resident has a right to be free of the deformity and pain that results from inadequate care. Contractures contribute to skin breakdown because of a change in the distribution of body weight. Residents with contractures are more difficult to move, position, bathe, and dress.

Contractures occur as a result of improper support and positioning of joints affected by arthritis, injury, inadequate movement, and exercise. **Edema** (swelling) of tissue or a joint for any reason contributes to the development of contractures. The fluid that produces edema becomes like glue and limits movement of the swollen joint. Residents who are dependent on others are especially prone to developing contractures. Special range of motion exercises must be given to residents as a preventive measure. Learning how to perform these exercises is an important part of your training.

SECTION 2 NURSING CARE RELATED TO THE MUSCULAR SYSTEM

OBJECTIVES/WHAT YOU WILL LEARN

When you have completed this section, you will be able to:
- Correctly perform range of motion for a dependent resident
- List four observations to be made, reported, and recorded while performing range of motion
- List the "steps" depicting readiness for ambulation
- Ambulate a resident using the step-by-step procedure
- List the safety precautions for ambulation devices
- List four reasons why dependent residents must be repositioned frequently
- Properly position a dependent resident in a wheelchair
- Correctly position a dependent resident in the:
  a. Supine position
  b. Semisupine position
  c. Prone position
  d. Semiprone position

RANGE-OF-MOTION EXERCISES

Nursing care of dependent residents is aimed at the prevention or reduction of the effects of disuse on the body through:

- Range-of-motion exercises

- Assisting with **ambulation** (walking)
- Positioning residents properly

Range of motion means that each joint is put through its normal range of activity. The exercises may be either **passive** (done for the resident by the nursing assistant) or **active** (done by the resident independently).

Regardless of whether the exercises are active or passive, there are several guidelines to be followed:

- Exercise in an organized systematic way
- Never exercise a swollen, reddened joint
- Be gentle—never exercise beyond the point of pain
- Support the limb at the joint as it is exercised
- Put each joint through each movement three times

TYPES OF MOVEMENT

The following terms are used to describe the many types of motion that are included in range-of-motion exercises.

- **Adduction**—to move an arm or leg toward the center of the body
- **Abduction**—to move an arm or leg away from the center of the body
- **Extension**—to straighten an arm or leg
- **Hyperextension**—beyond the normal extension
- **Flexion**—to bend a joint (elbow, wrist, knee)
- **Plantar flexion**—to extend the ankle (toward the sole of the foot)
- **Dorsiflexion**—to flex the ankle (away for the sole of the foot)
- **Rotation**—to move a joint in a circular motion around its axis
  —internal rotation—to turn in toward center
  —external rotation—to turn out away from center
- **Pronation**—to turn palms down
- **Supination**—to turn palms up
- **Radial deviation**—toward the thumb side of the hand
- **Ulnar deviation**—away from the thumb side of the hand

As you read through the procedure, put your own joints through their range of motion by closely following the illustrations.

PROCEDURE

PERFORMING
RANGE-OF-MOTION
EXERCISES

1. Wash your hands.
2. Identify the resident.
3. Explain to the resident what you are going to do.
4. Pull the curtain around the bed for privacy.
5. Place the resident in a supine position with knees extended and arms at the side.
6. Lower the side rail on the near side of the bed.
7. Exercise the neck.

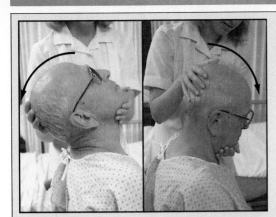

Head Flexion and Extension: With body straight, gently move head down, up, and backward, then straighten neck again.

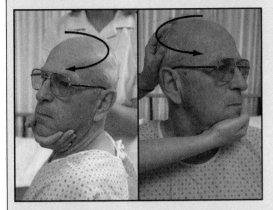

Right/Left Rotation: With head and body straight, gently rotate head to the right. Come back to the starting position, then rotate head to the left.

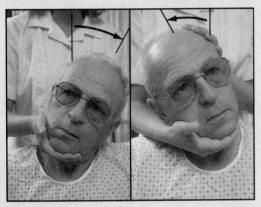

Right/Left Lateral Flexion: With body and head straight, move head gently toward the right shoulder. Come back to the starting position, then move head toward the left shoulder. Use the weight of the head to help move it.

8. Hold the extremity to be exercised at the joint (i.e., knee, wrist, elbow).
9. Exercise each shoulder.

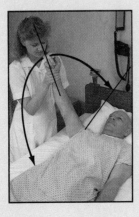

Shoulder Flexion: With elbow straight, raise arm over head, then lower, *keeping arm in front of you.*

PERFORMING RANGE-OF-MOTION EXERCISES (CONTINUED)

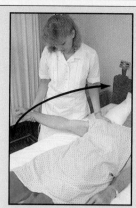

Shoulder Abduction and Adduction: With elbow straight, raise arm over head, then lower, *keeping arm out to the side.*

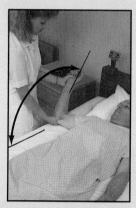

Shoulder Internal and External Rotation: Bring arm out to the side. Do *not* bring elbow out to shoulder level. Turn arm back and forth so forearm points down toward feet, then up toward head. With arm alongside body and elbow bent at 90°, turn arm so forearm points across stomach, then out to the side.

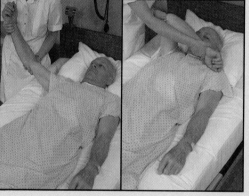

Shoulder Horizontal Abduction and Adduction: *Keeping arm at shoulder level*, reach across chest past opposite shoulder, then reach out to the side.

10. Exercise each elbow, wrist, and forearm.

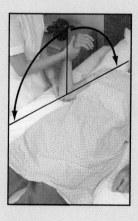

Elbow Flexion and Extension: With arm alongside body, bend elbow to touch shoulder, then straighten elbow out again.

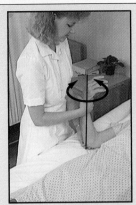

Forearm Pronation and Supination: With arm alongside the body and elbow bent to 90°, turn forearm so palm faces first toward head, then toward feet.

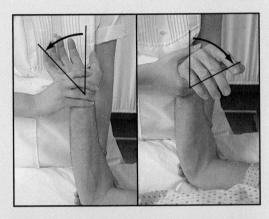

Wrist Flexion and Extension: Bend wrist up and down.

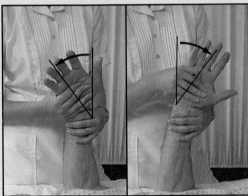

Ulnar and Radial Deviation: Bend wrist from side to side.

11. Exercise each finger.

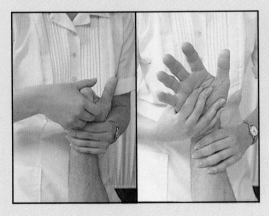

Finger Flexion and Extension: Make a fist, then straighten fingers out together.

PERFORMING
RANGE-OF-MOTION
EXERCISES
(CONTINUED)

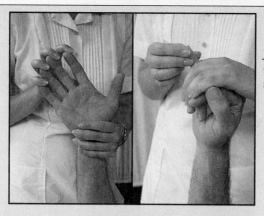

Individual Finger Flexion and Extension: Move each joint individually. Touch tip of each finger to its base, then straighten each finger in turn.

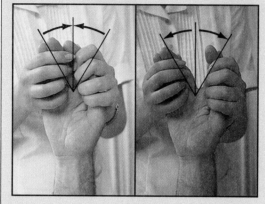

Finger Adduction and Abduction: With fingers straight, squeeze fingers together, then spread them apart.

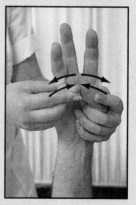

Finger/Thumb Opposition: Touch thumb to the tip of each finger to make a circle. Open hand fully between touching each finger.

12. Exercise the hip.

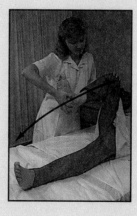

Hip/Knee Flexion and Extension: Bend knee and bring it up toward chest, keeping foot off bed. Lower leg to bed, straightening knee as it goes down.

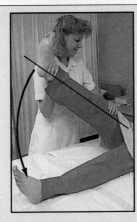

Straight Leg Raising: Keeping the knee straight, raise leg up off the bed. Return slowly to the bed, keeping the knee straight.

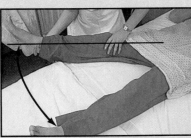

Hip Abduction and Adduction: With leg flat on bed and knee kept pointing to ceiling, slide leg out to the side. Then slide it back to touch across the other leg.

Hip Internal and External Rotation: With legs flat on bed and feet apart, turn both legs so knees face outward. Then turn them in so knees face each other.

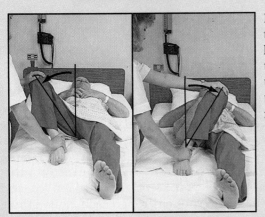

Hip Internal and External Rotation (Variation): With one knee bent and foot flat on bed, turn leg so knee moves out to the side, then inward across the other leg. Do each leg separately.

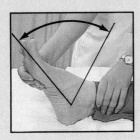

Ankle Dorsiflexion and Plantar Flexion: Bend ankles up, down, and from side to side.

13. Exercise the toes.

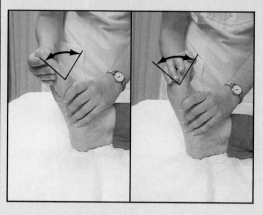

Toe Flexion and Extension:
Bend and straighten each toe.

14. Make the resident comfortable.
15. Be sure the signal cord is within easy reach.
16. Raise the side rails.
17. Wash your hands.
18. Record in the chart that you have completed range-of-motion exercises with the resident, and how the exercises were tolerated. Also record and report your observations of anything unusual.

The time spent in performing range of motion exercises gives the nursing assistant the chance to observe for special problems and communicate with the resident. You should note and report:

- Swollen joints
- Reddened skin over a joint
- Complaints of pain on movement
- Painful joints
- Weakness

ENCOURAGING ACTIVE RANGE OF MOTION

Those residents who are able should be encouraged and instructed in active range of motion. Active exercise has the additional benefit of increasing muscle strength as well as maintaining range of joint movement.

Many residents will enjoy the increased responsibility and independence that comes from performing their own exercises. Some see it as an activity that occupies time and interest during the day. Some residents may get "carried away" and exercise too much. Tell the resident to go through each motion three times and to exercise each extremity two or three times a day.

Even when residents do their own range-of-motion exercises, the nursing assistant needs to verify that the exercises are being done and to record that fact in the chart. Ask the residents to show you how they exercise and remind them during the day to exercise. Compliment their efforts: "You're doing a great job, Mr. Green. I can see the improvement in just one week."

As strength and movement in the joints increase, self-care activities will begin to substitute for the exercises in providing range of joint motion. Encourage self-care such as brushing hair and assisting with bathing and dressing.

Residents confined to wheelchairs may quickly develop hip and knee contractures. In addition to range-of-motion exercises, they need to stand frequently during the day and be positioned with hips and legs extended when in bed.

AMBULATION

Another skill that the nursing assistant will use to promote proper body functioning, exercise, and activity is assisting residents to ambulate. *Ambulation* means walking or moving about in an upright position.

Frequently, residents who need help with ambulation are weak or unsteady on their feet, or they experience dizziness. These residents are more likely to slip or fall. In order to protect yourself and the resident from injury, you will need to understand and use good body mechanics. Review the principles of body mechanics in Chapter 2. Ambulation has positive effects on body systems:

- Circulation is stimulated
- Muscles are strengthened
- Pressure on certain body parts is relieved
- Joints are extended and moved
- Weight is borne on the large bones
- The urinary and digestive systems work more efficiently
- Independence is increased, leading to a more positive self-image

Most residents want to be able to ambulate. The physican, along with input from the physical therapist and nurse, will determine the resident's readiness to ambulate and prescribe how and under what conditions the resident will ambulate. To be ready to ambulate, the resident needs strength and balance (Fig. 8-3). There is a natural progression of abilities needed.

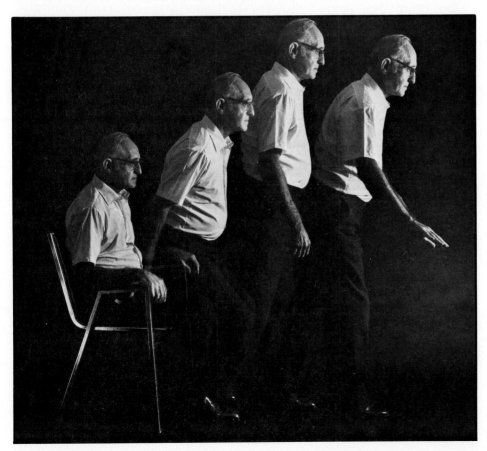

FIGURE 8-3
Ambulation requires both strength and balance.

The first time a resident ambulates after a period of illness is very important in building confidence and increasing motivation. The first ambulation is often performed or supervised by a physical therapist, a specially trained rehabilitation aide, or a restorative nursing assistant. Safety is essential! It is wise to use two people to reassure the resident that there is no danger.

PROCEDURE

ASSISTING THE
RESIDENT TO
AMBULATE

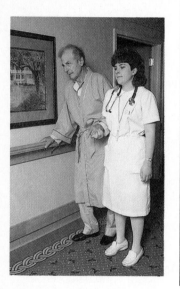

1. Identify the resident.
2. Explain what you are going to do, as well as what is expected of the resident.
3. Assist the resident to a sitting position and allow the resident time to gain balance.
4. Assist in dressing and putting on appropriate shoes (firm support with rubber heels are best).
5. Assist to stand. You may either stand directly in front or to one side.
6. Again, give the resident time to gain balance.
7. Stand on the *unaffected* (stronger) side to begin ambulation.
8. Remind the resident to stand up straight, with the chin parallel to the floor.
9. As you walk, observe the resident for signs of fatigue, such as difficult breathing, sweating, dizziness, and rapid heart rate. Allow the resident to rest if these signs occur.
10. Be on the alert for hazards such as untied shoes, objects on the floor, and wet spots.
11. Return the resident to bed or a chair.
12. Record in the chart the distance ambulated and the response of the resident. You may estimate distance by number of feet or number of steps. You may also describe from one place to another, such as "ambulated from the bed to the bathroom door" or indicate the time spent, "ambulated in hallway for 10 minutes."

Sometimes a resident can fall due to leg collapse or loss of balance. When this happens, gently ease the resident to the floor (Fig. 8-4), being careful to protect yourself by using good body mechanics (bending your legs instead of your back).

FIGURE 8-4
Easing the resident to the floor.

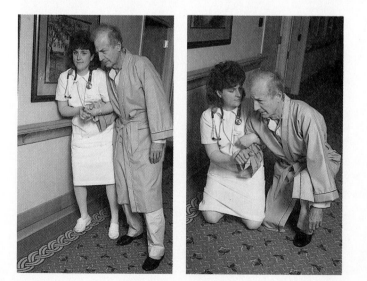

Stay with the resident and call for help. Before moving, the resident should be examined for injury by a licensed nurse. You will need additional help to lift a resident from the floor to the chair or bed.

AMBULATION DEVICES

Sometimes a **gait belt** is used for ambulation. This belt (made of leather or nylon webbing) is placed around the resident's waist (Fig. 8-5). The nursing assistant stands behind the resident with one hand holding onto the belt. The belt allows residents better control over their center of gravity.

As residents progress in their ability to ambulate, they may graduate from needing the assistance of another person to use of an ambulation device. Ambulation devices include braces, canes, crutches, and walkers. Although a wheelchair is not a true ambulation device, it is included here since it provides mobility for about 35 percent of LTC facility residents. Also, some residents use a wheelchair somewhat like a walker. They stand behind it, pushing the wheelchair for balance and support.

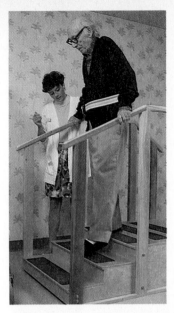

FIGURE 8-5
Using the gait belt.

TABLE 8-1: AMBULATION DEVICES

Devices	Purpose	Users	Safeguards
Back brace Short leg brace	To promote or limit movement of a body part	Residents with a weak or unstable back, knee, ankle, etc.	Observe the skin under brace for irritation or injury. Report needed repairs such as missing or loose screws. Note if device fits properly.
Conventional cane "Quad cane"	To provide balance and confidence or to decrease weight borne by one foot or leg	Residents who have strength but lack balance or confidence in their activity; used on the opposite side of affected part	Rubber tip(s) must be checked for wear. Report changes in resident which would indicate that cane is no longer appropriate. Inspect rubber tip(s) for wear. Should not be used if resident is weak, unsteady, or unable to maintain balance.
Conventional crutches Canadian crutches	To decrease weight borne by one or both feet and legs; to provide stability	Lower-extremity amputees; resident who is normally ambulatory but has suffered a sprain or fracture; someone with lower extremity paralysis or weakness	
Wheeled walker	To provide stability and support	Residents with poor backward/forward balance (Parkinson's disease); resident with general weakness (arthritis)	Be sure wheels turn properly. Check brakes.

TABLE 8-1 (continued)

Devices	Purpose	Users	Safeguards
Pick-up walker 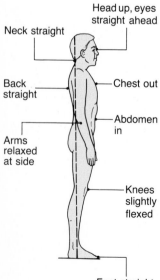	To provide stability	Resident with weakness or balance problems; frequently, those recovering from a hip fracture	Inspect rubber tip(s) for wear. Report increased weakness.
Standard wheelchair Battery-powered wheelchair	To provide mobility for nonambulatory resident	Residents unable to stand due to weakness, paralysis, amputations, contractures, serious illness; residents unable to propel their own chair; generally used with younger, disabled people	Inspect brakes for proper function. Report needed repairs on torn upholstery.

POSITIONING DEPENDENT RESIDENTS

Positioning dependent residents properly is a very important nursing function. Improper positioning leads to serious complications, such as:

- Skin breakdown from prolonged pressure
- Development of contractures due to improper support
- Decreased circulation from lack of movement
- Pneumonia—secretions collect in the lungs when position is not changed
- Discomfort and pain
- Edema in limbs that are in dependent positions

The dependent or inactive resident must be repositioned at least every 2 hours. Many residents need position changes even more frequently. The healthy person changes positions as often as 30 to 50 times during an 8-hour period of sleep. This movement prevents prolonged pressure in any one area. Prolonged pressure causes decreased circulation and eventual skin breakdown. The dependent resident must trust those who provide care to assume this responsibility. The dependent resident must have position changes made on a 24-hour basis while in bed or when up in a wheelchair.

Maintaining proper body alignment is a fundamental principle of all positioning. **Alignment** means to put in a straight line (Fig. 8-6). We look better, feel better, and our bodies function more efficiently when in good alignment.

Head up, eyes straight ahead
Neck straight
Back straight
Chest out
Abdomen in
Arms relaxed at side
Knees slightly flexed
Feet straight, toes forward

Residents need positioning in wheelchairs for the same reasons they need repositioning when in bed—to reduce pressure, to promote increased circulation, and to increase comfort. Most facilities place cushions in wheelchairs to help reduce pressure on the buttocks.

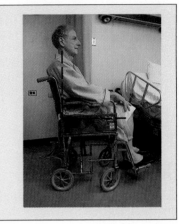

Once the resident is placed in the wheelchair, check alignment:

• Position the resident's hips well back in the chair.
• Make sure that the feet are resting on the foot rests or on the floor.
• The trunk of the body should be balanced.
• Be sure that male patients are not sitting on the genitalia.
• If necessary, place pillows at the resident's side to prevent sliding over to one side of the chair.
• Place arms on armrests or on a pillow placed across the lap.

Caution: Most dependent residents cannot tolerate sitting in a wheelchair for prolonged periods. These residents should be repositioned every 1 to 2 hours while in the wheelchair, and they should never be up in a wheelchair for more than 3 hours without being returned to bed for a rest period.

If the resident slips down in the wheelchair, reposition as follows:

• Lock the wheels of the wheelchair.
• Cross the resident's arms over the waist.
• Stand behind the resident, grasp wrists, and simply stand up straight. This moves the resident up in the wheelchair easily.

Whenever you reposition a resident, make sure that you consider nasogastric tubes, catheters, urinary drainage tubing, special dressings, and braces. Always turn and position the resident carefully to avoid dislodging or pulling on tubes, and always make sure that tubing is not obstructed or kinked.

There are special devices used to assist with positioning residents properly. Some of these are presented in Table 8-2.

TABLE 8-2: POSITIONING DEVICES

Device	Purpose	Users	Precautions
Pillows Sandbags	To assist in positioning, provide support and alignment; used to elevate, pad, protect	All residents who require assistance with positioning	Pillows or sandbags should be placed to support joints and to provide comfort. Improper placement can cause redistribution of pressure, discomfort, and pain.

TABLE 8-2 (continued)

Device	Purpose	Users	Precautions
Trochanter roll (placed next to the greater trochanter—the tip of the thigh bone)	To prevent external rotation of the hip, which results in permanent disability and interferes with ambulation	Residents in the supine position—especially the dependent resident	The rolls should be placed properly to prevent external rotation. They must be removed and the area massaged to avoid prolonged pressure. *Note:* A trochanter roll may be made by rolling up a towel or small blanket and placing it against the hip as shown.
Abduction splint (device designed to keep the thighs apart)	To keep thighs apart to maintain proper alignment of the hip joints, and to prevent skin-to-skin contact	Residents who have had hip surgery or who have skin breakdown on knees or thighs	It is very important to keep this splint properly placed after hip surgery until healing has occurred. The areas of splint contact must be massaged and observed to reduce chance of skin breakdown.
Palmer splint (device designed to keep the hand in a functional position)	To prevent contractures of the hand, fingers, and wrists	Used for residents with paralysis of the hand or wrist	The splint must be properly applied and checked frequently to avoid pressure from straps or frame of splint. The splint must be removed to allow for exercises, cleansing, and massage each shift.
Hand roll (round device made up of different materials, placed in the palm of the hand)	To prevent contracture and to maintain hands in a functional position; to prevent fingers and nails from pressing into palm of hand, creating pressure and skin breakdown	Residents who have contractures of the hand or may develop contractures	Hand rolls must be removed several times daily and the hand area cleaned. Air circulation in the hand area is reduced and moisture collects, which contributes to bacterial growth and skin breakdown.
Foot board (padded board placed or affixed to the foot of the bed)	To prevent foot drop, a type of contracture of the foot that impairs ambulation	Residents in the supine position who are non-ambulatory and who are dependent	The bottom of the foot must be placed securely against the board so that pressure is exerted against the bottom of the foot (similar to the pressure the resident would feel if standing). Make sure that pressure is off the heels, to avoid skin breakdown.

POSITIONING THE RESIDENT IN BED

Four basic positions are used for most residents:

- Supine
- Semisupine
- Semiprone
- Prone

Note: Some textbooks refer to right side-lying and left-side-lying positions. Research has shown that these direct side-lying positions should be avoided in the elderly or chronically ill because of the increased pressure on the bottom leg and hip. The right and left semisupine and semiprone are used in place of any direct side-lying position.

The Supine (Face Up) Position (Fig. 8-7)

The placement of the pillow is important. It should come to the tip of the shoulder, not under the shoulders. Too many pillows or pillows placed under the shoulders over a prolonged period causes too much flexion of the neck. This results in contracture of the neck and increased pain.

The arms should be placed at the side of the body allowing enough space for air to circulate around the axilla (armpits). They may be up or down. When arms are placed across the chest or against the body, air circulation is reduced and moisture collects, which contributes to bacterial growth and skin irritation. A general rule to follow is to avoid skin-on-skin contact when you are positioning a resident.

When a resident is in the supine position, there is a natural tendency for the legs to roll outward (called *external rotation*). If this external rotation is allowed to persist over a prolonged period, the hip joint becomes "fixed" and ambulation is very difficult. A rolled towel or blanket (**trochanter roll**) should be placed at the hip joint to prevent external rotation.

A resident who is unable to move the hands and fingers due to paralysis should have a hand roll placed in his or her hand to prevent contractures.

The feet need to be properly placed against a padded footboard to prevent foot drop, a type of contracture that occurs quickly in residents who do not stand.

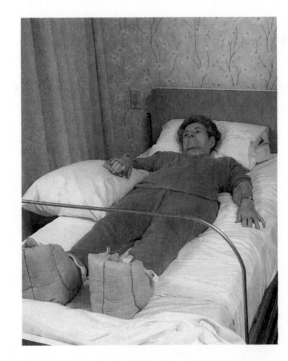

FIGURE 8-7
The supine (face-up) position.

In bed, the feet tend to point downward. The weight of the bed coverings contributes to this problem. This can be avoided by the use of a foot cradle.

Just as you move the arms slightly away from the body, you should position the legs so they are slightly apart to reduce irritation in the perineal area.

The heels need to be protected from pressure. A small roll, made with a towel, a piece of foam, or sheepskin, can be used to elevate the heels and keep them from touching the bed.

Caution: Never place a pillow or blankets under the heels. These are too large, causing redistribution of body weight and increased pressure on the sacrum or coccyx area and contributing to skin breakdown there.

The Semisupine (Tilt) Position (Fig. 8-8)

In the semisupine or tilt position, the resident is positioned so that body weight is supported by a pillow placed behind the back and another pillow folded in half under the top leg. Both legs are extended (not flexed). The top leg is placed a little behind the bottom leg and supported on the folded pillow so it is level with the hip joint. Make sure the lower shoulder is brought forward so that pressure is distributed over the back of the shoulder. Place the lower arm away from the body and support the upper arm on a pillow as necessary.

This position replaces the direct side-lying position and can be used on either right or left side. Note how this position prevents pressure on the sacrum and coccyx, yet does not place direct pressure on the hip, where skin breakdown frequently occurs.

Some residents who have experienced a recent stroke may need to have the paralyzed side flexed due to spasticity. Follow the directions of your physical therapist to determine whether this is necessary.

The Semiprone Position (Fig. 8-9)

The semiprone position is a reversal of the semisupine. The resident is tilted forward with one pillow supporting the chest and shoulder. Both legs are extended. The lower arm is usually placed behind the resident and the upper arm on a pillow in front of the resident. Semisupine and semiprone are positions that most residents find comfortable. They are excellent positions to reduce pressure and prevent contractures.

FIGURE 8-8
The semisupine (tilt) position.

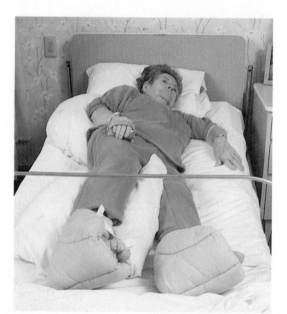

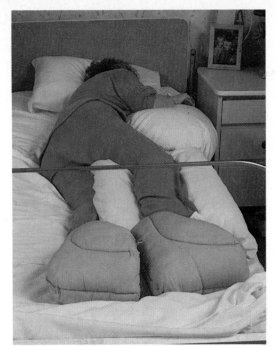

FIGURE 8-9
The semiprone position.

The Prone Position (Fig. 8-10)

The prone position is an important position that is not used often enough. There are some residents who cannot or will not tolerate this position so check with your charge nurse if you are unsure.

- The resident's head is turned to one side and placed against the mattress. No pillow is used.
- Position the resident so that the spine is in good alignment.
- Place a small or flat pillow under the lower abdomen to reduce strain on the back. However, some residents are more comfortable without the pillow.

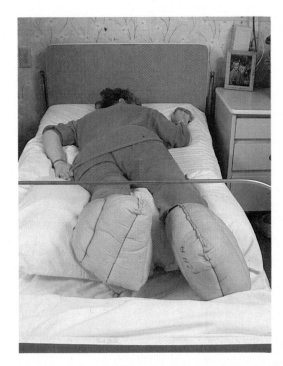

FIGURE 8-10
The prone position.

- If the shoulders roll forward, use a small rolled-up towel to support the shoulders.
- The arms may be positioned at the sides with the palms up, or one arm may be flexed and placed next to the head with palm down and the other down at the side with palm up.

  Caution: It is generally not advisable to place both arms up next to the head, as this produces strain across the shoulders and causes pain.
- The best way to position the feet is to allow the toes to fall between the end of the mattress and the end of the bed. If this is not possible, place a small rolled towel under the ankles to reduce pressure on the toes.

To some residents, the prone position is a little frightening because they feel so dependent. Some even fear suffocation in the face-down position. Explaining the procedure to the resident, having a call light in reach, and leaving the resident in the prone position only for short periods of time at first may make this position more acceptable.

Notice how this position prevents pressure on the major pressure points of the body. For this reason, it is very helpful in reducing pressure on the coccyx, sacrum, heels, hips, and shoulder blades.

Certain residents may require modifications of positioning techniques. These are residents who have **spasticity** (tightening of the muscle with short jerking movements), contractures, or pressure sores. With spasticity, it is more difficult to keep a limb extended, and you will need to reposition more often. With contractures, the joints must always be supported.

When pressure sores exist, care must be taken to avoid pressure on the involved area. This can be done through a technique called **bridging.** Bridging is accomplished by supporting the areas above and below the pressure sore with foam or pillows (Fig. 8-11). The involved area is thus free of pressure as it rests between the supports.

Positioning residents properly is a very important nursing responsibility. Good positioning reduces pain and helps to prevent both skin breakdown and joint deformities.

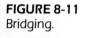

FIGURE 8-11
Bridging.

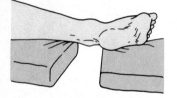

CHAPTER 9

The Digestive System

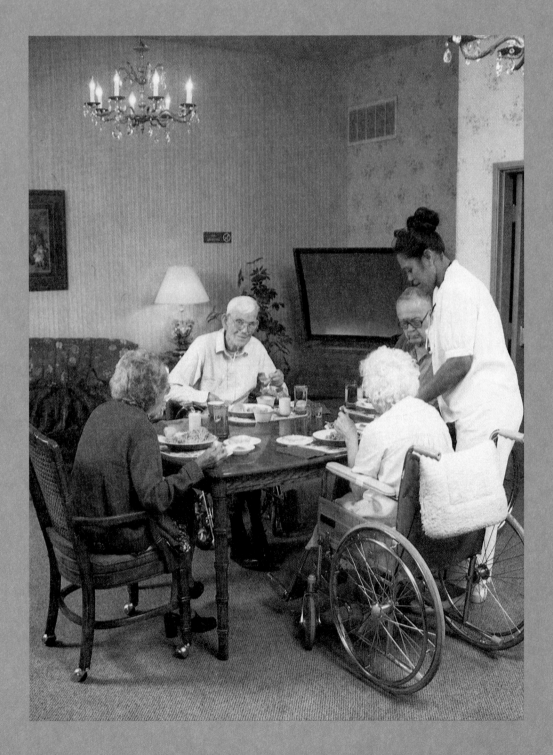

OBJECTIVES/WHAT YOU WILL LEARN

When you have completed this section, you will be able to:

■ List three basic functions of the digestive system
■ Label the components of the digestive system
■ Match the organs in the digestive system with their functions

THE DIGESTIVE SYSTEM

The digestive system (Fig. 9-1) is composed of:

- Teeth
- Tongue
- Salivary glands
- Esophagus
- Stomach
- Pancreas

- Appendix
- Liver
- Gallbladder
- Small intestine (including duodenum)
- Large intestine (including colon)
- Anus

Functions of the digestive system are to:

- Ingest food
- Prepare food for use by the body
- Excrete body wastes

The digestive system is responsible for the process of breaking down food that is eaten and changing it so that it can be used by the cells of the body. This process is both chemical and mechanical. The **alimentary tract** (route taken by food as it passes from the mouth to the anus) is about 30 feet long. Each part of the alimentary tract has special functions.

Digestion begins in the mouth, where food is chewed and mixed with saliva secreted by the salivary glands. When we swallow, moisturized food travels down the esophagus to the stomach. The stomach churns and mixes the food while it is being changed chemically by special digestive secretions **(enzymes).**

Water is essential to the chemical process of changing food into its final form. Most of the digested food particles are absorbed (taken into the bloodstream for use by the body) in the area of the **duodenum** the first loop of the small intestine and the most important area of digestion. Here partially digested food from the stomach mixes with digestive secretions from the duodenum, the pancreas, and the liver to complete the process of digestion. One of the liver's many functions is to manufacture a substance called **bile,** which is stored in the gallbladder and released into the duodenum to be mixed with other digestive enzymes. Bile is important in breaking down fats eaten so that the digestive enzymes of the pancreas and liver can further complete the digestive process.

THE DIGESTIVE PROCESS

The duodenum is composed of thousands of fingerlike projections called **villi.** Each of these projections (villus) absorbs digested food particles and

The digestive system includes the digestive tract and various supportive structures and accessory glands. The tract begins at the oral cavity with the teeth and tongue. The salivary glands release saliva into the mouth to moisten food for swallowing. The tract continues down the throat to the esophagus, through the cardiac sphincter, and into the stomach. Acid and digestive enzymes are added to the food to produce chyme. The chyme passes through the pyloric sphincter to enter the small intestine. Digestive enzymes from the pancreas and bile from the liver are added to the chyme. The process of digestion and absorption are completed in the small intestine. Wastes are carried through the ileoceccal valve into the large intestine. The wastes are moved to the rectum, from where they can be expelled through the anus.

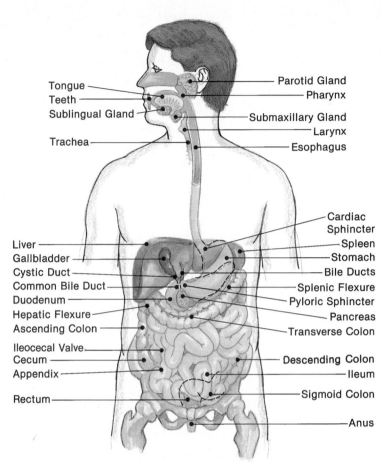

Organs of the Digestive System

Tongue
Teeth
Sublingual Gland
Trachea
Parotid Gland
Pharynx
Submaxillary Gland
Larynx
Esophagus

Cardiac Sphincter
Liver
Gallbladder
Cystic Duct
Common Bile Duct
Duodenum
Hepatic Flexure
Ascending Colon
Ileocecal Valve
Cecum
Appendix
Rectum
Spleen
Stomach
Bile Ducts
Splenic Flexure
Pyloric Sphincter
Pancreas
Transverse Colon
Descending Colon
Ileum
Sigmoid Colon
Anus

Liver, Stomach, and Pancreas

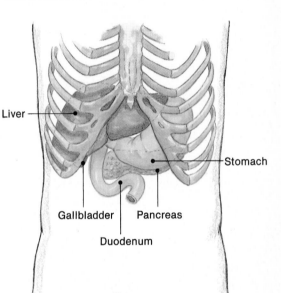

Liver
Stomach
Gallbladder
Pancreas
Duodenum

Large Intestine

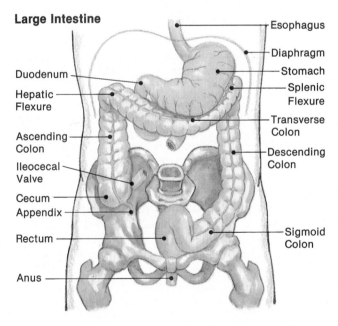

Duodenum
Hepatic Flexure
Ascending Colon
Ileocecal Valve
Cecum
Appendix
Rectum
Anus
Esophagus
Diaphragm
Stomach
Splenic Flexure
Transverse Colon
Descending Colon
Sigmoid Colon

Small Intestine

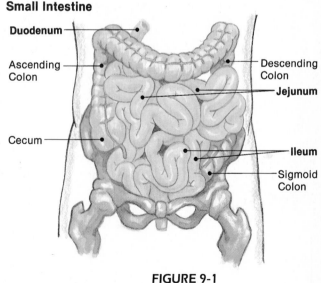

Duodenum
Ascending Colon
Cecum
Descending Colon
Jejunum
Ileum
Sigmoid Colon

FIGURE 9-1
The digestive system.

releases them into the bloodstream. Some digestion continues to occur in other parts of the small intestine.

The remainder of the digested food is moved by rhythmic contractions (**peristalsis**) through the large intestine.

The **appendix** is a small projection of tissue located where the small and large intestine meet. The appendix has no digestive function but frequently becomes infected, causing fever and pain. An appendectomy is the surgical removal of the appendix.

The lower portion of the large intestine curves in an S shape. This area is called the **sigmoid colon.** The sigmoid colon leads directly into the rectum. In the large intestine, water is reabsorbed by the body. Excess water is removed from the remaining digested material. Semisolid waste **(feces)** is created. Feces are excreted from the body through the rectum. The **rectum** is composed of delicate tissues surrounded by **sphincter muscles** (muscles that squeeze down). This allows the contents of the rectum (feces) to remain in the rectum until voluntary elimination (bowel movement) occurs.

Another organ important in the digestive process is the **liver.** The liver is a very complex organ and has many functions. The most important functions of the liver are:

- Storage area for simple sugar (glucose). This form of sugar is stored and released in large amounts when the cells need it.
- Storage of vitamins and proteins essential for proper circulation of the blood.
- Removal of poisons or toxins from the blood through a filtering function.
- Carrying out metabolic functions essential for the blood-clotting process.

ABNORMALITIES OF THE DIGESTIVE SYSTEM

Abnormalities of the digestive system include the following:

- **Ulcer** is a cavity that develops, creating an open wound. There are many factors related to the development of stomach ulcers, but prolonged stress and pain are the most common. Ulcers are very painful and require special medications, special diets, and sometimes surgical removal.
- **Gastritis** is inflammation of the stomach caused by bacteria, viruses, vitamin deficiency, excessive eating, or overindulgence in alcoholic beverages. Gastritis is often associated with nausea and vomiting.
- **Gallstones** are cholesterol crystals that settle out of the bile stored in the gallbladder. Stones form and often block the secretion of bile. This condition causes pain, nausea, and vomiting, especially following meals. Surgical removal of the gallstones or the gallbladder may be necessary.
- **Hemorrhoids** are enlarged blood-filled vessels that surround the area of the rectum. These enlarged blood vessels are painful, especially during a bowel movement. They may bleed, causing the stool to become blood tinged.
- **Cirrhosis** is an inflammation of the tissue of an organ, particularly the liver. The normal liver tissue is replaced by fibrous (tough) tissue, and liver function is decreased or lost. Cirrhosis is commonly associated with excessive drug or alcohol abuse. Poor nutrition over a long period of time also leads to cirrhosis.

SECTION 2 BASIC NUTRITION

OBJECTIVES/WHAT YOU WILL LEARN

When you have completed this section, you will be able to:

- Describe what a well-balanced diet should contain
- Describe the basic bodily functions of:
  — Carbohydrates
  — Proteins
  — Fats
- Explain why water is considered an essential nutrient
- List the four basic food groups and give three examples of foods found in each group.
- Correctly calculate percentages of food eaten

PRINCIPLES OF NUTRITION

Nutrition is the science of foods and their actions or relationship to health. The body depends on food for:

- Growth and repair of tissue
- Energy
- Maintenance and regulation of body functions

In this section you will learn what a well-balanced diet consists of as well as how different nutrients (substances) are essential to good health.

NUTRIENTS

The following table of nutrients, their bodily function, and food sources should be studied so that you understand what good nutrition means to you as well as to the LTC resident.

Calories in a normal diet are provided through eating:

Carbohydrates	58 percent
Proteins	12 percent
Fatty acids	30 percent
Calories	100 percent

A WELL-BALANCED DIET

- *Sufficient carbohydrates to meet the individual's energy requirements*

Nutrient Class	**Bodily Function**	**Food Sources**
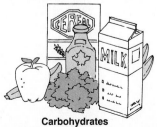 **Carbohydrates**	Provides work energy for body activities, and heat energy for maintenance of body temperature	Cereal grains and their products (bread, breakfast cereals, pasta products), potatoes, sugar, fruits, milk, vegetables, nuts.

There are no essential carbohydrates; however, it is important to have a good balance of the various carbohydrate sources.

- *Sufficient protein to supply the body with the nine essential amino acids.* (**Amino acids** are the units of structure in proteins.)

Nutrient Class

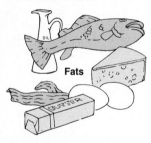

Proteins

Bodily Function

Build and renew body tissues; regulate body functions and supply energy. Complete proteins: maintain life and provide growth. Partially complete proteins will maintain life, but they lack sufficient amounts of some amino acids necessary for growth. Incomplete proteins are incapable of replacing or building new tissues and therefore cannot support life.

Food Sources

Complete proteins: derived from animal foods — meat, milk, eggs, fish, cheese, poultry. Partially complete proteins: derived from vegetable foods — soybeans, dry beans, peas, some nuts and whole-grain products. Incomplete proteins: gelatin from Jello.

- *Sufficient fatty acids to include the essential fatty acids.*

Nutrient Class

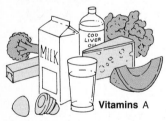

Fats

Bodily Function

Give work energy for body activities and heat energy for maintenance of body temperature. Carriers of vitamins A and D, provide fatty acids necessary for growth and maintenance of body tissues.

Food Sources

Some foods are chiefly fat, such as lard, vegetable fats and oils, and butter. Many other foods contain smaller proportions of fats — nuts, meats, fish, poultry, cream, whole milk.

- *Adequate amounts of vitamins*

Nutrient Class

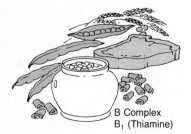

Vitamins A

Bodily Function

Necessary for normal functioning of the eyes, prevents night blindness. Ensures a healthy condition of the skin, hair, and mucous membranes. Maintains a state of resistance to infections of the eyes, mouth, and respiratory tract.

Food Sources

One form of vitamin A is yellow and one form is colorless. Apricots, cantaloupe, milk, cheese, eggs, meat organs (especially liver and kidney), fortified margarine, butter, fishliver oils, dark green and deep yellow vegetables.

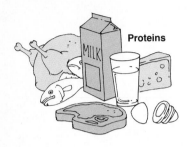

B Complex
B₁ (Thiamine)

Maintains a healthy condition of the nerves. Fosters a good appetite. Helps the body cells use carbohydrates.

Whole-grain and enriched grain products; meats (especially pork, liver, and kidney), dry beans and peas.

Bodily Function	Food Sources	Nutrient Class
Keeps the skin, mouth, and eyes in a healthy condition. Acts with other nutrients to form enzymes and control oxidation in cells.	Milk, cheese, eggs, meat (especially liver and kidney), whole-grain and enriched grain products, dark green vegetables.	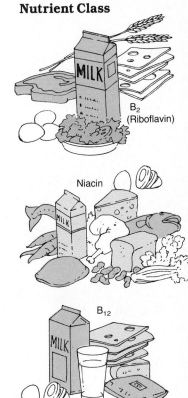 B₂ (Riboflavin)
Influences the oxidation of carbohydrates and proteins in the body cells.	Liver, meat, fish, poultry, eggs, peanuts, dark green vegetables, whole-grain and enriched cereal products.	Niacin
Regulates specific processes in digestion. Helps maintain normal functions of muscles, nerves, heart, blood — general body metabolism.	Liver, other organ meats, cheese, eggs, milk.	B₁₂
Acts as a cement between body cells, and helps them work together to carry out their special functions. Maintains a sound condition of bones, teeth, and gums. Not stored in the body. Protects vitamins A and E. Helps in the absorption of iron.	Fresh, raw citrus fruits and vegetables — oranges, grapefruit, cantaloupe, strawberries, tomatoes, raw onions, cabbage, green and sweet red peppers, dark green vegetables.	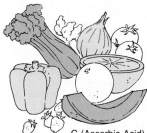 C (Ascorbic Acid)
Enables the growing body to use calcium and phosphorus in a normal way to build teeth and bones.	Provided by vitamin D fortification of certain foods, such as milk and margarine. Also fish-liver oils and eggs. Sunshine allows the body to make its own vitamin D.	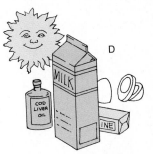 D
The vitamin helps the liver produce substances that are essential to blood clotting.	All green leafy vegetables, egg yolk, soy bean oil, liver, alfalfa, lettuce, spinach, cauliflower.	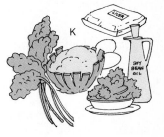 K

• *Essential elements — minerals.* There are many known essential elements. Some of the most common are shown.

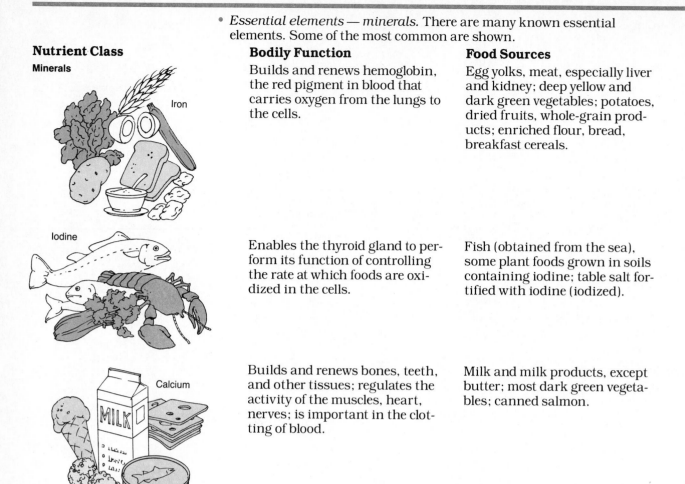

Nutrient Class	Bodily Function	Food Sources
Minerals		
Iron	Builds and renews hemoglobin, the red pigment in blood that carries oxygen from the lungs to the cells.	Egg yolks, meat, especially liver and kidney; deep yellow and dark green vegetables; potatoes, dried fruits, whole-grain products; enriched flour, bread, breakfast cereals.
Iodine	Enables the thyroid gland to perform its function of controlling the rate at which foods are oxidized in the cells.	Fish (obtained from the sea), some plant foods grown in soils containing iodine; table salt fortified with iodine (iodized).
Calcium	Builds and renews bones, teeth, and other tissues; regulates the activity of the muscles, heart, nerves; is important in the clotting of blood.	Milk and milk products, except butter; most dark green vegetables; canned salmon.

THE FOUR BASIC FOOD GROUPS

FIGURE 9-2
The four basic food groups.

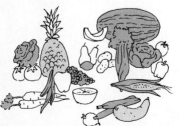

Now that you understand what a well-balanced diet consists of, it is important to understand in what amounts these substances need to be consumed daily to provide adequate nutrition (Fig. 9-2).

Group 1: Dairy Products

Milk

• 3 to 4 cups (children)
• 4 or more cups (teenagers)
• 2 or more cups (adults)

Cheese, ice cream, and other milk-made foods can be substituted for part of the milk requirement

Group 2: Vegetables and Fruit

• 4 or more servings

Include dark green or deep yellow vegetables; citrus fruits or tomatoes

Associated with calcium in some functions needed to build and renew bones and teeth. Influences the oxidation of foods in the body cells; important in nerve tissue.

Widely distributed in foods, especially cheese, oat cereals, whole-wheat products, dry beans and peas, meat, fish, poultry, nuts, and eggs.

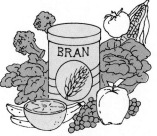

Phosphorus

- *Sufficient dietary fiber — roughage or indigestible material.* Only recently has dietary fiber been considered an essential component of a balanced diet.

Nutrient Class

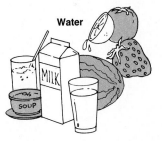

Bodily Function
Associated with prevention of constipation, hemorrhoids, and other digestive diseases, as well as cancer of the colon.

Food Sources
A widely varied diet that contains unprocessed grains, vegetables, nuts, and fruits.

Roughage
Nutrient Class

- *Sufficient fluid intake.* Although water does not furnish calories or vitamins, it is as essential as any nutrient. Water comprises 70% of an individual's body weight. Six to eight glasses (1 1/2 to 2 quarts) per day is essential to good health.

Water

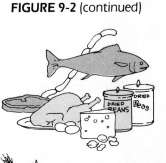

Bodily Function
Regulates body processes. Aids in regulating body temperature. Carries nutrients to body cells and carries waste products away from them. Helps to lubricate joints. Water has no food value, although most water contains mineral elements. More immediately necessary to life than food — second only to oxygen.

Food Sources
Drinking water and other beverages; all foods except those made up of a single nutrient, such as sugar and some fats. Milk, milk drinks, soups, vegetables, fruit juices, ice cream, watermelon, strawberries, lettuce, tomatoes, and cereals.

Group 3: Meat and Fish

FIGURE 9-2 (continued)

- 3 servings

Meats, fish, poultry, eggs, or cheese, with dry beans, peas, nuts as alternates

Group 4: Breads, Cereals, and Potatoes

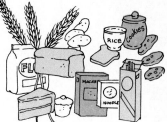

- 4 or more servings

Enriched or whole-grain breads and cereals. Added milk improves nutritional value

NUTRITION AND THE ELDERLY

Nutrition for the elderly is not much different from that needed by everyone. However, there are age-related changes that affect their nutritional status:

- The elderly require fewer calories because they are less active.
- Elderly residents require more vitamins and minerals because they have

more digestive disturbances, which affect how nutrients are absorbed and utilized.

- Elderly people take more drugs than any other age group in America. Many commonly used drugs affect how nutrients are absorbed and utilized.
- Poor oral hygiene or loose, poorly fitted dentures will contribute to poor nutrition.
- The elderly have a diminished sense of taste, which may make foods less appealing and cause residents to eat less.
- Many elderly suffer from chronic diseases that decrease energy or the ability to eat independently. Studies show that approximately 70 to 80 percent of all residents in skilled nursing facilities require some assistance with eating, and approximately 20 to 30 percent need assistive eating devices.

Some residents are affected by physical conditions that impair the resident's ability to chew and swallow. Others experience states of depression, loneliness, and dependency which affect appetite. Nutritional deficiencies can lead to changes in behavior such as:

- Anxiety (fear)
- Apathy (lack of interest)
- Fatigue (being overly tired)
- Loss of appetite
- Loss of memory
- Irritability

Food is very important to all of us. We usually get a great deal of pleasure from eating; eating is a social activity for most people. We also associate food with recreational activities, such as hot dogs with ball games, and turkey with holidays such as Thanksgiving and Christmas. Food is a source of pride and accomplishment for many — being a good cook and meal planner takes practice and skill. Food has religious importance, and special foods are prepared for certain religious occasions.

Most people follow dietary habits they have established early in life based on their cultural, social, and religious background. Some residents will refuse certain foods that are in conflict with their religious beliefs. These religious preferences should always be honored and a substitution made.

In order to help the resident adjust to the changes in dietary habits, the staff must be very sensitive to the resident's likes and dislikes. Research has shown that when residents are able to keep their normal food habits, eating behaviors improve, and nutrition is better.

CALCULATING AND RECORDING FOOD INTAKE

It is very important to assist residents in meeting their nutritional needs. You will need to learn how to evaluate the resident's intake accurately and how to report and record intake. Remember that the food percentages you calculate and record must be accurate. Important decisions related to the resident's medical care and treatment may be based on this documentation.

The most accurate way to chart intake is to observe the resident's tray after eating and chart exactly what was eaten. "For the dinner meal, Mr. Jones ate all the roast beef, half the potato, none of the vegetables, all the roll and margarine, dessert, milk, and coffee." However, most facilities require the nursing assistant to chart only the percentage of calories consumed at each meal, utilizing the guidelines on page 225.

If the resident consumes all the food and fluids served, he or she has eaten 100 percent of that meal. If the resident consumes none of the food or fluids served, he or she has eaten 0 percent of that meal.

In order to accurately chart partial percentages of food or fluids eaten, you must use the guides that have been developed by the dietician for the specific menus used in your facility. The following are samples taken from a typical menu.

SAMPLE CHARTING GUIDES

	Food Item	Percent of Calories
Breakfast	Juice	10
	Cereal	20
	Egg	20
	Toast/marg.	30
	Milk	20
		100
Lunch or dinner	Main dish*	40
	Starch	10
	Vegetable	5
	Bread/margarine	20
	Dessert	10
	Milk	15
		100

This breakdown shows the percentage of calories of each food item served in a meal. Simple arithmetic is used to calculate the total percentage of calories the resident consumes each meal. You must observe how much of each food item is consumed and add the percentages together. If the resident eats only half of a food item, add only half of the percentage of that food item.

*Note: When the main dish consists of a casserole or a combination of foods, add the percentages of each item to get the total percentage for the casserole or combination dish. Example: Chicken noodle casserole would be a total of the chicken and sauce (40 percent) and the noodles or starch (10 percent), which equals 50 percent of the calories from the tray. Coffee has no calories and is therefore not counted in the food percentages. *Remember* that if the resident ate half of the food on the tray, he or she did not necessarily receive half of the calories.

At first you may wish to check out your results with your instructor or charge nurse. Be sure to write down the information as soon as possible so that it is not forgotten.

Study the example below to see how the process works.

Meal	Percent of Calories	Resident Ate	Percentage Consumed
Roast beef	40	All the roast beef	40
Baked potato	10	Half the potato	5
Mixed vegetables	5	No vegetables	0
Roll/margarine	20	All the roll/margarine	20
Cake with icing	10	All the cake	10
Milk	15	Half the milk	7.5
Coffee	0	All the coffee	0
		Total percent consumed	82.5

Report to the charge nurse any time residents refuse a meal or their eating habits change. You must never ignore poor intake!

SECTION 3 THERAPEUTIC DIETS

OBJECTIVES/WHAT YOU WILL LEARN

When you have completed this section, you will be able to:
- Define the term *therapeutic diet*
- List two ways the nursing assistant can verify the resident's diet order
- Match the appropriate description of a diet with the correct terminology
- Explain why it is important for each resident to receive the diet ordered by the physician

THERAPEUTIC DIETS

Eating properly to provide the body with essential nutrients is always important. When a person has a disease, is weak, or sick, it becomes even more important. Remember, it is through the digestive process that all the cells of the body are nourished!

Many illnesses and diseases interfere with proper nutrition. Because of this, the physician will modify or restrict the resident's diet. The physician determines and orders the kind of diet that will best meet the resident's nutritional needs. These diets are frequently referred to as:

- Special diets
- Restricted diets
- Modified diets
- Therapeutic diets

Therapeutic means pertaining to or effective in the treatment of disease. The purpose of a therapeutic diet is to provide the resident with a diet that will help in the medical treatment of a particular disease or illness.

For example, a resident who has diabetes will generally be on a diet in which the total calories are limited and the amounts of protein, fat, and carbohydrates are specified. You will study more about the diabetic resident in Chapter 14.

A resident with heart disease or **hypertension** (high blood pressure) will generally be on a diet that is salt (or sodium)-free or salt-restricted.

Sodium (abbreviated Na) is contained in salt and is the primary element that is restricted. Therefore, the amount of sodium is specified in the metric system of grams, that is, 1-gm Na diet.

The proper diet is a very important part of the resident's treatment plan. You will need to understand the basic difference between the types of diets served so you can verify that the residents are receiving the diet ordered by their physician.

You can determine what the diet order for each resident is by:

- Checking the diet tray card (Fig. 9-3)
- Verifying the diet order on the resident's chart or health-care plan

```
Resident's name   Mary Smith                                    Rm. No. 210 A
Diet order        Regular mechanical soft
Food allergies    Strawberries, green beans
Breakfast         Likes prune juice, scrambled eggs only
Beverage          Coffee
Lunch             Likes soup often and fruit plate
Beverage          Coffee, juice
Dinner            No fish or rice
Beverage          Coffee

Likes/Dislikes         no rice — no fish — no gravy
                       Likes fruit plates, soups
Special Instructions      Needs plate guard each meal
```

FIGURE 9-3
A diet tray card.

In many facilities, residents who have special diet orders are given different-colored arm bands to remind those providing care of the modified or restricted diet order. Be sure you know what the color-coded arm bands mean in your facility; examples are:

- Red arm band — diabetic diet
- Yellow arm band — low sodium

Calorie Controlled • Low calorie • High calorie • Diabetic (The American Dietetic Assoc. ADA has established specific diets with appropriate balances of carbohydrates, proteins, and fats for diabetic residents)	Specifies the total number of calories allowed and the precise balance between carbohydrates, proteins, and fats.	Frequently ordered for residents who are on a weight reduction program and also for diabetic residents who require restricted calorie intake and balance. In the calculation of the type of calorie-restricted diabetic diet, the intake is balanced with the resident's insulin requirements and exercise. High-calorie diets may be ordered for residents who would benefit from weight gain or residents who are younger or more active and would require additional calories to maintain their weight.
No concentrated sweets and no added sugar	Excludes candies, pastries, and baked goods containing sugar. No sugar is served with meal. Fruit juices and alcoholic beverages are usually avoided.	May be ordered for some residents who do not require a calorie-controlled diet but who because of adult diabetes need to control simple carbohydrates. Is easier to follow and closer to a regular or normal diet.
Bland	Nutritionally adequate diet with food mixed in flavor. Does not contain highly seasoned or gas-forming foods (i.e., beans, onions, cabbage). Generally contains foods that are easily digested.	Easily digested foods that avoid irritation of the digestive tract for residents who have ulcers, colitis, or gallbladder disease.

(continued)

USE OF ASSISTIVE EATING DEVICES

There are many assistive devices available. These are special feeding utensils designed to help residents perform tasks that would otherwise be impossible for them (Figs. 9-9 and 9-10). Usually, an assistive eating device is necessary due to lack of mobility or disability due to weakness. Use of any assistive device requires training of the resident and consistent encouragement from the staff. In the beginning, it may take more time for the resident to use an assistive device than it takes for you to perform the task for the resident. Keep in mind the importance of encouraging independence and allow the time necessary for learning.

Most LTC facilities employ an occupational therapy consultant to evaluate and work with residents who require special assistance in performing activities of daily living (Fig. 9-11). The occupational therapy consultant will also assist the staff in learning how to help the resident use special assistive devices.

Many residents of LTC facilities require a nutritional supplement. This supplement is frequently necessary for residents to receive adequate nutrition. The most commonly used type of nutritional supplement is a high-protein drink.

If the resident requires a nutritional supplement, the physician's order will contain:

- The name of the supplement to be given
- The amount to be given
- How often it should be given

.Because the nutritional supplement is part of the physician's treatment plan, it is very important to see that the resident not only receives but also eats or drinks the nourishment provided. Residents on restricted diets will also have specific orders for the kinds and amounts of between-meal snacks they may have.

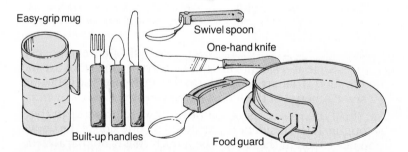

FIGURE 9-9
Assistive eating devices.

FIGURE 9-10
A food guard in use.

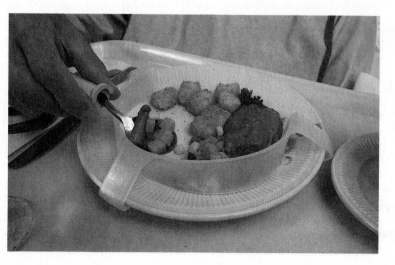

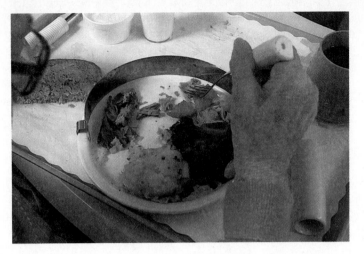

FIGURE 9-11
Resident using assistive devices.

SECTION 5 ELIMINATION

OBJECTIVES/WHAT YOU WILL LEARN

When you have completed this section, you will be able to:
- Define the term *defecation*
- List four important observations related to bowel elimination
- Describe why accurate recording of the resident's bowel function is essential
- List three nursing measures used to decrease constipation in the elderly or chronically ill
- Identify one complication related to constipation that requires the immediate attention of the licensed nurse
- Insert a rectal suppository
- Administer a cleansing enema
- Define the term *colostomy*
- Change the colostomy bag
- Collect a stool specimen
- List four ways the nursing assistant can assist a resident regain bowel control

THE PROCESS OF ELIMINATING WASTES

As you know, the foods you eat contain various nutrients that are absorbed and used by the body. Some elements of food cannot be used and are eliminated as waste material. These various waste products are eliminated through the skin, lungs, kidneys, and the bowel. The bowel is the most important excretor of solid wastes of the body. **Defecation** is the process of eliminating waste material from the bowel. The waste product itself is called **feces** (stool, BM). Normally, the stool is about three-quarters water by weight and one-quarter solid waste materials. This waste material is about 30 percent dead bacteria and 70 percent undigested roughage from food. The normal color of feces is brown, caused by bile which is stored and released from the gallbladder. The characteristic odor of the stool is produced by the action of intestinal bacteria on food eaten.

The appearance and composition of feces are important indications of whether or not the digestive system is functioning normally. Changes in bowel habits may also be an indication of illness or disease. If the bowel becomes obstructed or blocked, it is a medical emergency and must be treated immediately.

You should report and chart the following related to bowel elimination:

- Changes in the color of the stool. (*Note:* The color of the feces can change when certain drugs or vitamins are taken. For example, drug preparations containing iron give the stool a black color, and some green vegetables or foods may cause the stool to be green.) You should always report changes in color to the charge nurse.
- Presence of blood. Blood in the stool should always be reported immediately. Save the specimen for observation by the licensed nurse.
- Presence of large amounts of undigested foods or mucous.
- Presence of parasites (worms).
- Change in bowel habits.
- Complaints of pain related to bowel movement.
- Constipation or diarrhea.
- Uncharacteristic odors.
- **Diarrhea** is defined as semifluid feces. It may occur as a result of bacterial or viral infections, from eating spoiled and irritating foods, or from emotional upsets. Persistant diarrhea can lead to severe loss of fluids and loss of chemicals necessary for normal body functions. The nursing assistant must report to the charge nurse when any resident has diarrhea.

CONSTIPATION

Constipation is the buildup of fecal material in the large intestine that is not easily passed through the rectum. Constipation occurs as a result of several factors. Nursing measures effective in decreasing the likelihood of constipation include: encouraging adequate intake of the right kinds of foods/fluids; encouraging exercise and ambulation, if possible; helping residents protect the need for privacy when toileting; and helping residents to reduce fears of incontinence by responding promptly to their needs.

Constipation is a common problem of the elderly and chronically ill. The nursing assistant must immediately report a lack of bowel movement or complaints of pain or discomfort.

A serious complication related to constipation is the development of a **fecal impaction.** Feces stay in the S-shaped area of the colon and rectum where water is absorbed, causing the feces to become dry and hard. This condition is very serious. It may block the intestinal passages, and it is very painful for the resident. This condition requires the immediate attention of a licensed nurse. Any complaints of pain, absence of bowel movements, or liquid movements should be reported to your charge nurse immediately.

Remember, it is the digestive system that prepares food for use by the body. Whenever a disruption in the normal process occurs, it can be very serious. Nausea, which causes a resident to reject food, can be serious and should never be taken lightly by the nursing assistant. Report all complaints of nausea or episodes of vomiting, constipation, or diarrhea to your charge nurse immediately. Episodes of flu, abdominal distress, or diarrhea can be life-threatening to a weak or seriously ill resident.

LAXATIVE MEDICATIONS

There are some special medications and treatments ordered by the physician to treat problems related to elimination. The purpose of enemas, laxative medications, and suppositories is to empty the bowel of its contents. A **laxative** is a medication that loosens the bowel contents and encourages evacuation.

Laxative medications and treatments may only be given when the physician orders them as there are dangers associated with overuse. Frequently, the physician will order laxative medication administered by the licensed nurse. Many times the only way the licensed nurse can determine a resident's need for laxative medication is by the records and reports the nursing assistant makes. For this reason, it is essential to record each bowel movement. You will need to question those residents who have independent bowel function to gather this information.

In some facilities, the licensed nurse will be responsible for insertion of laxative suppositories; in other facilities the nursing assistant is trained to insert them. Make sure you follow your facility's policies and procedures regarding insertion of suppositories.

THE USE OF RECTAL SUPPOSITORIES

A rectal **suppository** is a cone-shaped semisolid medicated substance that frequently contains glycerin. It is about $1\frac{1}{2}$ inches long. The rectal suppository works to stimulate the inner surface of the rectal lining, creating an urge to empty the bowel as well as lubricating and coating the stool for easier evacuation.

PROCEDURE

INSERTING RECTAL SUPPOSITORIES

1. Assemble your equipment:
    - A suppository as ordered
    - Lubricant
    - Bedpan with cover
    - Disposable gloves
    - Toilet tissue
2. Wash your hands.
3. Identify the resident.
4. Provide privacy.
5. Explain to the resident what you are going to do.
6. Raise the bed to a comfortable working position.
7. Position the resident or ask the resident to turn on one side and raise one knee toward the chest. Assist as necessary.
8. Lift the sheet and expose the buttocks.
9. Put on disposable gloves.
10. Open lubricant and apply to gloved index finger.
11. Apply lubricant around anal area.
12. Holding the suppository between the thumb and index finger, spread the buttocks. Slowly and gently insert the suppository with a rotating motion, as far as your lubricated index finger will reach (2 to 3 inches).
13. It will help the resident relax the anal sphincter if he or she "pants" while you insert the suppository.
14. Withdraw the finger and hold toilet tissues against the anus briefly.
15. Remove gloves by turning them inside out.
16. Reposition the resident and encourage him or her to retain the suppository as long as possible (15 to 20 minutes).
17. Provide a bedpan for use, if necessary, or assist to the bathroom.

18. Discard disposable gloves, toilet tissue, and suppository wrapper and wash your hands.
19. Monitor the resident every few minutes.
20. Assist the resident to clean up.
21. Reposition and make comfortable, lower the bed, and replace the call signal.
22. Return or discard used equipment appropriately.
23. Wash your hands.
24. Record the time and type of suppository given, as well as the results.
    - Example: 9:15AM Glycerin suppository inserted S. Smith N/A
      9:45AM Large amounts of soft brown formed stool eliminated, resident stated he feels much better. S. Smith N/A

ENEMAS

An **enema** is the introduction of fluid into the rectum and colon. Enemas are given to stimulate the bowel and cause the contents to be released. The kind of solution and the amount of fluid used for the enema are prescribed by the physician. The most common solutions are:

- Tap water
- Commercially prepared (Fleets, oil retention)
- Saline (salt solution)
- SSE (soap suds enema)

Commercially prepared enemas are the most common types used in LTC facilities today.

The amount of solution varies between 500 cc (2 cups) to 1000 cc (4 cups). The solution should be a comfortable temperature (40 to 50°C or 105°F). Always check the temperature against the inside of your wrist. Solutions that are too cold cannot be retained, and solutions that are too hot can cause irritation, pain, and damage to the rectal tissues. The container holding the solution, if not the commercially prepared type, should not be higher than 18 inches above the anus. Any height greater than that creates too much pressure, causes discomfort, and increases the urge to expel the contents immediately.

The resident receiving an enema should be positioned on the side or the back as tolerated. The side-lying position is the most common position. If the resident can be positioned on the left side with the hips slightly elevated, the flow of the solution is better.

Residents should not be given enemas while seated on a toilet or commode, as the sitting position does not allow the solution to flow up into the colon. It merely collects in the rectum, causing dilation and the urge to defecate immediately.

1. Assemble your equipment:
   - Disposable enema unit or reusable enema, bucket bag, tubing, clamp
   - Solution ordered by the physician at warm temperature (105°F, 40.5°C)
   - Disposable gloves   • Toilet tissue   • Lubricating jelly
   - Bed protector   • Bedpan

2. Close the clamp on the enema tubing and fill the enema bucket with the specified type and amount of solution.

3. Test the temperature of the solution to ensure that it is neither too hot nor too cold. It should feel warm when run across the inside of your wrist (105°F, 40.5°C).

4. Open the clamp and allow the solution to fill the tubing to remove air. Close the clamp.

5. Wash your hands.

6. Identify the resident.

7. Provide privacy.

8. Explain to the resident what you are going to do.

9. Raise the bed to a comfortable working position.

10. Position the resident on the left side with the left knee and hip flexed, if possible, or in the supine (back-lying position) with knees flexed, if the side lying position cannot be used.

11. Protect the bed with disposable pads or linens.

12. Have the bedpan within easy reach.

13. Keep the resident covered, exposing only the buttocks.

14. Put on gloves.

15. Lubricate the tip (2 to 4 inches) of the enema tubing by rotating it in lubricant jelly which has been placed on toilet tissue.

16. Lift the upper buttock to expose the anal area, then gently and slowly insert the tip of the tubing 2 to 4 inches. Never push against resistance. Use a gentle rotating movement. Have the patient "pant" while you insert the enema tubing, as this will help the resident relax.

17. Open the clamp and raise the enema bucket about 12 to 15 inches above the anus and let the solution flow in slowly.

18. If the resident is uncomfortable, you may need to clamp the tubing and wait a minute or so before allowing the flow of solution to continue. Encourage the resident to take all the solution ordered; however, stop if the resident is too uncomfortable.

19. When the solution is almost gone, clamp the tube and slowly withdraw the tubing. Place the tubing into the enema bucket. Avoid bringing the contaminated tip into contact with the bed or floor.

20. Assist the resident onto the bedpan, toilet, or bedside commode. Encourage the resident to retain the solution as long as possible.

21. Monitor the resident every few minutes.

22. Assist the resident to clean up.

23. Reposition and make the resident comfortable, lower the bed, and replace the call signal.

24. Return or discard equipment appropriately.

25. Wash your hands.

26. Record the time and type of enema given, as well as the results.

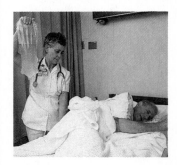

position patient on patient left side.

ADMINISTERING THE COMMERCIALLY PREPARED ENEMA

The disposable commercially prepared enema is commonly used. The administration is simple. Whenever you use any disposable product, read the directions printed on the container carefully. You will follow the basic procedure for administering a cleansing enema, with the addition of:

- Removing the protective cover
- Inserting the prelubricated tube slowly and gently
- Squeezing the bottle to expel the solution slowly
- Replacing the tube and restoring it in the original container to discard in the appropriate waste container

THE OIL RETENTION ENEMA

The oil retention enema is given in the same manner; however, the resident needs to be encouraged to retain the solution for a longer period, 10 to 20 minutes, if possible. Frequently, the physician will order a cleansing enema after an oil-retention enema.

There are occasions when the physician will order laxative medications and "enemas until clear." This is done to cleanse the bowel prior to diagnostic procedures or surgery. You would follow the physician's order for the type of solution and the amount of solution to be used. Clarify any questions regarding this procedure with your charge nurse. **Enemas until clear** means that there is no solid fecal material present when the solution is expelled. The solution, however, will be discolored and particles of feces will be present.

Elderly or seriously ill residents may become very fatigued after receiving an enema. For this reason check with the charge nurse before giving more than two enemas, even when the results are not yet clear.

OSTOMIES

An **ostomy** is a surgical opening made on the surface of the abdomen to release waste from the body. The opening is called a **stoma.** An ostomy becomes necessary when the ileum, colon, or urinary tract becomes diseased or injured to the extent that normal passage of waste materials is impossible. The most frequent reason for an ostomy is the removal of tumors or obstructions. Sometimes the surgery is done to permit the colon to heal following an injury. This is referred to as a *temporary ostomy.* Once healing has taken place, surgery is performed to reconstruct the normal passage for the waste materials. Permanent ostomies are performed when reconstruction is impossible due to diseased tissue. The location (site) of the ostomy and stoma depend on where the disorder is located (Fig. 9-12):

- **Colostomy** — opening into the colon
- **Ileostomy** — opening into the ileum
- **Ureterostomy** — opening into one of the ureters

There are thousands of people with permanent ostomies who live normal lives. Most residents with ostomies have made their initial adjustment prior to admission to the LTC facility because the surgery and patient teaching is part of most acute hospital programs. For some residents, the adjustment is very

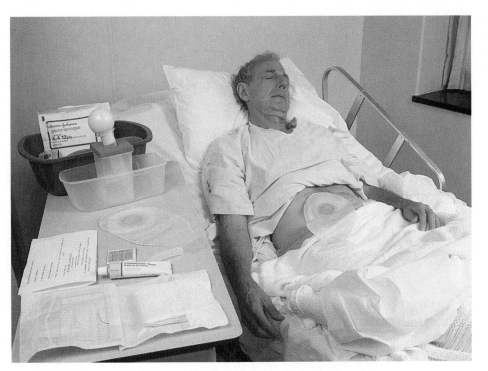

Colostomy—transverse colon:
stool is toothpaste consistency,
controlled by irrigation every
one to two days

Colostomy—ascending colon:
frequent, liquid, semi-liquid;
difficult to control

Ileostomy sites:
liquid, runny stool;
no control

Colostomy—descending colon:
solid stools, controlled by
irrigations

FIGURE 9-12
Common ostomy sites.

FIGURE 9-13
An ostomy device in place
over a stoma, and
equipment.

difficult. When possible, ostomy residents are encouraged to perform their ostomy care independently.

Some individuals wear only a small gauze pad over their stoma, but most ostomy residents wear an appliance that covers the stoma and collects waste material released (Fig. 9-13). There are many different types of appliances used, depending on the size and location of the stoma as well as the sensitivity of the resident's skin to the various adhesive substances.

Three very important nursing functions are associated with providing care to the resident with an ostomy. They are to:

- Protect the skin around the stoma from breakdown or irritation.
- Assist in reducing odors.
- Observe to ensure that the ostomy is functioning properly.

1. Assemble your equipment
   - Bedpan
   - Clean ostomy appliance, adhesive, and belt (optional)
   - Toilet tissue
   - Skin protector or cream as ordered by the physician
   - Bed protector
   - Disposable gloves
   - Basin of water and soap
   - Washcloth, towel
2. Wash your hands.
3. Identify the resident.
4. Provide privacy.
5. Explain to the resident what you are going to do.
6. Raise the bed to a comfortable working position.
7. Position the resident in the supine position with the head elevated, if possible.
8. Protect the bed with a bed protector on the side of the stoma.
9. Place the bedpan within easy reach.
10. Expose the abdomen, taking care to keep the genital area covered.
11. Fill basin with moderately hot water (115°F, 46.1°C), have washcloth and soap nearby. Put on disposable gloves.
12. Carefully open belt and remove the soiled or full ostomy bag, taking care to peel it away from the stoma gently. Use toilet tissue to protect the skin around the stoma from coming into contact with fecal material.
13. Place the soiled ostomy bag in the bedpan. Remove the belt if it is soiled, and cleanse the area around the ostomy stoma with soap and water.
14. Apply lubricant, skin protector, or skin cream, as ordered, around the stoma. Observe for any skin irritation or breakdown.
15. Place a clean belt around resident and place a clean bag over the stoma. Make sure that it is attached securely.
16. Assist the resident as necessary to clean up.
17. Observe the contents of the ostomy bag for blood, undigested food particles, or for changes in form consistency. Report anything unusual to your charge nurse immediately.
18. Dispose of the full ostomy bag according to your facility's policies. Most facilities consider waste material that is not flushed away as **infectious waste,** which requires special handling.
19. Remove your gloves.
20. Return or discard equipment appropriately.
21. Wash your hands.
22. Record changing the bag and any unusual observations.
23. Reposition and make the resident comfortable, lower the bed, and replace the call signal.

The ostomy bag may be changed in the bathroom with the resident seated on the toilet. For some residents, this is preferred because the problem of odor is confined to the bathroom, and privacy is maintained. The bag itself should not be discarded in the toilet. Follow the basic procedure for changing the bag in bed.

There are occasions when residents may require an ostomy irrigation. This is done to help the resident establish a regular pattern of elimination. Ostomy irrigation is a procedure much like that of giving an enema. Before attempting this procedure, you must find out if nursing assistants in your facility are permitted to perform the irrigation, and you must receive specific instructions and supervision.

COLLECTION OF A STOOL SPECIMEN

There are times when it is necessary to collect specimens for laboratory analysis. You will be instructed by the charge nurse when a stool specimen has been ordered by the physician.

1. Assemble your equipment
   - Bedpan and cover
   - Stool specimen container and label
   - Wooden tongue depressor
   - Disposable gloves (optional)
2. Wash your hands.
3. Identify the resident.
4. Provide privacy.
5. Explain to the resident that you need to collect a specimen. Ask the resident to call you when he or she feels the need to move the bowels. If the resident is unable to cooperate, check frequently and have equipment ready for collection of the specimen when defecation occurs.
6. Once the resident has had a bowel movement, take the covered bedpan into the bathroom and use the wooden tongue depressor to remove one to two tablespoons of fecal material from the bedpan. Place this into the labeled stool specimen container.
7. Cover the container immediately.
8. Wrap the tongue depressor in a paper towel and discard.
9. Empty the bedpan, clean it, and return it to its proper place.
10. Wash your hands.
11. Follow the instruction of the charge nurse for storage of a stool specimen prior to collection by the laboratory.
12. Assist the resident as necessary to clean up.
13. Reposition and make the resident comfortable, lower the bed, and attach the call signal.
14. Record and report collection of the stool specimen, along with any unusual observations.

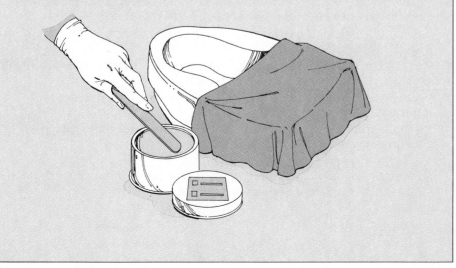

BOWEL INCONTINENCE

When normal nerve pathways that control the release of the contents of the bowel are affected, incontinence may result. This embarrassing condition may be caused by stroke (CVA), spinal cord, or brain injury, in addition to many other diseases or medications.

Incontinence may occur during an episode of serious illness or hospitalization. Regardless of the cause, it is always important to assist the resident to regain control if possible. Incontinence occurs most often with residents who are not fully aware of their surroundings. However, even residents who are confused or unaware realize when they have soiled themselves. Incontinence promotes feelings of embarrassment, humiliation, and loss of self-respect and self-esteem. For these reasons, it is never appropriate to scold or make fun of the incontinent resident. A matter-of-fact attitude is the best way to reduce negative feelings.

The physician and the licensed nurse will evaluate the nature of the resident's bowel incontinence as well as their food and fluid intake pattern and habits of elimination. A plan will then be developed to assist the resident in regaining bowel control. The specific plan for bowel retaining should be recorded on the health-care plan. Your charge nurse will give you further instructions.

BOWEL RETRAINING

As a nursing assistant you can play a major role in helping residents regain bowel control by:

- Encouraging the resident to consume adequate amounts of food and fluids. Fluid intake of between 2000 cc (8 cups) and 3000 cc (12 cups) daily is needed to provide the average adult with good hydration and to prevent constipation.
- Reporting signs of constipation so that medication can be administered.
- Following carefully and consistently the bowel retraining plan found on the resident's health care plan. *Note:* The bowel retraining plan should be based on the individual resident's problem and his or her bowel habits as well as the resident's ability to communicate and comprehend.
- Answering the call signal promptly as well as checking with residents frequently to assist them to use the bathroom or bedpan. Some residents are considered incontinent because they are unable to get the help they need fast enough!
- Identifying the residents' normal bowel evacuation times and assisting them to use the bathroom or bedpan prior to that time.
- Assisting residents to exercise in and out of bed. Exercise helps maintain muscle tone necessary for good bowel function.
- Helping the resident get adequate rest and sleep is important. Confusion and incontinence result when the resident is overly tired.
- Praising the resident for successful efforts to regain continence and ignoring accidents.
- Providing the resident and family with emotional support and encouragement.

Assisting a resident to regain bowel control is a very important accomplishment. It builds self-esteem and self-confidence.

CHAPTER 10

The Urinary System

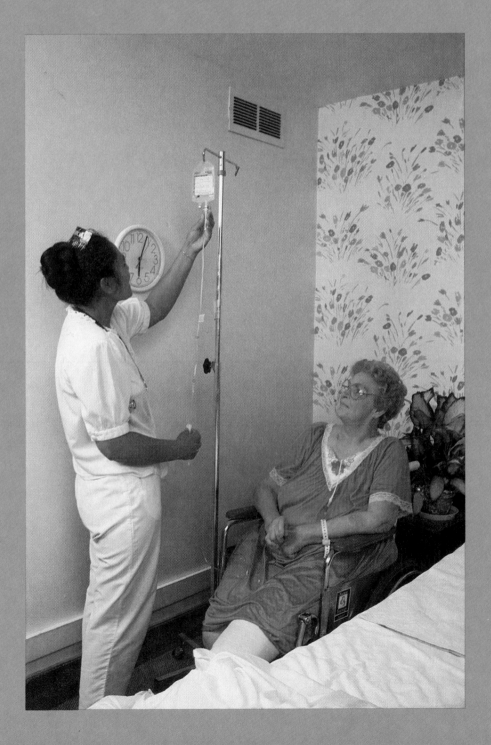

OBJECTIVES/WHAT YOU WILL LEARN

When you have completed this section, you will be able to:

- List three important functions of the urinary system
- Correctly label the components of the urinary system
- Identify the average adult urinary output for 24 hours
- List three common age-related changes affecting the urinary system
- List three contributing factors related to the development of urinary tract infections

THE URINARY SYSTEM

The urinary system (Fig. 10-1) is composed of:

- Kidneys
- Ureters
- Bladder
- Urethra

Functions of the urinary system are:

- Remove wastes from the bloodstream
- Produce urine
- Maintain homeostasis

The urinary system removes waste products from the body by producing and eliminating urine. Other organs that assist in the elimination of waste products are the lungs, intestinal tract, and sweat glands.

FIGURE 10-1
The urinary system.

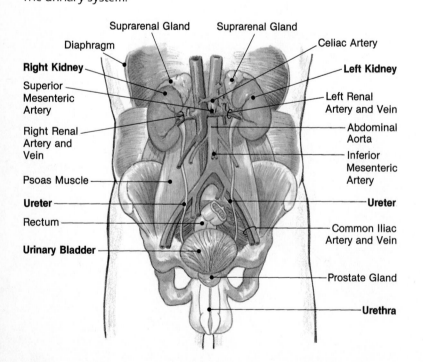

The urinary system is part of the body's excretory structures (urinary system, lungs, sweat glands, and intestine). The kidneys remove the wastes of chemical activities (metabolism) in the body. These wastes are removed from the blood to produce urine. At the same time, the kidneys remove certain excess compounds, regulate the blood pH (acid-base balance), and the concentration of sodium, potassium, chlorine, glucose and other important chemicals.

THE KIDNEYS

The **kidneys** are two bean-shaped organs that lie just below the diaphragm and posterior abdominal wall on either side of the lumbar region of the spine (Fig. 10-2). In an adult, the kidney is about 4 inches long, 2 inches wide, and 1 inch thick. Each kidney weighs 4 to 6 ounces. In this tiny organ, there are over a million microscopic filtering units called **nephrons** (Fig. 10-3). One of the amazing examples of the body's reserve is that we can lose large amounts of nephrons to age or disease and still live normally. Many people live with only one kidney.

Blood enters the kidney from the **renal artery,** where it is distributed through arterioles into millions of capillaries that lead to the nephrons. Fluids and other substances pass through the thin capillary walls and are collected in the central part of the nephron, the **glomerulus,** which is found inside Bowman's capsule. This special network of capillaries acts like a filter. Materials not needed by the body are filtered out and carried through a series of tubules. These tubules make up the rest of the nephron. When this filtered material from the blood flows through the tubules, the tiny capillaries surrounding the tubules selectively reabsorb (take back into the blood) substances needed by the body. Other substances not needed, such as drugs, some vitamins, and excessive fluids, are not reabsorbed. Combined with excess water, these substances create the waste product, urine.

Once urine is formed, it moves into a collecting "funnel" called the **renal pelvis,** where it passes into the right and left ureters attached to the right and left kidneys. The **ureters** are tiny tubes about 10 inches long that start at the renal pelvis and empty into the bladder. Here special **stretch-receptor** nerve cells in the walls become stimulated when the bladder is full. A message is sent to the brain, which results in **urination** (emptying of the bladder).

The bladder has a tube (the **urethra**) that leads outside the body. It is through the urethra that urine passes from the body. The urethra in the male is about 8 inches long because it runs through the penis. In the female, it is about $1\frac{1}{2}$ inches long. Because this tube opens to the outside, there is always

FIGURE 10-2
The kidney.

FIGURE 10-3
The nephron.

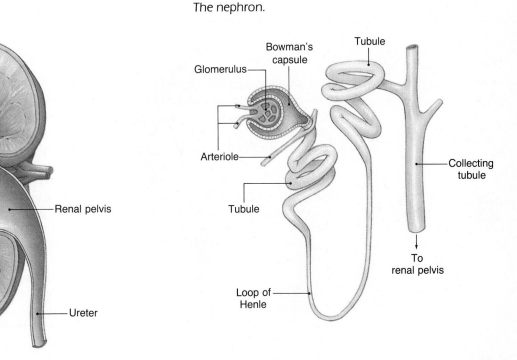

a threat of infection. When infection develops, it travels up into the bladder and sometimes into the kidney itself, causing very serious complications.

In the average adult, about $1\frac{1}{2}$ quarts of urine is produced each 24 hours. The kidney is a very efficient organ when functioning normally. It has the capacity to filter 1 quart of blood per minute or 360 gallons each day. Normal urine is straw-colored and clear. Urine that is dark, bloody, or filled with sediment (flecks or particles) or mucus is not normal and should be reported immediately. Urine has a characteristic odor, but this changes when it is very concentrated or when infection is present. One of the most important factors in maintaining normal kidney function is to ensure that residents have adequate fluid intake. You will study problems related to dehydration and will learn how to measure intake and output later in this chapter.

AGE-RELATED CHANGES

The kidney and its specialized tissues function to maintain homeostasis. The kidney actually determines the water and chemical composition of the blood, which in turn determines the content of the tissue fluid that surrounds the cells.

There are a number of age-related changes that affect the urinary system. As an individual ages, the kidneys function less efficiently. A person 80 years old will have about half the nephrons of the newborn infant. If only half the nephrons are available, their efficiency will decrease greatly. For this reason, an elderly resident is more likely to have a drug reaction than the middle aged or young adult. The kidney is less efficient in removing the drug from the bloodstream. Reactions to medications must be observed for and reported to the charge nurse.

Arteriosclerosis can affect the blood vessels that supply the urinary system. When circulation is poor, there is a greater chance of developing infection as well as decreased ability to recover from illness or injury. There are age-related changes that decrease the elasticity of the ureters, bladder, and urethra. The muscle tone decreases, and the amount of urine the bladder can hold is reduced. Sometimes the elderly resident will not be aware of the need to urinate until the bladder is almost full. This leads to:

- **Frequency** — the need to urinate often
- **Urgency** — an immediate need to urinate
- **Nocturia** — waking at night to urinate

These problems, along with chronic illness and some types of medications, may lead to incontinence. **Urinary incontinence** is the inability to control urination. It is a very distressing and embarrassing problem for most residents. Residents with neurological disease or injury frequently have no control of the bladder functions because the brain is unable to receive signals that control urination.

Urinary tract infections are a common problem in all ages. However, the elderly resident who is confined to bed or has an **indwelling catheter** (a tube inserted into the bladder that drains urine into a collection bag) is especially vulnerable. Immobility has serious effects on the urinary system primarily due to the incomplete emptying of urine from the kidneys and bladder. When urine is retained too long, bacteria grow, resulting in infection and development of kidney stones. Stones (called **calculi**) may develop in either the kidneys or the bladder, and they are extremely painful. Incomplete emptying of the bladder may be related to the position of the body when urinating. When the resident is confined to bed and is in a reclining or semireclining position, it is almost impossible to empty the bladder completely (Fig. 10-4).

FIGURE 10-4
Contrast in degree of bladder emptying.

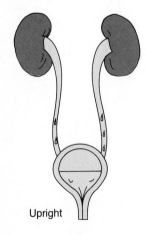

Upright

Recumbent

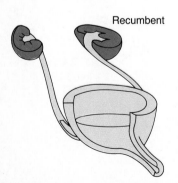

Urinary tract infections will also develop when good hygiene measures are not practiced after urination and defecation. Bacteria normally present in the bowel are very frequently the source of the infection. Poor fluid intake is also a cause of urinary tract infections. Repeated infections damage the kidneys and are a major cause of fever and serious illness in the elderly. There are many important nursing measures that can help reduce the incidence of infection.

SECTION 2 FLUID BALANCE — INTAKE AND OUTPUT

OBJECTIVES/WHAT YOU WILL LEARN

When you have completed this section, you will be able to:

- Describe what is meant by "fluid balance"
- Identify those items that should be calculated as fluid intake
- Compute intake accurately
- Compute output accurately
- List three ways the nursing assistant can help residents meet their fluid needs
- Identify three observations of a resident with an IV that must be reported promptly to the charge nurse
- Describe the guidelines to be followed when caring for the resident with an IV.

FLUID BALANCE

The nursing assistant assists residents in maintaining normal fluid balance. Water is essential to human life. Next to oxygen, water is the most important substance the body takes in. A person can lose half of the body protein and almost half of the body weight before death occurs. Yet if an individual loses about one-fifth of the total body fluids, death usually results.

Through eating and drinking the average healthy adult will consume between $2\frac{1}{2}$ and $3\frac{1}{2}$ quarts in a 24-hour period. **Fluid intake** is the amount of fluid consumed by:

- Mouth
- Special feeding tubes
- The **parenteral** routes (into a vein and under the skin)

FLUID INTAKE AND FLUID OUTPUT

The same average healthy adult will eliminate between $2\frac{1}{2}$ and $3\frac{1}{2}$ quarts in a 24-hour period. **Fluid output** is the total amount of fluid eliminated from the body through:

- The kidneys as urination, also referred to as voiding or passing water (approximately $1\frac{1}{2}$ quarts in 24 hours).
- The skin through perspiration and the lungs through respiration (approximately 1 quart in 24 hours).
- The intestinal tract where fluid is absorbed and discharged as part of the feces or stool (less than 1 cup).

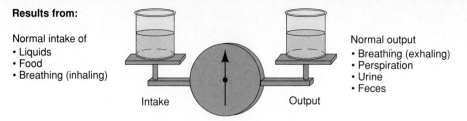

FIGURE 10-5
Fluid balance: intake equals output.

Results from:

Normal intake of
- Liquids
- Food
- Breathing (inhaling)

Intake   Output

Normal output
- Breathing (exhaling)
- Perspiration
- Urine
- Feces

- Other ways, such as **emesis** (vomiting), wound drainage, severe perspiration, severe diarrhea, or **hemorrhage** (bleeding).

Fluid balance means that the person eliminates about the same amount of fluid that is taken in (Fig. 10-5).

FLUID IMBALANCE

An **imbalance** of body fluids occurs when fluid intake exceeds fluid output (Fig. 10-6). Fluid is retained in the body, leading to **edema.** Symptoms of edema or fluid retention are:

- Swelling of feet, ankles, face, hands, fingers
- Weight gain
- Collection of fluid in abdomen and lungs
- Decreased urine output

Another type of imbalance exists if fluid intake is less than fluid output (Fig. 10-7). This results in a condition called **dehydration.** Dehydration is one of the most common medical problems of the long-term care resident. Dehydration is due to consuming insufficient quantities of liquids. Dependent residents may be reluctant or unable to ask for water of may simply "forget." Incontinent residents may stop drinking to reduce the chance of having an "accident."

Eliminating too much fluid also causes dehydration. Examples are:

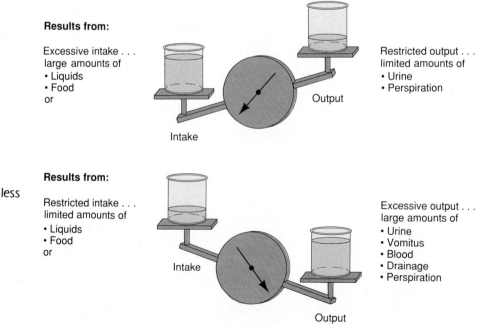

FIGURE 10-6
Fluid imbalance: intake more than output.

Results from:

Excessive intake . . . large amounts of
- Liquids
- Food
or

Output

Restricted output . . . limited amounts of
- Urine
- Perspiration

Intake

FIGURE 10-7
Fluid imbalance: intake less than output.

Results from:

Restricted intake . . . limited amounts of
- Liquids
- Food
or

Intake

Excessive output . . . large amounts of
- Urine
- Vomitus
- Blood
- Drainage
- Perspiration

Output

vomiting, bleeding, perspiring profusely, or losing fluid through diarrhea or wound drainage. The symptoms of dehydration are:

- Thirst
- Decreased urine output
- Dry-looking, nonelastic skin tone
- Parched or cracked lips and tongue

Dehydration affects all systems of the body; it is a life-threatening problem. Although the physician will prescribe treatment for the cause of dehydration, you play a vital role in helping residents meet their fluid needs. You do this by:

- Keeping fresh water within the resident's reach at all times.
- Offering fluids and reminding residents to consume fluids. A good habit to follow is to offer residents fluids each time you enter the room unless there is a fluid-restriction order.
- Providing encouragement to the resident so that all fluids served with meals or as between-meal nourishments are consumed. Menus are planned to provide the resident with a substantial portion of their required fluid intake.

Each facility has established policies and procedures for providing residents with fresh water. This is usually done each shift so that there is a constant supply of fresh drinking water available to residents. In some facilities, each water pitcher is taken to a clean area and filled with ice and fresh water. In other facilities, water pitchers are reprocessed and filled in the dietary department and returned to the resident. You will need to follow the policies and procedures established in your facility.

UNDERSTANDING FLUID INTAKE AND FLUID OUTPUT

In order to determine the resident's intake, you must measure and record everything a resident consumes by mouth that is a fluid, including water, milk, juice, coffee, tea, soups, and so on. Food items that become liquid at room temperature, such as Jello and ice cream, must also be included. Although solid foods contain some liquid, most of the fluid intake comes from what a person drinks in the form of actual liquids (Fig. 10-8).

Some residents who are unable or unwilling to drink fluids by mouth may receive them **parenterally** either through a vein (intravenous or IV) or through a catheter placed into the atrium of the heart (**central line**). The licensed nurse is responsible for recording fluids administered parenterally.

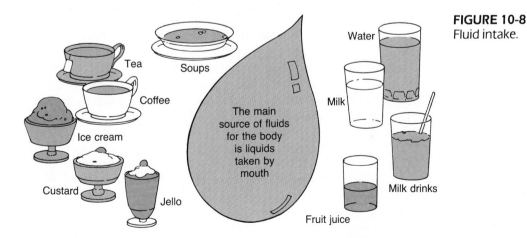

FIGURE 10-8
Fluid intake.

Tea
Soups
Water
Coffee
Milk
Ice cream
The main source of fluids for the body is liquids taken by mouth
Custard
Jello
Milk drinks
Fruit juice

To determine the resident's fluid output, you must measure and record all urinary output and vomitus and report hemorrhage, excessive wound drainage, or excessive perspiration. You will measure urinary output of the resident with an indwelling catheter by emptying and measuring the contents of the urinary drainage bag. If the resident is incontinent, you will not be able to collect or measure urine output. It is important to record on the intake and output record the number of times the resident is incontinent each shift.

If vomiting, hemorrhage, excessive wound drainage, or excessive perspiration occur, notify your charge nurse at once. The charge nurse will help you estimate the amount of fluid lost and will take other corrective actions. Never discard vomitus or drainage before the charge nurse has a chance to observe it.

Severe diarrhea can result in excessive fluid loss. Any observations or complaints of diarrhea should be reported to the charge nurse at once. When a fluid imbalance is suspected, you may be instructed to measure and record the resident's fluid intake and output. LTC facilities have written policies and procedures on how to measure and record intake and output. Be sure you follow the specific procedures outlined in your facility.

Measuring and recording fluid intake and output is very important! Many times the physician will use the data recorded on the intake and output record to determine which medications or treatments the resident needs.

The time for the nursing assistant to record fluid intake is when the resident consumes it. Fluid output should be recorded when urination or vomiting occurs. Do not try to remember — this is not the time for guesswork. Most facilities total the resident's intake and output at the end of each shift. The 24-hour total is generally calculated and recorded on the night shift.

Another method of finding out if a fluid imbalance exists is by measuring the specific gravity of the urine. This may be done by using a test tape and following the manufacturer's directions or by using a piece of equipment called a hydrometer. The hydrometer includes a glass tube that holds the urine and a measuring device similar to a thermometer that floats in the urine and gives the reading. If your facility uses this equipment, ask for a demonstration and instructions. The specific gravity shows how concentrated or how dilute the urine is. The specific gravity is an indicator of too much or too little fluid in the body.

USING THE METRIC SYSTEM

The most commonly used system of measurement in all hospitals is the metric system. In the past, the facilities in the United States used a system called the U.S. customary system, made up of ounces, pints, quarts for measuring liquids, and inches, feet, yards, and miles for measuring distance. However, there is increasing reason to use the metric system of measurement because scientists, engineers, and health-care personnel almost always use this system.

Fluids are measured in cc's or cubic centimeters. A cubic centimeter is simply a square block with each edge of the block 1 centimeter long (Fig. 10-9). If the block is filled with water, there would be 1 cubic centimeter (1 cc) of water inside the block. The accompanying conversion chart lists the U.S. customary liquid measure with equivalent metric measurements.

Containers, graduates, or measuring cups are used to measure fluid intake and output. Notice that the side of the graduate is **calibrated** (marked) with a row of short lines and numbers. This shows measurement in both cubic centimeters (cc) and ounces (oz).

FIGURE 10-9

Size contrast: cubic inch versus cubic centimeter.

cc = cubic centimeter
ml = milliliter
oz = ounce
1 cc = 1 ml
$\frac{1}{4}$ teaspoon = 1 cc
1 teaspoon = 4 cc
30 cc = 1 oz
60 cc = 2 oz
90 cc = 3 oz
120 cc = 4 oz
150 cc = 5 oz
180 cc = 6 oz
210 cc = 7 oz
240 cc = 8 oz
270 cc = 9 oz
300 cc = 10 oz
500 cc = 1 pint
1000 cc = 1 quart
4000 cc = 1 gallon

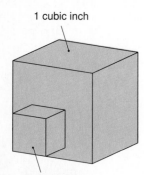

1 cubic inch

1 cubic centimeter

- Obtain a list of the most commonly used fluid containers in your facility, along with a listing of how many ounces or cc's it will hold. If this is not available, you will need to measure the amount of liquid each container holds and make a list for yourself.
- Obtain the forms used for recording intake and output in your facility.
- Measure and record all fluids consumed by the resident during your shift of duty. (Calculate the difference between the full amount of the container and the amount left in the container.) Observe and record fluids consumed from the resident's meals, water pitchers, and between-meal snacks.
- Convert (change) amounts such as half a bowl of soup, half a glass of juice, or a quarter cup of coffee into cubic centimeters for recording. For example: Mrs. Jones's water pitcher contained 1 quart (liter), which equals 1000 cc. At the end of the shift, you would measure what remained (in this case, 250 cc) and subtract the difference: 1000 cc minus 250 cc equals 750 cc. In addition, Mrs. Jones drank half a glass of juice (4-ounce juice glass equals 120 cc) (120 cc divided by 2 equals 60 cc) and a quarter cup of coffee (8-ounce cup equals 240 cc) (240 cc divided by 4 equals 60 cc).

Water	=	750 cc
Juice	=	60 cc
Coffee	=	60 cc
Total	=	870 cc

- Record intake after each meal before the tray is removed.
- Record other intake as it is consumed.

It is not possible to measure accurately the amount of fluid eliminated through the intestinal tract, the respiratory tract, or the skin. Therefore, the urinary output is the most reliable measurement of fluid output.

PROCEDURE

MEASURING URINARY OUTPUT

1. Assemble your equipment in the resident's bathroom:
   - Bedpan, urinal, or special container
   - Disposable gloves
   - Graduate or measuring cup
2. Put on your gloves.
3. Pour the urine into the measuring graduate.
4. Place the graduate on a flat surface at eye level and read the amount of urine in the graduate.
5. Observe the urine for any abnormalities, such as blood, dark color, large amounts of mucus or sediment, or changes in the characteristic odor. Report any abnormalities to your charge nurse immediately before discarding the urine.
6. Discard the normal urine into the toilet or hopper.
7. Rinse the graduate, bedpan, urinal, or special container and return to their proper places.
8. Remove your gloves.
9. Wash your hands.
10. Record the amount of urine (cc) on the intake and output record. Record the time of each entry.

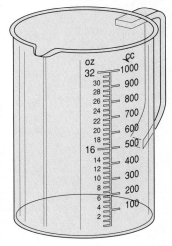

Calibrated Graduate

PROCEDURE

EMPTYING THE URINARY DRAINAGE BAG

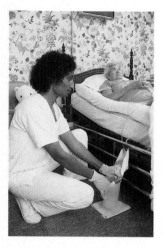

1. Assemble your equipment:
   - Graduate or measuring cup
   - Disposable gloves
   - Bedpan or urinal
2. Put on your gloves.
3. Carefully open the drain outlet from the urinary drainage bag, making sure the *drain outlet does not touch the container or the floor.* Bacteria can be introduced into the drainage bag, causing infection.
4. Allow the bag to drain competely and reattach the drainage outlet securely to the drainage bag.
5. Pour the urine from the bedpan or urinal into the measuring graduate.
6. Place the graduate on a flat surface at eye level and determine the amount of urine in the graduate.
7. Discard urine into toilet or hopper.
8. Rinse graduate, bedpan, or urinal and return to their proper places.
9. Remove your gloves.
10. Wash your hands.
11. Record the amount of urine in cc and the time collected on the Intake and Output Record.
12. Report any unusual observations, such as blood in the urine, a change in the color, or characteristic odor of the urine, to the charge nurse immediately.

Some residents are able to assist in keeping track of their fluid intake. Allow the resident to help as much as possible, being sure their accuracy is verified. The following procedure should be used when emptying a urinary drainage bag.

ENCOURAGE FLUID INTAKE

When residents need to have their fluid intake increased, the physician or nurse will give instructions to "force fluids." More accurately stated, the term **force fluids** would be "encourage fluids." Sometimes a resident will need continuous encouragement and persuasion to consume adequate fluids. On some occasions the physician will even specify the amount of fluids the resident is to receive: "Give 2000 cc each 24 hours." Ways you can help residents consume more fluids are:

- Follow the plan for carrying out the physician's order. For example: "Give 2000 cc each 24 hours. Total of 1300 cc contained on meal trays, encourage to consume all. Give 350 cc additional on 7–3 shift and 350 cc on 3–11 shift."
- Offer liquids each time you enter the room.
- Find out what kind of liquids the resident prefers and notify the charge nurse so that they are available when the diet order permits.
- Have the family assist in encouraging the resident to take more fluids. Suggest that they bring in special fluid treats, as the diet order permits.

INTRAVENOUS FLUIDS

Intravenous (IV) therapy includes any medication or fluid that is prescribed by a physician to be given directly into a person's bloodstream. IVs are given to provide more effective medication administration, to increase fluid intake, to provide nutrition, or to replace fluid or other necessary elements in the blood that have been lost through prolonged vomiting, diarrhea, or bleeding.

The fluid to be given is contained in a bottle or plastic bag that hangs on a pole above the resident's bed (Fig. 10-10). Most often there is a pump or rate control machine that is attached to the pole. The pump controls the rate (speed) at which the fluid goes from the bag, through the tubing, and into the resident. There is either a needle or plastic tube inserted into the resident's vein that provides the opening into the bloodstream. Usually the needle or tube is covered with a transparent (see-through) dressing. The fluid and medication may be given continuously (all of the time) or intermittently (part of the time).

The role of the nursing assistant is primarily one of observing and reporting as well as protecting the IV from becoming dislodged. You have already learned how to change the gown of the resident with an IV. Regardless of what you are doing for the resident with an IV, use caution so that there is no tension or pulling on the tubing.

Observe for and report to the charge nurse immediately any of the following:

- Alarm ringing on the pump
- Resident complaints of pain or burning at the IV site
- Swelling or redness at the IV site
- Signs of fever
- Difficulty breathing
- Bleeding or leakage of fluid onto the bed or floor

The resident with an IV requires the same good nursing care as every other resident. Don't allow your concern about dislodging the tubing to cause you to avoid providing necessary care to the resident.

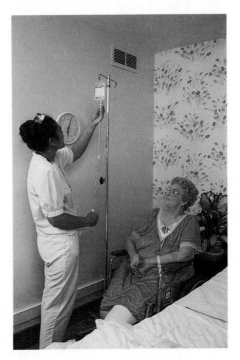

FIGURE 10-10
Giving intravenous fluids.

- Wash hands thoroughly before caring for the resident.
- Reassure the resident that you have been instructed in the proper care of a resident with an IV.
- Observe the resident carefully and often.
- Report anything unusual.
- Do not take the blood pressure in the arm the IV is in.
- Do not reconnect any tubing that does become disconnected. It is contaminated and must be replaced by the licensed nurse to prevent a serious infection.
- Admit any mistakes that you make so that prompt corrective action can be taken.

RESTRICTING FLUID INTAKE

There are times when it is necessary for the physician to order that fluids be restricted. Residents who have congestive heart failure or kidney disease may need to have their fluid intake limited. Residents on kidney **dialysis** (the use of a machine that performs the basic functions of the kidney) almost always require some type of fluid restriction. The physician's order may read "Give no more than 1500 cc in 24 hours." It is always important to explain the reasons for fluid restrictions to the resident and family. Follow the instructions of your charge nurse and measure all fluids accurately. If liquid restrictions are not followed, the resident may suffer severe consequences.

There are some occasions when a physician will order a resident to be **NPO** (consume nothing by mouth). NPO is taken from the Latin *nils per os*, which means "nothing by mouth." This is usually ordered prior to surgical or laboratory procedures. The NPO resident may not eat or drink anything at all — not even water! For example, the physician's order might say "NPO until lab work done in A.M." After the lab work has been drawn, normal intake may be resumed. Since residents who are NPO can become irritable, explain why the order is necessary.

SECTION 3 NURSING MEASURES RELATED TO THE URINARY SYSTEM

OBJECTIVES/WHAT YOU WILL LEARN

When you complete this section, you will be able to:

■ Place a resident on a bedpan and offer a urinal to a male resident
■ Give perineal care to a resident with a catheter
■ Identify four places where bacteria can enter the urinary drainage system
■ Identify activities necessary for collecting a "clean-catch" urine specimen

PROVIDING PRIVACY

Elimination of waste products is a natural process, and most healthy people have regular elimination habits. When someone becomes ill, these habits are disrupted. Sometimes control is lost. Most people regard elimination as a very personal function, and when it becomes necessary to ask for assistance, they are embarrassed.

Consider the feelings of residents when you are assisting them with their elimination needs. You can help preserve dignity by providing care with an accepting, matter-of-fact attitude. Remember, your body language and facial expressions convey many messages.

When you are assisting the resident to use a bedpan, urinal, or bedside commode, provide as much privacy as possible. Put yourself in the resident's place and consider how you would feel.

The female resident will use the bedpan for both urination and bowel elimination, while the male resident will generally use the bedpan for bowel elimination and the urinal for urination. The regular-sized bedpan is most commonly used (Fig. 10-11). Some residents who have difficulty moving (especially following hip fracture) will need to use the smaller, flatter "fracture" bedpan.

FIGURE 10-11
A urinal and bedpan.

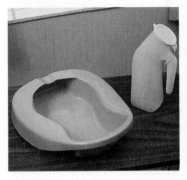

PROCEDURE

OFFERING THE
BEDPAN OR URINAL

1. Assemble your equipment on the bedside table:
   - Bedpan and cover, or fracture bedpan and cover, urinal
   - Toilet tissue
   - Disposable gloves
2. Wash your hands.
3. Provide privacy.
4. Lower the side rails.
5. Fold back the top sheets so that they are out of the way.
6. Raise the resident's gown, but keep the lower part of the body covered.
7. Ask the resident to assist by bending the knees and placing the feet flat on the mattress. Then ask the resident to raise the hips. Assist as necessary by slipping your hand under the lower back and lifting slightly. Place the bedpan in position, with the seat evenly under the buttocks.
8. If the resident is unable to assist, turn the resident to one side and place the bedpan against the buttocks, pushing downward into the mattress as you gently turn the resident back onto the bedpan.

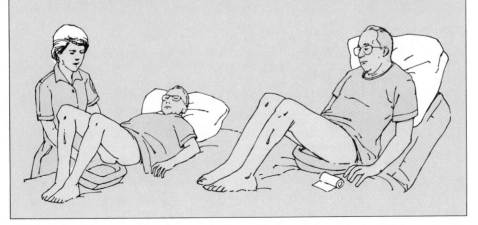

9. Give the urinal to the resident or assist as necessary in placing the urinal between the legs, with the penis inside the opening.
10. Replace the sheets over the resident.
11. Elevate the head of the bed and the knees slightly if allowed, so the resident can assume a sitting position.
12. Put toilet tissue and the call signal within easy reach of the resident.
13. Ask the resident to signal when finished.
14. Raise the side rails to the up position.
15. Wash your hands and leave the room to provide the resident with privacy.
16. When the resident signals, return to the room. If the resident is unable to signal, *check frequently*. Never leave a resident sitting on a bedpan for a prolonged period or with the urinal where pressure can be created.
17. Put on your gloves.
18. Assist the resident to raise the hips so that you can remove the bedpan.
19. Cover the bedpan or urinal immediately. You can use a disposable pad or a paper towel if no cover is available.

PROCEDURE

USING THE PORTABLE BEDSIDE COMMODE

1. Assemble your equipment:
   - Portable bedside commode next to the bed
   - Bedpan and cover, or the container used in your facility
   - Toilet tissue
   - Disposable gloves
2. Wash your hands.
3. Provide privacy.
4. Tell the resident you will assist with transferring onto the bedside commode, if necessary.
5. Place the commode next to the resident's bed. Open the cover and insert the container under the toilet seat.
6. Assist the resident to sit on the side of the bed. Put slippers on the resident before transferring onto the bedside commode.
7. Place toilet tissue and the signal cord within the resident's reach.
8. Ask the resident to signal when finished.
9. Wash your hands and leave the room to provide the resident with privacy.
10. Put on your gloves.
11. When the resident signals, return to the room and assist the resident as necessary to clean and wipe. Make sure that the anal area is clean.
12. Assist the resident in transferring back to bed.
13. Close the cover on the commode.
14. Remove the container from under the commode. Cover it and take it to the bathroom.
15. Check the feces or urine for abnormal appearance.
16. Measure the output if the resident is on intake and output. If a specimen is required, collect it at this time.
17. Empty the bedpan into the toilet and flush.

20. Assist the resident to clean and wipe as necessary. Make sure the anal area is clean. Turn the resident to the side for easier cleaning.
21. Remove the bedpan or urinal to the bathroom.
22. If a specimen is required, collect it at this time. Measure urine if the resident is on intake and output.
23. Check the feces or urine for abnormal appearance.
24. Empty the bedpan or urinal into the toilet and flush.
25. Follow your facility's procedure for cleaning the bedpan or urinal.
26. Remove and dispose of your gloves.
27. Wash your hands.
28. Put the clean bedpan or urinal and cover back into the bedside table.
29. Assist the resident with handwashing.
30. Make the resident comfortable. Lower the head of the bed as necessary and replace the call signal.
31. Wash your hands.
32. Report and record when a specimen is collected and any unusual observations.

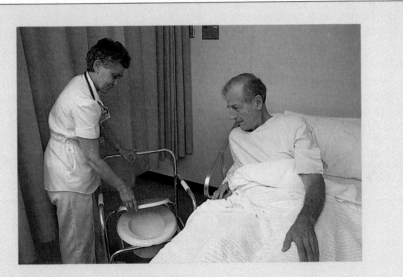

18. Follow the procedures for cleaning the bedpan in your facility.
19. Remove and dispose of your gloves.
20. Wash your hands.
21. Put the clean bedpan back in the bedside table. Put the commode in its proper place.
22. Assist the resident with handwashing.
23. Make the resident comfortable, lower the head of the bed as necessary, and replace the call signal.
24. Wash your hands.
25. Report and record if a specimen was collected and any unusual observations.

Assisting the residents to practice good hygiene following urination and defecation is very important in preventing urinary tract infections. The female resident is much more likely to develop infection than the male, due to the shortness of her urethra. It is easier for bacteria to travel up the short urethra into the bladder and kidneys. For residents who provide their own care, help them remember:

- Always wipe from front to back after urination and defecation.
- Wash the perineal area thoroughly with soap and water when bathing.

Some residents have indwelling catheters (Fig. 10-12). Catheters may only be inserted on the orders of a physician. An indwelling catheter is a tube inserted through the urethra into the bladder. It is used to drain urine from the bladder. The catheter is connected to the drainage tubing, allowing the urine to flow uninterrupted into the urinary drainage bag or collection unit. This is called a **closed urinary drainage system.**

An indwelling catheter is often necessary for residents with neurological (nerve) injury following a stroke or spinal cord injury. These residents are unable to tell when the bladder is full and have no control of urination. Some incontinent residents may require a catheter to avoid tissue damage or skin breakdown resulting from constant exposure to urine. There is an increased risk of developing infection when a catheter is present (Fig. 10-13), so indwelling catheters should only be used when absolutely necessary. First you must understand where bacteria can enter the urinary drainage system. Contamination of any of these areas can lead to urinary tract infection.

The **indwelling catheter** (often referred to as a Foley catheter) is designed to be held in position in the bladder by an inflatable balloon located along the tip of the catheter. The catheter is inserted by a licensed nurse using strict aseptic technique and the balloon is inflated with sterile water so that it will not come out. Once a catheter is inserted, special catheter care must be given daily. There are some very important guidelines that must be understood and followed in order to provide safe care to residents with indwelling catheters.

FIGURE 10-12
A catheter with balloon.

FIGURE 10-13
Sites where bacteria can enter.

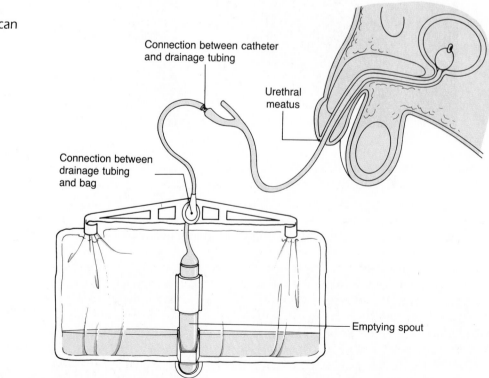

Connection between catheter and drainage tubing

Urethral meatus

Connection between drainage tubing and bag

Emptying spout

1. Assemble your equipment:
   - Antiseptic solution (packets)
   - Disposable bed protector (optional)
   - Disposable gloves
2. Wash your hands.
3. Identify the resident.
4. Provide privacy.
5. Explain to the resident what you are going to do.
   Note: Make sure that the genital/perineal area is clean. Provide perineal care as necessary prior to providing catheter care. See Chapter 6.
6. Place disposable bed pad under resident.
7. Observe the area around the catheter for lesions (sores), crusting, leakage, or bleeding. Report any unusual observations to your charge nurse immediately.
8. Open antiseptic solution packet.
9. Put on disposable gloves.
10. Remove the antiseptic applicator from the packet. Apply antiseptic solution around the entire area where the catheter enters the urethra. On female residents, gently separate the labia with your thumb and forefinger and apply the antiseptic solution. On the uncircumcised male resident, retract the foreskin and apply the antiseptic solution to the entire area.
11. Apply antiseptic solution to the 4 inches of catheter tubing nearest the resident.
12. Apply antiseptic ointment (if ordered) around the catheter tube at the urethra according to your facility's policies.
13. Position the resident so that the catheter and tubing are free of kinks or pulling.
14. Remove the disposable bed protector.
15. Cover the resident.
16. Discard disposable equipment.
17. Wash your hands.
18. Reposition and make the resident comfortable and replace the signal cord.
19. Wash your hands.
20. Report and record care given and any unusual observations.

Make sure that the catheter tubing and drainage tubing are free of kinks or obstruction. Many facilities use a strap that goes around the resident's thigh to secure the catheter and prevent pulling or sliding in and out of the urethra. The strap has a loop or Velcro fastener that attaches to the catheter tubing. The strap must not be so tight as to injure the skin or interfere with circulation. Always check the strap to be sure that it is not too tight or causing irritation of the skin.

Report to the charge nurse if there is any leaking around the catheter. This is often a sign of infection, bladder spasms, or obstruction. Observe for, report, and document any swelling, discoloration, skin irritation, or complaints of pain in genital or perineal area.

Measure and record urinary output as required as well as the color, odor, and appearance of the urine. As urine collects in the drainage bag and tubing, it begins to break down or decompose. Bacteria multiply very quickly under

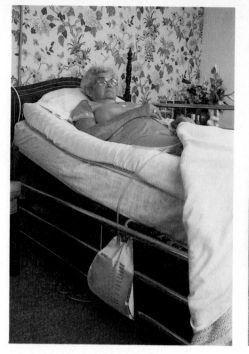

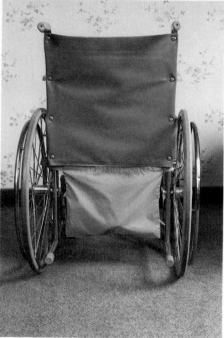

FIGURE 10-14
Positioning of catheter with resident
in bed.

FIGURE 10-15
Positioning of catheter with resident
in wheelchair.

these conditions. For this reason the collection bag must always be kept below the level of the resident's bladder (Fig. 10-14). This prevents urine collected in the bag from running back up the tubing and into the bladder. This is called **reflux.**

When the resident is in a wheelchair, the collection bag should be passed below or under the wheelchair seat and fastened behind the wheelchair at a point below the level of the resident's bladder (Fig. 10-15). There are special decorative bags available that fasten to the chair. The drainage bag slips into the container. Use of this type of container helps to protect the privacy and dignity of the resident.

If the resident is ambulating, carefully disconnect the tubing and collection bag from the bed or wheelchair. Fasten the coiled tubing and bag to the resident's clothing below the level of the bladder. It is important to drain the urine prior to ambulation.

The closed urinary drainage system should not be disconnected unless absolutely necessary. Each time the system is opened, the chance of infection increases greatly. If the system must be disconnected and a catheter plug used, follow aseptic technique while:

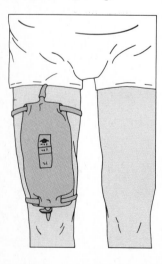

FIGURE 10-16
A leg drainage bag.

- Disconnecting the catheter from the tubing
- Inserting the sterile catheter plug
- Covering the drainage tubing with the sterile cap

The drainage collection bag and drainage tubing should never come in contact with the floor. The floor is always considered contaminated, and this equipment should be protected to avoid the possibility of infection.

Some residents, such as those who have spinal cord injury with neuromuscular loss of bladder control, may prefer to have their catheters attached to a leg drainage bag (Fig. 10-16). Notice that the leg drainage bag is positioned so that the inlet of the bag is at the top.

The straps are always attached to the collection bag prior to applying it to the resident's leg. They are applied next to the resident's leg. Review your facility's policy for emptying, cleaning, and storing leg bags if reusable bags are used.

When providing care to residents with indwelling catheters, you must:

- Make sure the system is open (urine is flowing into the collection bag). If the catheter becomes plugged with sediment or mucus, the licensed nurse must be notified immediately.
- Observe for decreased urinary output. This is a serious problem that must be reported to the charge nurse immediately. The normal healthy adult will produce between 1500 and 2000 cc in 24 hours (approximately 50 to 80 cc each hour).
- Make sure that the catheter tubing and drainage tubing are free of kinks or obstructions.
- Report to the charge nurse if there is any leaking around the catheter. This is often a sign of infection, bladder spasms, or obstruction.
- Observe for, report, and document any swelling, discoloration, skin irritation, or complaints of pain in genital or perineal areas.
- Measure and record urinary output as required as well as the color, odor, and appearance of the urine.

The entire urinary drainage system (catheter, drainage, tubing, and bag) should be changed together. If the drainage bag is changed by itself, strict aseptic technique must be followed.

Some residents with catheters have a physician's order to irrigate the catheter as necessary if drainage is slow or if it becomes obstructed. The irrigation order is carried out by a licensed nurse using strict aseptic technique. You can help the resident with a catheter by encouraging adequate intake of fluids. Many times irrigations or replacement of the catheter would be unnecessary if fluid intake were increased.

GUIDELINES FOR USE OF AN EXTERNAL CATHETER

Incontinent male residents may have a physician's order for the application of an external catheter (a condom connected to a tube that drains urine into a collection bag). The collection bag may be a leg bag for ambulatory residents or a urinary drainage bag.

An external catheter must be properly applied to prevent skin breakdown, cutting off circulation or closing off the urethra, leading to stopping the flow of urine. Use the following guidelines when applying the external catheter.

- Wear gloves.
- Wash and dry the penis.
- Special surgical adhesive may be used.
- Roll the condom over the penis, leaving 1/2 to 1 inch extending beyond the tip of the penis.
- Apply elastic tape spirally around condom and penis. Never completely encircle the penis, as this could interfere with circulation.
- Apply tape snugly enough to prevent leakage but not tight enough to restrict circulation.

Because the condom is flexible, it tends to twist around itself after application. The nursing assistant must check the resident with an external catheter frequently to ensure that the urine flow is not obstructed and there is no injury or cutting off of circulation. Usually, the external catheter is reapplied daily or more frequently if it is necessary.

The nursing assistant is usually responsible for the collection of urine specimens. It is very important to remember to wash your hands carefully before and after you collect specimens. One of the most frequently ordered tests is a urinalysis, which requires a routine urine specimen. Follow the procedure below when collecting a routine urine specimen.

COLLECTING A
ROUTINE URINE
SPECIMEN

1. Assemble your equipment:
   - Resident's bedpan and cover, or urinal
   - Disposable gloves
   - Graduate used for measuring output
   - Urine specimen container and lid
   - Label, if your facility's procedure is not to write on the lid
   - Laboratory request slip, which should be filled out by the charge nurse
   - Paper bag
2. Wash your hands.
3. Identify the resident by checking the identification bracelet.
4. Provide privacy.
5. Tell the resident a urine specimen is needed and explain the procedure. Some residents may be able to collect the specimen themselves.
6. Have the resident urinate into the clean bedpan or urinal.
7. Ask the resident not to put toilet tissue into the bedpan or urinal and to use the paper bag provided.
8. Prepare the label immediately by copying all necessary information from the resident's identification bracelet. Record the time and date.
9. Put on your gloves.
10. Take the bedpan or urinal to the resident's bathroom and pour the urine into a clean graduated container.
11. Pour urine from the graduate into a specimen container and fill it three-fourths full, if possible.

12. Place the lid on the specimen container. Check to ensure that the correct label is on the container.
13. Pour the leftover urine into the toilet and flush.
14. Clean and rinse the graduate. Put it in its proper place.
15. Clean the bedpan or urinal and put it in its proper place.
16. Remove and dispose of your gloves.
17. Wash your hands.
18. Make the resident comfortable and replace the signal cord.
19. Assist the resident in hand washing.
20. Take the labeled specimen container to the charge nurse.
21. Wash your hands.
22. Report and record that a specimen was obtained and any unusual observations.

A special method is used to collect a resident's urine when the specimen must be free from contamination. This kind of specimen is called a **midstream clean-catch** urine specimen. In most health facilities, a disposable midstream cleaning kit is available.

All the equipment, supplies, and instructions necessary for this type of specimen are found in the kit. Midstream means catching the urine specimen between the time the resident begins to urinate and the time urination stops. **Clean catch** refers to the fact that the urine is not contaminated by anything outside the resident's body. The procedure requires careful washing of the perineal area.

There are a number of ways to recognize abnormal function of the urinary system. You should be familiar with the following in order to report problems promptly.

- Inadequate urinary output — if resident does not void or voids very small amounts frequently, there is a serious problem that requires immediate attention
- Changes in color, consistency, and odor of the urine
- Poor skin turgor — the skin becomes limp or dry and nonelastic
- Fever, complaints of burning, frequency, urgency
- Unusual discharge, swelling, redness at the urethral opening
- Change in excretory habits — a continent resident becomes incontinent

The excretory function is very important. Be sure you observe carefully and report problems promptly!

SECTION 4 CARE OF THE INCONTINENT RESIDENT

OBJECTIVES/WHAT YOU WILL LEARN

When you have completed this section, you will be able to:
- Define the term *incontinence*
- List four possible causes of urinary incontinence
- Describe proper use of disposable briefs
- List four nursing measures that can increase a resident's chance of successful bladder retraining

CHAPTER 11

The Nervous System

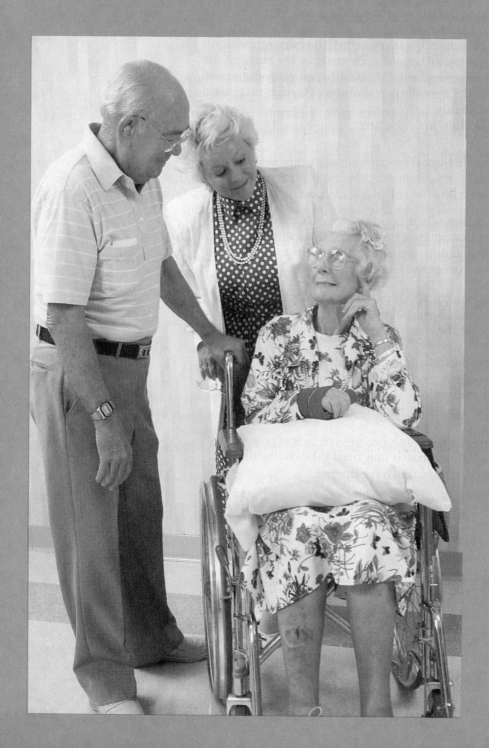

SECTION 1 ANATOMY AND PHYSIOLOGY

OBJECTIVES/WHAT YOU WILL LEARN

■ Describe two functions of the nervous system
■ Briefly explain how damage or disease of the nervous system differs from damage and disease of other body systems
■ Give the primary function of the four areas of the brain
■ Explain the basic function of the spinal cord

Level III,

THE NERVOUS SYSTEM

The nervous system (Fig. 11-1) consists of:

- The central nervous system
  — the brain
  — the spinal cord

- The peripheral nervous system *or Autonomic*
  — Thirty-one pairs of spinal nerves
  — Twelve pairs of cranial nerves

The nervous system controls and organizes all body activities. The nervous system and the endocrine system function together to maintain a balance among the various body activities. The nervous system is composed of billions of specialized cells called **neurons** (Fig. 11-2). The neuron is the most complex cell in the body, and it differs from other body cells in a very important way — it does not reproduce. If nerve cells or neurons are destroyed, they are not replaced.

Neurons and nerve fibers are present all over the body. Special types of neurons work together to carry out their important functions. Remember, it is the nervous system that coordinates and controls all of the body's activity. The nervous system makes it possible for you to speak, hear, taste, smell, see, think, act, learn, and remember.

One of the most important functions of the nervous system is to receive signals from inside or outside the body and send these signals to the brain. The brain interprets these signals and sends a message back to the appropriate body part or system.

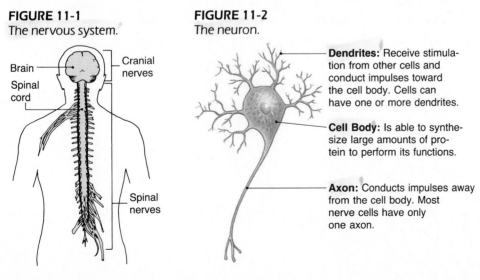

FIGURE 11-1
The nervous system.

Brain
Spinal cord
Cranial nerves
Spinal nerves

FIGURE 11-2
The neuron.

Dendrites: Receive stimulation from other cells and conduct impulses toward the cell body. Cells can have one or more dendrites.

Cell Body: Is able to synthesize large amounts of protein to perform its functions.

Axon: Conducts impulses away from the cell body. Most nerve cells have only one axon.

THE BRAIN

The brain is a very complex organ that has many functions. It is surrounded by the skull and in an adult weighs about 3 pounds. The brain is divided into specific areas, all of which have specialized functions (Fig. 11-3).

The **cerebrum,** in the upper portion of the skull, is divided into **hemispheres** or halves by a deep groove. The right hemisphere controls most of the activity on the left side of the body, and the left hemisphere controls most of the activity on the right side of the body. It is in the cerebrum that all learning, memory, and associations are stored. It is here, too, that decisions are made for voluntary actions. Certain areas of the cerebrum perform special activities.

- Occipital lobe — the place where what you see is interpreted
- Frontal lobe — the primary area of thought, reason, and speech
- Temporal lobe — the auditory (hearing) area
- Parietal lobe — the area for awareness of sensations of heat, cold, touch, pressure, and pain

The **diencephalon** is the area of the brain where a specialized structure (hypothalmus) exercises great control over the body's activities, including regulation of body temperature and the endocrine glands. This area screens all impulses going to the brain, either speeding them up or slowing them down.

The **cerebellum** is the part of the brain that coordinates voluntary movement. It is essential for normal movement and works with parts of the inner ear so that equilibrium (balance) is maintained.

The **midbrain, pons,** and **medulla** are primary pathways through which nervous impulses reach the brain from the spinal cord. The medulla is called

FIGURE 11-3
The brain.

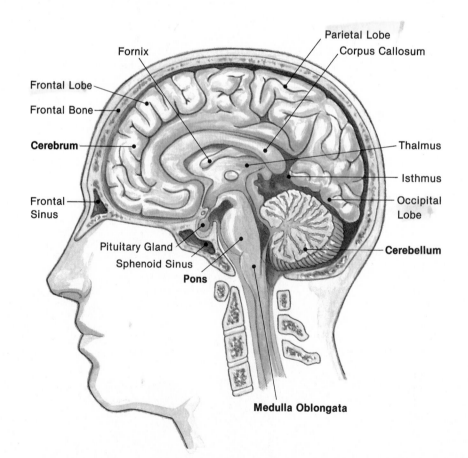

the "vital center" because it controls breathing, swallowing, sleep, and the heartbeat.

THE SPINAL CORD AND PERIPHERAL NERVOUS SYSTEM

The **spinal cord** is a long cable of nerves that extends from the area below the medulla to the level of the second or third lumbar vertebra (Fig. 11-4). The spinal cord serves to relay messages to and from the brain and is the center for reflex activity. **Reflexes** are automatic responses of the muscles or skin to stimulation. There is no thought involved. Most reflexes occur without a message going all the way to the brain. An example would be the knee-jerk reflex. When a doctor taps a particular area of the knee with a rubber hammer, the knee jerks.

The spinal cord is oval in shape and runs through the **vertebral column**. Thirty-one pairs of spinal nerves exit from successive levels of the spinal cord. These nerves have specific functions.

The peripheral nervous system consists of the 31 pairs of spinal nerves and 12 pairs of cranial nerves arising principally from the brain stem. The nerves of the peripheral nervous system have many branches, which extend to all parts of the body.

FIGURE 11-4
The spinal cord.

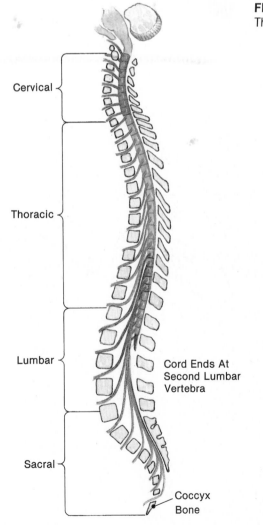

Cervical

Thoracic

Lumbar

Cord Ends At
Second Lumbar
Vertebra

Sacral

Coccyx
Bone

The peripheral nervous system has a special division called the **autonomic nervous system.** The autonomic division supplies structures and organs of the body not under voluntary control. Some examples of involuntary activities are:

- Digestion
- Heart beating
- Glands secreting

The autonomic nervous system has two divisions, the **sympathetic** and the **parasympathetic.** The neurons that make up the sympathetic division become active during stress, danger, excitement, or illness. These neurons cause the pupils of our eyes to become larger so that we can see more clearly. These neurons also cause the heart to beat more strongly and to send more oxygen to the large muscles of the body in case it is necessary to fight or run. Sometimes when we experience frequent or prolonged stress, the action of the sympathetic system causes changes in the structure or function of some of our vital organs, causing illness.

The neurons that make up the parasympathetic division are in control when we are relaxed or when we are sleeping. They help us conserve energy.

We are fortunate that there is a check and balance system between the two divisions; when one has been active for too long, the other automatically switches on. The autonomic nervous system plays a vital role in maintaining homeostasis.

ABNORMALITIES OF THE NERVOUS SYSTEM

in aging

After age 25 there is a gradual and steady loss of neurons. In general these losses do not cause changes in behavior or performance unless disease, injury, or nutritional deficiencies occur.

Cerebral vascular accident (CVA or stroke), organic brain syndrome, seizure disorders, Parkinson's disease, Alzheimer's disease, and multiple sclerosis are among the more common abnormalities of the nervous system. There are also many long-term care residents who have conditions that they were born with or that resulted from trauma at some other point in their lives. Examples are the developmentally disabled resident and residents who have sustained spinal cord or brain injuries. Because the nervous system is so highly specialized, each of these conditions affects people in a unique way. Not only is each condition or disease unique, but each person who has the condition or disease has particular signs and symptoms as well as specialized needs.

SECTION 2 THE RESIDENT WITH A NERVOUS SYSTEM ABNORMALITY

OBJECTIVES/WHAT YOU WILL LEARN

When you have completed this section, you will be able to:
- List three common symptoms of Parkinson's disease
- Describe the nursing care of the resident with Parkinson's disease
- Identify the age group most often affected by multiple sclerosis
- Describe why the nature of multiple sclerosis makes adjustment more difficult for the victim
- Define the terms *remission* and *exacerbation* in relationship to multiple sclerosis
- Define the terms *paraplegic* and *quadriplegic*

- Give one example of how spinal cord injury affects each of the body systems
- Describe the measures to be taken when the emergency called "autonomic dysreflexia" occurs
- Explain the nature of a CVA or stroke
- Select a stroke victim and write a case study
- List four tips for improving communication with the aphasic resident
- Identify five conditions that increase the frequency of seizures
- Identify which statements about epilepsy are true and which are false
- Describe emergency measures to be taken when a resident experiences a seizure
- Define the term *chronic brain syndrome*

PARKINSON'S DISEASE

Parkinson's disease is a disease of the brain that usually occurs in people in middle to later life. It progresses slowly and does not shorten life. The intelligence is not affected. The typical symptoms are:

- Rigid muscles
- Tremor (shaking)
- Weakness

These symptoms combine to cause the following problems:

- Difficulty swallowing, which results in drooling as well as eating problems and weight loss.
- Speech problems; speech is very slow and without expression.
- Constipation.
- Difficulty moving.
- Difficulty in ambulation. The typical resident with Parkinson's walks with body leaning forward on tiptoes. The steps taken are very small. The speed increases to the point where the person has trouble stopping. Falls are common.
- Lack of facial expression or "masklike" face.
- Depression due to loss of ability to function normally.

Although no cure is known, many residents receive medications to reduce or control their symptoms. Nursing care is directed toward preventing complications and managing the disabilities resulting from the condition.

The following chart indicates common problems, goals of care, and nursing measures to be followed with a resident who has Parkinson's disease. This is not a plan of care as you studied earlier because it does not consider each resident's individual problems and needs. In addition, the goals described are nursing goals rather than resident goals.

CARE OF RESIDENTS WITH PARKINSON'S DISEASE

Problem	Goal of Care	Nursing Care
Drooling	Protect the skin from breakdown	Keep skin clean; apply protective cream or ointment
Slowness in eating	To provide adequate nutrition	Keep food from becoming cold by using warming dish. Give time enough to eat. Assist with finishing, if resident becomes too tired.
Difficulty speaking. Speech very slow and without expression	To establish communication	Be patient! Take time to listen. Do not ignore.

Problem	Goal of Care	Nursing Care
High risk for contractures	To prevent contractures	Encourage self-care; give range-of-motion exercises.
Constipation	To eliminate constipation	Encourage to take fluids. Encourage intake of roughage in diet (fruits, vegetables, cereals).
High risk for falls, due to propulsive gait	To prevent falls	If assisting to ambulate, walk in front or have resident push a straight chair. May use pick-up walker. Encourage to stand as straight as possible.
Depression, shown by withdrawal from contact with others	To decrease depression	Promote self-care. Spend time with resident. Encourage to talk about feelings. Listen.

MULTIPLE SCLEROSIS

Multiple sclerosis, or MS as it is often called, is a chronic degenerative disease of the nervous system. In MS there is a destruction of the insulating material, or **myelin,** that surrounds the nerve fibers. Multiple sclerosis is neither hereditary nor contagious, and although it may cause severe disability, it does not usually shorten life.

MS is called "a disease of young adults" because it usually begins between the ages of 20 and 40. At the present time, no cure is known and the cause is still unknown. About 250,000 people in the United States have been diagnosed as having MS. There is no particular laboratory or X-ray test that will establish that the disease is present. The physician usually makes the diagnosis by eliminating other possibilities and by studying the symptoms described by the person over a period of time.

Symptoms include:

- Lack of coordination
- Visual disturbances, such as double vision, blind spots, blurriness, loss of color vision
- Difficulty in speech
- Bowel and bladder disturbances
- Paralysis
- Loss of sexual functioning
- Weakness
- Tremors
- Array of unusual sensations, such as numbness, tingling, burning

Only rarely are there mental disabilities. The intelligence is not affected. Some MS victims experience mood changes, which cause them to be chronically depressed or constantly **euphoric** (experiencing an exaggerated feeling of well-being).

The symptoms tend to come and go for no apparent reason. One of the characteristics of MS is that although there is usually steady deterioration, the course is one of **remission** (symptoms go away) and **exacerbation** (symptoms return). This fact makes MS victims particularly vulnerable to rumors of magic cures. Since symptoms seem to disappear for no apparent reason, it is difficult to connect a particular treatment with remission of symptoms.

There are some things that seem to cause a return of symptoms. They include infections of any kind, especially respiratory (colds, pneumonia) and bladder infections, and very warm weather, fatigue, stress, and anxiety. The MS victim is so sensitive to heat that a hot bath may cause return of symptoms, including weakness that prevents them from getting out of the bathtub.

Some special emotional or psychological factors are common with MS. Some of these problems have to do with the difficulty in determining the diagnosis and the lack of predictability about the course of the disease. The MS victim is unable to make plans for the future. He or she may become depressed due to loss of control and the need to be more dependent on others.

Most MS victims continue to live outside institutions. Usually, those seen in LTC facilities are those whose symptoms have progressed to a point where they require nursing care. It is important to remember that you may be caring for those who are most severely affected.

Nursing care of the resident with multiple sclerosis must be individualized due to the great variety of symptoms. The goals include prevention of complications of inactivity (contractures, pressure sores, pneumonia, kidney and bladder infections, and kidney and bladder stones) and helping the person to be as independent as possible for as long as possible.

SPINAL CORD INJURY

Every year more than 10,000 people experience injury to the spinal cord. About 85 percent are men between the ages of 18 and 25. Most spinal cord injuries result from automobile, motorcycle, and sports injuries.

Injury to the spinal cord is one of the most catastrophic events that can affect the human body. Because of the fact that cells within the nervous system do not repair themselves, spinal cord injury is permanent. Scientists are looking for a way to repair injured spinal cord tissue, but they have not been successful so far.

In describing a person with a spinal cord injury, the terms *quadriplegic* and *paraplegic* are used. A **quadriplegic** has paralysis of all four limbs and the trunk of the body. A **paraplegic** has paralysis of the lower limbs and lower trunk. The part of the spinal cord that is injured determines the amount of paralysis. The term **level of injury** identifies the location of the injury in relationship to the vertebrae that surround the cord. There are seven cervical, twelve thoracic, five lumbar, five sacral (fused into one sacrum), and five coccygeal vertebrae (fused). The level of injury will be stated in the diagnosis such as "quadriplegia, C-5 (cervical 5)" or "paraplegia with injury at the L-1 (lumbar 1) level."

Other important terms are *complete* and *incomplete.* These terms describe the degree of damage to the cord itself. If complete, all functions below the level of injury are lost. If incomplete, some functions may be retained.

Since the spinal cord acts as a relay station, sending impulses or messages to and from the brain, injury causes this process to stop. The impulses from the brain to the rest of the body include impulses for fine skillful movement, balance, respiration, and flexor motor activity.

The impulses from the rest of the body to the brain that can be lost include:

- Pain
- Temperature
- Pressure
- Touch
- Vibration
- Knowledge of location of body parts (called **proprioception**)

INITIAL TREATMENT OF SPINAL CORD INJURIES

The first phase of medical treatment of a spinal cord injury is emergency life-saving care. For about the first six weeks after injury, a condition known as spinal shock exists. During this time, all function below the level of injury is lost, including reflex activity. The paralyzed limbs are **flaccid** or limp. The bladder, the bowel, and the sexual organs are also paralyzed and flaccid. All sensation below the injury is also lost. Due to injury to the autonomic nervous system, the blood pressure is low, there is no perspiring below the level of injury, and there is decreased activity in the gastrointestinal tract.

Once spinal shock has subsided, there is a return of reflex activity below the level of injury. This is involuntary movement, which may give the victim false hopes of a return of voluntary activity. Many times the reflexes are overactive or **hyperactive,** which is shown by **spasm** (sudden uncontrolled jerking movements). These spasms may be so strong that they cause the individual to fall out of a wheelchair or off the toilet. Spasms can be started by touching the bottom of the feet of the paralyzed person such as during dressing or bathing or when placing the feet on the wheelchair pedals.

Individuals who sustain a spinal cord injury have the best chance of recovery when they receive immediate treatment from a physician who is knowledgeable and experienced in treating spinal injuries. There are some medications and treatments that can decrease the damage to the spinal cord if administered promptly.

When a paraplegic or quadriplegic is admitted to an LTC facility, the acute phase of the injury will have passed and some rehabilitation may have begun. Nursing care is difficult and complex, requiring special knowledge and skill. The resident will often know more about the care required than the nursing staff. One important tip is to *listen* to the resident and allow him or her to participate fully in the care.

SPINAL CORD INJURY EFFECTS

Every system of the body is affected when a spinal cord injury occurs. The effects on each system and the required nursing care follow.

The Integumentary System

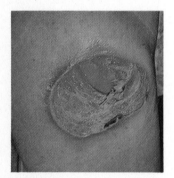

FIGURE 11-5
A pressure sore.

Due to immobility, the person with a spinal cord injury is at great risk for development of pressure sores (Fig. 11-5). Lack of sensation prevents awareness that a sore is developing, and the message to move or change position because of discomfort does not "get through" to the brain. Lack of ability to perspire below the level of injury interferes with the maintenance of body temperature. When the temperature outside the body goes up, the temperature inside the body does, too.

Nursing care of the skin not only involves keeping the skin clean, dry, and lubricated, but also includes pressure sore prevention measures. Tub baths are desirable because they improve circulation and reduce spasms. Since sensation may be absent, special care must be taken to avoid burns from hot bath water.

The Muscular System

Muscles that are not used **atrophy** (waste away). Below the level of injury, the paralyzed muscles will appear thin and lacking in bulk.

Nursing care related to the muscular system consists of passive range of motion and encouraging maximum independence in activities of daily living.

Residents often exercise their unimpaired muscles in order to take over the work done by the paralyzed muscles. A paraplegic often has highly developed arm muscles even though the legs may be atrophied.

The Skeletal System

Inability to bear weight on the long bones leads to a loss of calcium. Bones become porous and are weakened. Fractures can occur with only slight trauma. Nursing care related to the skeletal system includes gentle turning and repositioning as well as measures to prevent falls and injuries. Frequently, residents with a spinal cord injury will have a "standing frame" or long leg braces to allow them to bear weight on their legs in order to decrease the loss of calcium from the bones.

The Digestive System

The movement in the digestive system is slower and less efficient, leading to constipation. Lack of voluntary control contributes to the problem, making a bowel management program essential.

Residents are urged to eat a high-protein diet with ample bulk. High fluid intake is needed to reduce constipation. In addition, the routine for bowel management may include use of rectal stimulation from a lubricated, gloved finger, a suppository, or occasional enemas. As a rule, frequent enemas tend to stretch the bowel and cause it to lose tone. Due to the chronic nature of the bowel problem, enemas are discouraged.

The Urinary System

The calcium that leaves the bones is eliminated through the kidneys and bladder. This increases the risk of kidney and bladder stones. The loss of control of urination requires the use of an indwelling catheter, external catheter, intermittent catheterization, or wearing of protective clothing. Some paraplegics empty the bladder by **crede** (pressing on the area of the abdomen over the bladder to push the urine out.) Regardless of the method used, the spinal cord injury victim is very likely to retain urine in the bladder and to develop infection. In fact, the most common cause of death of the spinal cord injured is kidney disease.

Nursing care related to the urinary system begins with encouraging a high intake of fluids. A young, otherwise healthy quadriplegic should consume about 3000 cc of liquid every 24 hours. This individual may require catheter care to prevent infection if an indwelling catheter is used. Use of external urinary devices of a "Texas catheter" requires thorough care of the skin of the penis as well as frequent observation for impairment of circulation.

The Nervous System

Damage to the nervous system includes paralysis and loss of sensation. In addition to the inability to move independently, the resident is at risk for injury because of lack of ability to recognize pain, temperature, and location of body parts. The person might burn himself with a cigarette or spill a hot liquid and never know it. He may be positioned in a way that restricts the circulation to a part of his body and not notice until damage has been done. Nursing care focuses on protecting the person from harm through careful observation and monitoring.

The Cardiovascular System

The blood tends to pool due to the effects of inactivity and gravity. There is a greater risk of blood clot formation, and the person often experiences low blood pressure **(hypotension),** rapid pulse, and fatigue. Hypotension occurs most often when the person is sitting upright and may even cause loss of consciousness or fainting.

Nursing care to prevent hypotension includes gradual raising of the head of the bed to increase tolerance, use of antiembolic (TED) stockings or elastic bandage wraps, and with some individuals, use of a corsetlike abdominal binder. When the resident loses consciousness and is up in the wheelchair, simply pull the chair back against your body, tilting it at an angle. This will raise the blood pressure and return consciousness. If the resident is in bed, lower the head of the bed to raise the blood pressure.

The Respiratory System

If the level of injury is above the T-7 (thoracic 7) area, the respiratory muscles can be involved. Breathing is shallow, and the resident has difficulty in coughing. Combined with inactivity, this increases the risk for pneumonia.

The nursing assistant can help prevent respiratory complications by repositioning the resident and by encouraging deep breathing and coughing. Some quadriplegics are unable to cough or sneeze. There is a technique for assisting these residents to cough by applying manual pressure to the diaphragm. The resident will probably be able to instruct you. This should not be attempted without supervision from a licensed nurse.

The Reproductive System

Men with spinal cord injury are seldom able to father children. Generally speaking, a quadriplegic has erections that are reflex in nature. That is, the penis will become erect when stimulated physically, but not psychologically. There is rarely an ejaculation. Pleasurable sensations are experienced only above and at the level of injury, not below.

Paraplegics, particularly those injured at the lumbar level (L-1) or below, often have no erections. Although sexual intercourse may not be possible, they experience the same pleasure of closeness and intimacy as they did before they were injured. There are surgical procedures available called penile implants that either keep the penis permanently erect or have inflatable parts. Although this would permit intercourse, it cannot provide an ejaculation.

Some paraplegics and quadriplegics have injuries that are incomplete, that is, the spinal cord is not completely severed. They may have erections and ejaculations.

Women with spinal cord injury are still able to become pregnant and bear children. They usually do not experience orgasms but, like men, experience other physical and psychological pleasure.

SPINAL CORD EMERGENCY

The spinal cord-injured victim may experience an emergency condition called **autonomic dysreflexia.** This condition is *life-threatening* and results in severe high blood pressure. Causes are stimuli from the skin, the bowel, and the bladder. When the bladder is full, when there is trauma to the skin, or when the bowel is full, the body overreacts, resulting in dysreflexia. The person experiencing dysreflexia develops headache, goose pimples, sweating of the face, and stuffy nose. The blood pressure increases, and the heart rate slows.

This is an emergency and must be acted upon immediately! Treatment includes raising the resident's head (to lower the blood pressure) and finding and removing the cause. Commonly, the catheter is kinked or plugged, an arm or leg is positioned poorly or caught between the bed and side rail, or a fecal impaction exists. Appendicitis, kidney stones, and bowel obstruction can also cause dysreflexia. Report any signs of dysreflexia to the charge nurse immediately. When a resident complains of dysreflexia, believe him!

REHABILITATION OF THE SPINAL CORD INJURED RESIDENT

Rehabilitation consists of preventing complications and helping the individual to learn to cope with his disability. The resident is taught as much as possible about his or her condition and how best to live with it. The resident who has spent time in a rehabilitation program is usually very well informed. As in all rehabilitation, maximum independence is the goal. The resident should be given as much control as possible over his life. This person may exert his control by directing the nursing assistant in every activity he or she performs. It is best to accept his need for control and do things the resident's way whenever possible.

CEREBRAL VASCULAR ACCIDENT

The term **cerebral vascular accident** (CVA) means stroke. Stroke is the third leading cause of death in the United States. About 2 million persons in the United States are living with disabilities caused by stroke.

Stroke is caused by bleeding in the brain or by existence of a blood clot in a blood vessel of the brain (Fig. 11-6). This clot may originate in the brain **(thrombosis)** or travel to the brain from elsewhere in the body (called an **embolus**). Usually, the person has high blood pressure and arteriosclerosis, which increase the risk of stroke. Stroke or CVA is actually a disease of the circulatory system but is discussed here because the results of stroke affect the nervous system profoundly.

The type of symptoms and their severity are determined by the location of the problem and the amount of brain tissue destroyed due to lack of oxygen and other necessary nutrients. For our purposes, we will deal with some common results of stroke.

Frequently, the stroke victim is left paralyzed on one side of the body. This is called **hemiplegia.** Depending on whether the person's left or right side is

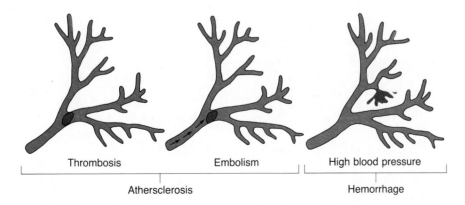

FIGURE 11-6
Mechanisms of stroke.

Thrombosis   Embolism   High blood pressure

Atherosclerosis   Hemorrhage

paralyzed, we use the term *left hemiplegia* or *right hemiplegia.* In addition to paralysis, sensation can be lost. This includes loss of ability to feel heat, cold, pressure, and pain in the areas affected. Some individuals seem to forget the paralyzed side and fail to dress, apply makeup, shave, or groom that side.

When the face is involved, there may be drooping of the eyelid or inability to close the eyelid. The eye may become dry and irritated because of decreased or absent tearing. There are often accompanying losses of vision in the affected eye. Drooping of the muscles on one side of the face may cause drooling on that side. There may be problems in chewing and swallowing on the affected side. There is often an inability to feel the food on the paralyzed side, which increases the risk of burns, choking, and accumulating food in the cheek.

Spasticity of paralyzed limbs can also occur. **Spasm** is an involuntary contraction of muscles. The stimulation of exercise or bathing and dressing may cause the muscles to spasm into a position of flexion or extension. Spasms are increased by nervous tension, cold temperature, and pain. This greatly increases the risk for contractures since the limb remains fixed in one position.

Paralysis of the arm and leg interferes with the ability to perform all activities of daily living, including eating, grooming, dressing, ambulation, and toileting. The inability to move increases the risk of contractures, pressure sores, pneumonia, urinary stones, and constipation.

Because certain brain fuctions are located only on one side of the brain, there are differences between individuals who have right brain injury (left paralysis) and left brain injury (right paralysis). It is important to know these differences so that your care can be most effective.

Right brain injury (left paralysis):

- Partial or complete paralysis of the left face, arm, and leg.
- Loss of, or changes in, sensation of pain, touch, and temperature on the left side. May not know location of body parts on the left side.
- Difficulty in judging size, distance, and rate of movement.
- May behave impulsively and unsafely. Tends to overestimate abilities.

Left brain injury (right paralysis):

- Partial or complete paralysis of the right face, arm, and leg.
- Loss of, or changes in, sensations of pain, touch, and temperature on the right side. May not know location of body parts on the right side.
- Loss of language (aphasia) may include speaking, understanding of speech, reading, and writing.
  Note: About 50 percent of left-handed people will not have loss of language with left brain injury because their speech area is on the right. That group may have loss of language when they have right brain injury.
- Tends to be very cautious and slow. Needs lots of encouragement to keep trying.

It has been estimated that out of every 100 people who survive a stroke, 10 will have no impairment, 40 will have mild disability, 40 will be severely disabled, and 10 will need institutional care. Some residents may experience significant recovery with a return of function, while others must learn to adapt to a permanent disability.

NURSING CARE OF THE RESIDENT WITH A CVA

Nursing care of the resident with a cerebral vascular accident is aimed toward protection from injury, prevention of disability, and achieving the maximum independence possible for the individual.

Protection from injury involves:

- Eye care. The eye may be taped shut, and a patch may be worn. Physician may prescribe eye drops.
- Supervision of feeding to prevent choking. Place food on unaffected side of mouth. Check mouth after meals to be sure food is not stored in the paralyzed side.
- Prevention of facial skin breakdown from drooling. Wash and dry gently. Use protective skin creams.
- Supervision of shaving and grooming. Absence of sensation may cause the resident to omit shaving or grooming the paralyzed side or to keep shaving over and over the same place, causing a burn or skin damage.
- Assist with ambulation to prevent falls. Lack of vision on affected side may cause falls or bumping into objects.
- Supervision of bathing to prevent falls and burns from water that is too hot. The ability to perceive temperature can affect judgment about how hot the shower or bath is.

Prevention of disability involves:

- Positioning in proper alignment using trochanter rolls, hand rolls, foot boards, and foot cradles to prevent contractures. Special positioning splints are often used to prevent contractures of the wrist and fingers.
- Providing good skin care to prevent pressure sores. This includes repositioning, keeping skin clean and lubricated, using pressure-reducing devices, and preventing injury.
- Giving passive range-of-motion exercises to strengthen and prevent contractures.
- Providing food and fluids to prevent bowel and bladder complications, such as constipation and dehydration. Food should be adequate in calories to meet needs and should include the four basic food groups, with sufficient protein, vitamins, and roughage.
- Preventing withdrawal and loss of hope by treating each individual as a unique, worthwhile person with potential to improve. Louis Pasteur, the famous French scientist of the 1800s, carried on most of his work after suffering a major stroke.

Achievement of maximum independence for the person who has suffered a stroke involves:

- Encouraging involvement in care through decision making and doing as much of the care as possible.
- Teaching self-care techniques such as how to feed, groom, bathe, and dress oneself.
- Obtaining special self-help devices for the stroke resident. These devices allow the resident to be more independent.
- Providing an environment where independence is praised and encouraged.
- Giving the resident time to do things.
- Enhancing ambulation and function through use of braces and splints (Fig. 11-7). These devices are used to stabilize the paralyzed limb. They are prescribed and fitted by specialists.

Self-help devices can be a great aid to the stroke victim. Some of these devices can be made by the staff or family while others may be purchased from medical supply companies. An occupational therapist is an excellent resource for recommending and obtaining self-help devices.

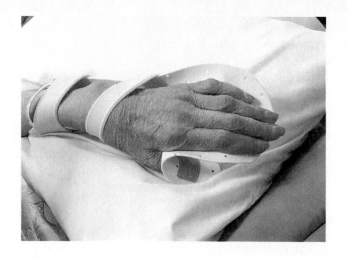

FIGURE 11-7
Positioning a splint.

EMOTIONAL REACTIONS TO STROKE

When individuals experience CVA or stroke, their lives change suddenly and drastically. The person grieves for the lost functions of the paralyzed limbs, loss of ability to communicate, loss of independence, loss of control over his or her life, and lost hopes and dreams for the future.

The denial, anger, depression, and eventual acceptance are often accompanied by emotional lability. **Emotional lability** is the overreaction to a stimulus. The person may burst into tears or laughter for no apparent reason. This is both frightening and embarrassing to the person, who may feel that he or she is going crazy. The nursing assistant must accept the behavior in a matter-of-fact way. Usually, it is best to ignore the inappropriate bursts of laughter or tears.

RESIDENTS WITH APHASIA

About one-fifth of adult stroke victims experience **aphasia.** The term *aphasia* refers to a loss of language. Aphasia occurs most commonly with the right hemiplegic, as the language area of the brain is on the left in most people. There are many types of aphasia. The resident may have difficulties in understanding what is heard, using numbers, reading, writing, or speaking. Some have difficulty in all these areas. Usually, automatic speech is retained. This means that the resident may swear or sing or use common phrases such as "yes," "no," "thank you," though not correctly or accurately. These words or phrases just come out automatically.

The ability to communicate is so important to our lives that the loss of this ability has severe effects on the resident. Anger, frustration, depression, and withdrawal are common responses. You must be able to recognize the problem in order to be most helpful. Probably the most important aspect of caring for the aphasic person is patience. Keep trying! Don't avoid the person or attempt to anticipate all her needs. Persons with aphasia usually need extra time to understand what is said and often take longer to express themselves. Speech may return completely or partially, but in either case, return takes work. Although a speech therapist may be involved, you, the nursing assistant, deal with the resident for longer periods of time on a continuous basis. You can make the difference!

Techniques for talking with an aphasic resident include:

- Get the attention of the resident before beginning to talk.
- Talk and work slowly.

- Use short sentences. Communicate one idea at a time.
- Repeat or rephrase instructions as often as necessary.
- Describe what you are doing as you perform tasks.
- Use body language (gestures, facial expression, tone of voice) to communicate your message.
- Try writing.

When listening to the resident, remember:

- Encourage writing or using a communication board if the resident is able (Fig. 11-8).
- Allow lots of time for a response.
- Avoid scolding the resident for swearing or making mistakes.
- Don't interrupt the resident when he tries to say something.
- Give clues to the words, instead of the words themselves.
- Trigger the word by saying the first sound. For example, "You want cr____ in your coffee." If the person can't find the word, tell her.
- Treat the person like an adult.

With patience and cooperation, communication may be established. Keys to communication with the aphasic resident should be written on the plan of care so that all staff can benefit from what is known to be effective with the individual resident.

SEIZURES

Seizures occur when a group of brain cells overreact, disrupting the normal conduction within the brain. The term *seizure* means "sudden attack." The individual has no control over the seizure, though some have a brief warning before the seizure begins. Seizures occur in all age groups. Sometimes the entire brain is involved; other times only part of the brain is involved.

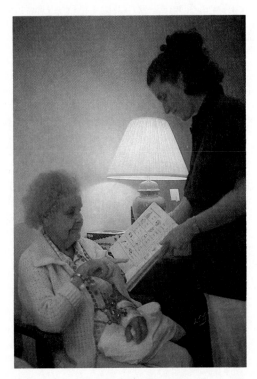

FIGURE 11-8
Using a communication board.

There are many causes of seizures:

- Injury before, during, or after birth
- Infection — **encephalitis, meningitis** (infection of the brain and surrounding membranes)
- High fever
- Pressure in the brain — from tumor or blood clot or bleeding
- Presence of toxic chemicals in the blood — poisons, drugs
- Lack of necessary substances, such as hormones, calcium, sugar

Everyone is capable of having seizures if their brain cells are irritated enough. There are several types of seizures. Some individuals experience more than one type.

Grand mal seizures include loss of consciousness followed by a **convulsion.** A convulsion consists of a tightening of the muscles (the tonic phase) followed by jerking movement (the clonic phase) of the arms and legs. There may be production of frothy saliva, and the person's color may change briefly due to lack of oxygen. There may be incontinence of bowel or bladder. Usually, the seizure lasts only 3 or 4 minutes and is followed by sleepiness, confusion, and headache. The person cannot remember the seizure.

Petit mal seizures are more common in children. The child does not fall but simply stares or stops whatever he or she is doing. There may be some jerking of a particular muscle group. All petit mal seizures end quickly and may occur many times each day.

Focal or Jacksonian seizures frequently begin as spasmodic movements of the hands, face, or foot and may spread to other areas of the brain, resulting in a grand mal seizure.

Psychomotor seizures usually consist of a temporary impairment of consciousness associated with loss of judgment or abnormal acts, but where automatic behavior, such as driving a car, typing, or eating, may continue as normal. As with all types of seizures, there is frequently an amnesia or no memory of the seizure.

When prone to seizures and no specific cause can be determined, a person is said to have **epilepsy.** Epilepsy can often be controlled by taking certain medications. There are many superstitions about epilepsy and those who have it.

The nursing assistant should know the facts about epilepsy:

- Epilepsy is not disfiguring.
- Epilepsy is not painful.
- Epilepsy does not shorten life.
- Epilepsy does not cause insanity.
- Epilepsy does not cause mental retardation or affect one's intelligence.
- Epilepsy is not contagious.

Many prominent individuals in the arts, science, and politics have had epilepsy. They have lived successful and productive lives.

In addition to taking the prescribed medication, the person with epilepsy can reduce the risk of seizures by avoiding these things:

- Illness of any type
- Lack of physical activity
- Fatigue
- Constipation
- Emotional stress

In an LTC facility, you will have residents who have epilepsy as well as those who might have a seizure due to tumor, stroke, or high fever. When a seizure occurs, it may frighten all concerned. It is important to rehearse the proper nursing actions.

NURSING CARE DURING A SEIZURE

The major concern is to protect the resident from injury. During a grand mal seizure, the jaw clamps down tightly. Because this results in an occasional biting of the tongue or cheek, "bite sticks" or padded tongue blades were used in the past. It has since been determined that the dangers of using the stick (injury to the teeth, choking, etc.) are greater than any possible benefits.

Do not leave the resident. There is no time. Use the call signal to summon help. Assist the person to lie down to prevent a fall. Move furniture out of the way to prevent injury. Protect the head with a pillow or other soft cushion. Never attempt to restrain the resident from moving. If possible, turn the resident to one side to allow secretions to drain from the mouth and nose.

Observe the seizure so that you can report the length, the presence of any warning, the part of the body where the seizure began, incidence of incontinence, and any injury. When the seizure is over, the resident should rest in bed. Side rails should be up at all times. Sometimes side rails may be wrapped with soft cloth to provide cushioning to prevent injury. Help the resident through the period of amnesia that may follow a seizure. Any seizures must be reported and recorded in the health record.

RESIDENT WITH DISEASE BRAIN SYNDROME

The term **brain syndrome** refers to a number of signs or symptoms that indicate brain disease is present. Other terms used to describe similar symptoms are dementia and senility. They include:

- Loss of memory
- Loss or decrease in orientation (awareness of person, place, time)
- Decrease in ability to do simple calculations
- Decrease in general information
- Impaired judgment

When these symptoms seem to be reversible or are able to be treated, the term *acute brain syndrome* is used. Acute brain syndrome may occur as the result of dehydration, high fever, pneumonia, or presence of infection. When the causing condition is treated, the symptoms leave.

When the symptoms are not reversible, they are said to be "chronic." The term used is *chronic brain syndrome.* Usually the symptoms develop slowly and gradually. Loss of cells in the cortex of the brain causes many of the symptoms. The cortex covers the entire brain and contains billions of cells. Each day we live, we lose many of these cells. Usually, the loss is not even noticed. Sometimes something happens that destroys large numbers of cells, such as an accident, poor health, malnutrition, stress, or diseases that cause high fever.

Two of the most common irreversible causes of mental impairment in old age are multiple minor strokes (called cerebral infarctions or multiple infarct dementias) and Alzheimer's disease. About 50 to 60 percent of all elderly persons with mental impairment have Alzheimer's disease. (See Section 3). Even though the disease is not reversible, such things as medication to reduce anxiety, agitation, and depression, proper nutrition, physical activity, and social contacts help improve the quality of life.

In order to diagnose the different types of dementias and brain syndromes, highly involved testing is required to measure the extent of memory loss, the ability to calculate, grasp of general knowledge, and orientation. Even then the physician may not be able to make a specific diagnosis.

ORIENTATION

Orientation refers to the ability to accurately describe person, place, and time. That is, most patients can state who they are or where they are and the day, date, and month. Many of us have experienced loss of orientation to place and time. When on vacation, we may forget the date or day of the week. When traveling to a new place, we might take a wrong turn or become lost. We are different from the disoriented resident, however, in our ability to find out rather quickly either the date or place. We might think back to a remembered date: "Let's see, Sunday was the twentieth so today, Wednesday, must be the twenty-third." If lost, we might notice a familiar street or landmark. Disoriented residents are unable to reorient themselves. The kinds of behavior seen will depend on the amount and type of brain damage, the personality of the individual, and the circumstances.

NURSING CARE OF RESIDENTS WITH CHRONIC BRAIN SYNDROME

Many residents are admitted to facilities because of chronic brain syndrome. Nursing care for them is directed toward providing a safe, caring, undemanding environment. This includes assistance in activities of daily living, assuring the intake of a nutritious diet, and providing for adequate rest. Other ways the nursing assistant can contribute to the well-being of the disoriented resident are communicating with the resident as care is given and encouraging the resident to do as much as possible for herself.

Those who wander from the facility present a special challenge. Because of your responsibility for protecting the residents from harm, they must not be permitted to leave alone. These residents must be checked on frequently. Some facilities have special alarms that ring or buzz when the doors are opened. It is not appropriate to restrain an individual just to prevent wandering. When a problem exists that jeopardizes the safety of the resident, a transfer to a locked facility may be the best solution.

Nursing care of the resident with chronic brain syndrome is based on the symptoms displayed. Whatever the type of brain syndrome involved, nursing care must be directed toward improvement of the symptoms and avoidance of any actions that would make them worse.

SYMPTOMS OF CHRONIC BRAIN SYNDROME

Symptom	Nursing Care
• *Lack of orientation to time*	Include time when talking with the resident. "It's 11:30, almost time for lunch!" Have clocks with large numbers available. Day of week and date announced daily on intercom. Calendars available.
• *Lack of orientation to place*	Name outside the door. Way to recognize own room. Remind where he or she is. Reality orientation board prominently placed.
• *Lack of orientation to person*	Address by name. Introduce self as often as needed.
• *Poor memory*	Repeat information as often as necessary in a pleasant tone of voice. Provide memory clues — "Remember me? I'm Susan, I took care of you yesterday."

Symptom	Nursing Care
• *Lack of judgment*	Provide a safe environment. Observe frequently in case resident wanders from facility.
• *Poor understanding*	Repeat information in simple terms. If one statement isn't understood, restate in a different way.
• *Changes in mood*	Provide consistency in the way you relate to the resident. Avoid reacting to the mood change. Continue to be pleasant and kind despite the resident's mood change.

REALITY ORIENTATION

The person who is disoriented needs an environment that has little change. Room changes should be avoided. If possible, the same staff members should care for the resident all the time. Such items as clocks and calendars should be available and prominently displayed. Sometimes it is helpful to identify the resident's room and bed in a special way. The physical layout of many facilities is confusing even to the staff! In these cases, a picture by the door or a large red bow, for instance, will single out a particular room.

The way you communicate with the resident is extremely important. Despite the resident's unusual or childlike behavior, always show respect. One way we show respect is by avoiding teasing or "playing along" with the disorientation. Residents may have a doll, for instance, that they refer to as their "baby." This baby may have a name and daily routines. Although the resident may never overcome the attachment to the doll, you must never add to the disorientation by saying "How is your baby today?" or "May I hold your baby?"

The concept of **reality orientation** is controversial at the present time. Reality orientation was developed by people working with elderly, mentally ill residents. Some say the results at bringing residents back to reality have been poor. The techniques of reality orientation must be practiced by all staff 24 hours a day. *Repetition is the key.* The disoriented resident usually attends a "class" daily during which the day, date, time, weather, place, and person's name are given repeatedly (Fig. 11-9). The information is also written and posted prominently in the facility.

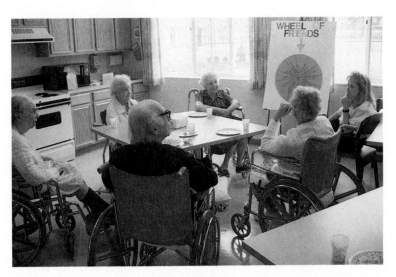

FIGURE 11-9
Using a reality orientation board.

Nursing staff remind residents frequently of who they are, where they are, and the date. Incorrect remarks made by the resident are corrected. For example, "No, Mr. Smith, your wife is not here. She died several years ago." Through consistency and repetition, the resident is supposed to regain orientation. Regardless of whether one believes that the person can regain his or her previous level of orientation, it would certainly never be appropriate to do anything that added to the existing disorientation. The attitude taken should be one of firm kindness. If the resident becomes angry or agitated when attempts are made to correct false statements, it may be best to simply ignore the statements.

Current research indicates that there are many benefits to the elderly when reminiscence therapy is used. *Reminiscence* is defined as "the act or habit of thinking about or relating to past experiences." The benefits include reducing loneliness, helping the person feel better about him or herself, and creating a positive attitude toward life. Most elderly residents conduct a type of life review in which they evaluate their past experiences and accomplishments and decide whether or not they reached their life goals. They often take great pleasure in talking about their life experiences. The nursing assistant can assist the resident in reminiscing by showing interest, asking questions, and listening.

SECTION 3 THE RESIDENT WITH ALZHEIMER'S DISEASE AND DEMENTIAS OF THE ALZHEIMER'S TYPE

OBJECTIVES/WHAT YOU WILL LEARN

When you have completed this section, you will be able to:
- Select the correct definition of Alzheimer's disease
- Identify which statements are true and which are false about Alzheimer's disease
- Categorize symptoms of Alzheimer's disease into appropriate stages of the disease
- Identify the three most important considerations when providing care to an Alzheimer's disease resident
- List four factors that worsen the behavioral problems in an Alzheimer's disease resident

Alzheimer's disease (AD) is an incurable disease affecting the brain. It is the most common cause of progressive *dementia* in older adults. **"Dementia"** means deprived of reason, mentally deteriorated. Alzheimer's is the fourth leading cause of death in the United States of those over 75, and it affects an estimated 1.5 million Americans. Projections indicate that by the year 2040, one in every three families will be directly touched by this devastating disease.

Several diseases can cause dementia besides Alzheimer's disease. They include:

- Huntington's disease
- Multi-infarct dementia
- AIDS-related dementia

These diseases of the brain may affect residents in different ways; however, loss of recent (short-term) memory, confusion, and lack of reasoning and poor judgment are the most common indicators (Fig. 11-10).

The deterioration of the brain seen in the AD resident is not part of the normal aging process. AD is more common in people over 65, but it also occurs in middle-aged and younger persons. It is a terminal illness that affects more women than men and is more common in countries where the life expectancy is longer. It was first identified by a German pathologist, Dr. Alois Alzheimer, and bears his name.

Current research supports the theory that a *genetic* (inherited) mechanism is evident in the development of Alzheimer's disease. There are also, however, many cases of Alzheimer's disease where there is no previous history of the disease within the family. There is no easy way to diagnose AD except by examining brain tissue after death, so diagnosis is done by excluding all other causes of curable and incurable memory loss.

During the course of the disease, the nerve cells in the brain that control memory, thinking, and judgment are damaged. There is disruption in the ability of nerve cells to transmit messages to one another, and one theory suggests that certain substances (called neurotransmitters) necessary for this transmission to occur are missing in AD victims. If you think of the brain as the body's master switchboard that processes information, receives calls, and sends calls, you can understand the result if the switchboard were to become defective and inoperable on certain lines; this is what happens to the AD resident.

The most important symptom in AD is memory loss for recent events. Memory impairment becomes so severe that the resident is eventually unable to carry on a conversation, follow a line of thought, or even recognize loved ones. This progressively devastating disease is unlike most other terminal illnesses where physical deterioration is the primary concern. The AD victim suffers a kind of psychological death — it is the personality of the AD victim that is lost. Once the AD resident's personality and memory deteriorate, the qualities that make each person a unique individual are gone. The AD resident is unable to provide necessary input which is essential to sustain any healthy relationship. The "loss of the person" while the body is physically intact is one of the most difficult adjustments for families and loved ones.

The entire health care team should be involved in providing information and support to the family and loved ones. There are community support groups (Alzheimer's Disease and Related Disorders Association, 1-800-621-0379), and many facilities offer special programs for families of the AD victim. The nursing assistant can offer the most important support to families and loved

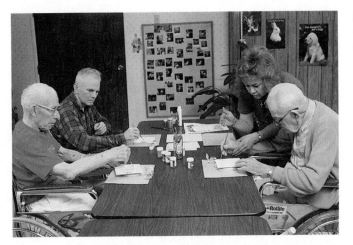

FIGURE 11-10
Residents in Alzheimer's unit.

ones by providing the resident with the best possible care. As they have to cope with their loss and grief, there is a lessened burden when they know the resident is receiving professional, compassionate care. It is important to understand that AD affects people in different ways and people react differently and do not progress through the various stages with any kind of uniformity. In some, the deterioration is more rapid than others.

The stages listed below have been adapted (with permission from *Care of Alzheimer's Patients: A Manual for Nursing Home Staff* by American Health Care Association and Alzheimer's Disease and Related Disorder Association). The stages are only a basic road map of the course of the disease, with each person following a slightly different route and time frame.

First Stage

Two to four years; this stage leads up to and includes diagnosis. Its symptoms are:

- Recent or short-term memory loss, which begins to affect everyday activities and if working, job performance
- Difficulty concentrating
- Unable to remember what they were just told to do
- Confusion about place — gets lost going to and from familiar places and misplaces and loses things
- Loses spontaneity — spark or zest for life, seems disinterested
- Loses initiative — cannot start anything
- Mood/personality changes — anxious about symptoms, withdraws from others
- Has poor judgment, makes poor decisions
- Requires more time to perform/accomplish routine tasks, unable to organize, plan things, and follow through
- Has difficulty handling money, paying bills
- May have thoughts of persecution and/or inappropriate outbursts of anger

Second Stage

Two to ten years after diagnosis; this is the longest stage. Will require supervision and assistance. The second stage will include all of the symptoms of the first stage plus those listed below.

- Has increasing memory loss and confusion along with a much shorter attention span
- Loss of some perceptive responses, seeing, hearing, and touch
- Makes repetitive statements and/or movements
- Becomes restless, especially in late afternoon and at night
- Experiences occasional muscle twitching or jerking motions, unsteady gait
- Has difficulty with perceptual-motor problems, is unable to get into a chair easily, and may be unable to set the table or use familiar objects correctly
- Has trouble expressing self with the right words and will often make up stories to fill in the blanks
- Finds reading, writing, and working with number combinations very difficult
- May become suspicious, irritable, fidgety, silly, and subject to mood swings, especially tears
- Loses some basic impulse-control behaviors; may not want to bathe, may undress in public; may forget table manners

- Has weight fluctuation, usually gains and then loses weight; will eat other people's food; will forget when last meal was and gradually loses interest in food
- May see or hear things that are not there and will be convinced they are real
- Often gets fixed ideas about something that is not real or true; repeats things over and over
- Generally requires full-time supervision
- Difficulty speaking, unable to understand and carry on conversation

Third or Terminal Stage

One to three years; requires constant supervision. The third stage includes all the symptoms of the first and second stages plus those listed below.

- Cannot recognize family, or self in mirror
- Will lose weight even with a balanced diet
- Has very little ability to provide any self-care, such as dressing, eating, and toileting
- Loses the ability to communicate with words; may groan, scream, or make strange sounds
- May revert to behaviors such as putting everything into the mouth or touching everything
- Loses control of bowel and bladder functions
- May experience seizures, difficulty swallowing, skin breakdown, and infection as a generalized debilitation occurs
- Will become totally dependent and will sleep more; gradually, body functions decline until death occurs

CONTROLLING DIFFICULT BEHAVIORS

After reviewing the symptoms of AD, it is understandable that one of the greatest challenges in providing nursing care is to manage difficult and disruptive behavior. It is this behavior that prompts most families to seek placement in a long-term care facility.

It is helpful to remember that the AD resident is not deliberately difficult. The behaviors are a result of the disease, and the resident is often unable to control angry outbursts, irrational, or childish behaviors. Some researchers believe that difficult behavior is related to some type of discomfort and that agitated and combative behavior is always a reaction to a stimulus. Frequently, staff can only guess the event that might have triggered an episode. There is an element of trial and error that allows staff to determine "this works with Mr. ____" and "this seems to agitate him more." What is effective in reducing undesirable behavior in one resident may be totally ineffective with another. Remember, it is how the AD resident perceives the event that triggers the behavior.

Example: You may tell a resident that you are going to take him to the shower, but by the time you get there he has forgotten what you are going to do. Then as you start to undress the resident, he may perceive this as a type of assault and become combative.

The AD resident will often overreact or experience exaggerated responses to many situations. These disruptive reactions are referred to as "**catastrophic reactions**" (sudden changes from baseline behavior that are socially unacceptable). Four factors seem to worsen behavioral problems with AD residents:

Fatigue

Residents with dementia tend to get tired easily, and as they fatigue, they are less able to function. The nursing assistant should be alert to signs the resident is getting tired and should plan ways to help conserve energy. Scheduling naps or rest periods, and reducing time in activities are just a few of the ways to help the AD resident conserve energy and avoid fatigue.

Change of Routine or Environment

The resident with any type of dementia usually finds any kind of change very disruptive. Change requires residents to think about how to do things — the more they have to think about a task, the harder it is for them to accomplish the task. Residents with dementia initially tend to develop specific routines — they do things the same way, at the same time, everyday. This way, function is almost automatic. When routines are changed and disrupted, the resident may experience increased anxiety, leading to behavioral problems. Allowing residents to do things in their own way and minimizing changes in routine and environment are ways the nursing assistant can help the AD resident to avoid behavioral outbursts.

Too Much Stimulation

As dementia increases, the AD resident has trouble understanding and processing all kinds of external stimuli (sights, sounds). What they see is often misinterpreted, and what they hear is confusing and irritating. Sometimes areas where there is a lot of activity and/or sound will increase the AD residents' anxiety level. Common signs of increased anxiety include fidgeting, picking at clothing, wringing hands, pacing, and wandering.

The nursing assistant can help minimize noise and activity levels when disturbing to the AD resident. Reporting signs of stress and anxiety responses to the charge nurse early may help to avoid episodes of difficult or disruptive behavior. Sometimes medications are ordered to help reduce anxiety.

Family, loved ones, and staff need to understand that it is inappropriate to push the AD resident to perform. AD residents are initially aware of their loss of function or ability. When others challenge them to try harder, they are less able to perform. Pressures and demands that force the resident to think or concentrate on a function almost always result in failure. The more a resident with dementia concentrates or thinks about a task, the more impossible it becomes.

Asking a resident with AD to "try harder" is like asking an amputee to walk without a prosthetic device or assistance. The family and facility staff must become the assistance device and the memory prosthesis for the AD resident.

Physical Pain, Discomfort, and Reactions to Medication

Whenever behavior becomes different or disruptive, the charge nurse should be notified so that a determination can be made whether or not physical problems such as constipation, a full bladder, arthritic pain, upper respiratory, or urinary tract infection exists. Even mild discomfort can cause increased anxiety in the AD resident. Because some medications cause behavioral changes, the licensed nurse should be made aware of any changes in order to assess the resident's response to prescribed medications.

The following principles are generally helpful in dealing with a resident with difficult or disruptive behaviors:

- Remain calm, get the resident's attention, try to establish direct eye contact
- Touch the resident gently, take his/her hand, speak slowly using as few words as possible
- Keep communication clear and simple, speak slowly

- Patting, rocking, holding hands may help to calm the resident
- If a resident shrinks away from touch, refrain from touching
- Assure the resident that he or she is safe
- Try to redirect or distract his or her attention to a different, less upsetting focus: "Come outside for a walk"; "Sit down and talk with me."
- When possible, remove the resident from the immediate surroundings and take to a quiet, less stimulating environment; because short-term memory is impaired, just the change may cause the resident to forget the reason for the outburst
- Use a calm unhurried approach; do not make unnecessary demands on the resident
- Use reflective terms like "you seem upset" — allow the resident to express angry or hostile feelings as long as talking about them decreases the behavior; if this intensifies the behavior, try to distract the resident using familiar words or objects: "It is lunch time, let's go to the table"; "The picture has beautiful flowers"; "What is your favorite song?"
- Avoid approaching the resident from the side or behind, intrusions into what they think of as personal space is viewed as loss of control of their environment and may lead to aggressive behavior
- Reassure the resident when behavior is related to feelings of persecution: "You are safe, no one can hurt you"; "We would never keep you from visiting with your wife"; "Your dog is safe, he is with your daughter"
- Help out when you observe frustration building such as difficulty buttoning a shirt or dress: "May I help you with that?"
- Avoid verbal battles — never argue or scold the resident, for even though they may be confused they are able to experience feelings of shame and embarrassment; it is not helpful and will not change the undesirable behavior
  For example, when a resident takes things from another resident's room:
  Do not say: "You know this is not your room, you should never go into someone else's room!"
  Do say: "Take my hand, I will take you to your room."
- Observe and identify *patterns* of behavior with your charge nurse; look for events or circumstances that might lead to undesirable behavior; when this is possible, removing or eliminating these events can markedly decrease difficult behavior

Other common behaviors seen in many Alzheimer's residents are depression and **apathy** (a lack of feeling or interest in things). This is particularly true of residents in the earlier stage of the disease as they recognize that something is not right. Alzheimer's residents suffering from depression function below their real abilities and there is a constant feeling of withdrawal and sadness.

The following strategies may be helpful in caring for depressed or withdrawn behaviors.

- Report observations of depressed behavior to the charge nurse so that an assessment can be made to determine if medications might be helpful.
- Identify events that might cause feelings of worthlessness, sadness, or apathy.
- Encourage residents to talk with staff and others. Find opportunities to assist residents in developing social relationships.
- Listen — help residents feel comfortable in your presence. Show them you are interested in them by listening. Very often they will share their feelings with you.
- Do not deny their feelings. Don't try to "cheer them up." Respect the residents right to feel sad and offer your support and concern.
- Encourage the resident to become involved in activity programs and to do physical exercise as possible.

Recent years have shown a definite trend toward development of special treatment units designed specifically to meet the unique needs of AD residents. Many people believe that AD residents function better longer when they are in a separate environment where special programs are used to maximize their functional abilities.

Because Alzheimer's is an incurable, terminal disease, goals for care of the AD resident must be directed toward improving the quality of life. We can:

- Develop programs to maximize resident's functional abilities — keep them as independent and as much in control of their lives as possible for as long as possible.
- Design environments that promote mobility and independence while safeguarding the welfare and safety of the residents.
- Reduce the complexity of both the daily routines and environment so that residents can be as effective (successful) as possible each day.
- Recognize the uniqueness of each resident and ensure that all residents are treated with respect and dignity.
- Provide families with accurate information regarding the resident, the disease process, the plan of care, and the facility routines.
- Recognize the family's need for emotional support and understanding as they watch the deterioration and loss of their loved one each day.

Three of the most important considerations in providing care to the AD resident will be referred to as the three C's:

Caution: protect from physical harm.
Communication: provide a clear understanding by using simple terms.
Comfort: physical, emotional, and environmental.

Caring for AD residents and providing the necessary support to the families is one of the most challenging responsibilities of the nursing assistant!

Problem	Goal of Care	Actions/Approaches
High risk for falls due to unsteadiness.	Decreased incidence of falls, no injuries by ____ (date).	Properly fitted nonskid shoes. Remind to use hand rail. Close supervision.
Wanders and rummages through drawers, unable to find room.	Decreased intrusions into other residents rooms by ____. Will rummage in specially prepared drawer by ____.	Identify room with colored ribbon — tie some color to wrist band. Provide a rummaging drawer. Distract with other activities.
Weight loss due to inability/refusal to feed self and swallowing difficulties.	No decrease in weight by ____.	Report intake less than 80% to charge nurse. Offer substitutes. Offer finger foods. Change consistency of foods to resident's tolerance.
Inappropriate behavior and catastrophic reaction to various daily routines.	Decrease number of catastrophic reactions by ____.	Reduce noise. Reduce contact with crowds. Break down tasks into simple steps. Plan rest periods. Report symptoms of pain or discomfort.
Family distress at resident's inappropriate behavior.	Family verbalizes understanding of disease process and its effect on resident's behavior by ____.	Listen, allow family to express feelings. Refer problems or questions to charge nurse. Invite to family night.

CHAPTER 12

The Respiratory System

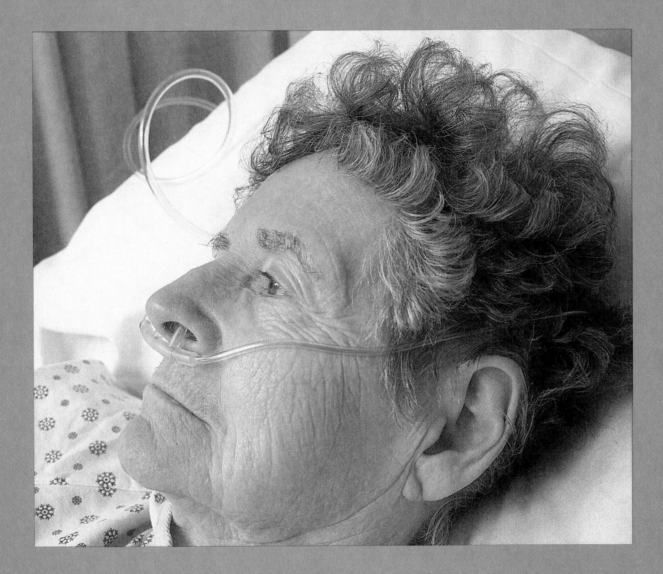

OBJECTIVES/WHAT YOU WILL LEARN

When you have completed this section, you will be able to:

■ Define the term *respiration*
■ Identify six major changes in respiratory function that would signal that a respiratory emergency exists
■ Describe the step-by-step procedures for removing airway obstruction (emergency choking)
■ Describe the step-by-step procedure for mouth-to-mouth ventilation (rescue breathing) and give the rate for delivering ventilations
■ List the three signs of cardiac arrest

RESPIRATORY SYSTEM

The respiratory system (Fig. 12-1) is composed of:

- Nasal cavity
- Oral cavity
- Pharynx
- Larynx
- Trachea
- Bronchi — right and left
- Bronchioles
- Alveoli
- Lungs — right and left
- Diaphragm

Functions of the respiratory system are to:

- Provide oxygen to the cells of the body
- Remove waste products in the form of carbon dioxide

The respiratory system provides a route or pathway for oxygen to get from the air into the lungs. In the lungs it is picked up by the blood and carried to the cells. The word **respiration** means an exchange of gases between an organism and the environment in which it lives.

The most vital work of the respiratory system is done at the cellular level, where the exchange of oxygen and carbon dioxide occurs. The respiratory system is mainly responsible for getting oxygen into the blood where it is carried to the cells of the body.

Breathing is regulated by a center in the medulla of the brain. If there is an injury or disease to this area, the respiratory function is affected.

The process of respiration consists of one inhalation (breathing in) and one exhalation (breathing out) (Fig. 12-2). Oxygen (O_2) is essential to life. When you inhale you take in air containing oxygen through the air passages into the lungs. Oxygen enters the blood through the millions of tiny air sacs called **alveoli** in the lungs.

The body uses this oxygen as well as food ingested as the fuel to supply energy for the activities of living. Carbon dioxide (CO_2) is formed as the waste product of the **metabolism** (breakdown) of food and oxygen at the cellular level.

The respiratory system is structured to help us keep the respiratory passages open at all times. The **trachea** and **bronchi** are kept open by incomplete cartilage rings that give structure to those important air passages.

The **larynx** or voice box contains the vocal cords that make speech possible. There is an important piece of cartilage that covers the opening to the trachea,

The airway consists of structures involved with the conduction and exchange of air. Conduction is the movement of air to and from the exchange levels of the lungs. Air enters through the nose (primary) and mouth (secondary) and travels down the pharynx to enter the larynx. After passing through the larynx, air enters the trachea. At its distal end, the trachea branches into the right and left primary bronchi. These bronchi branch into secondary bronchi, which then branch into the bronchioles. Some of the bronchioles end as closed tubes. Air movement in them helps the lungs expand. The rest of the bronchioles carry the air to the exchange levels of the lungs.

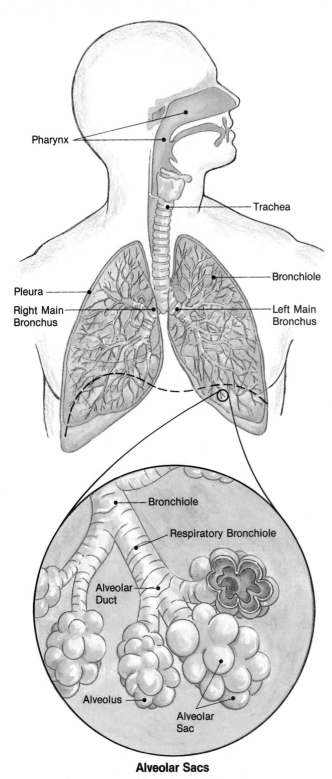

Pharynx

Trachea

Pleura

Right Main Bronchus

Bronchiole

Left Main Bronchus

Bronchiole

Respiratory Bronchiole

Alveolar Duct

Alveolus

Alveolar Sac

Alveolar Sacs

The respiratory bronchioles turn into alveolar ducts. These form alveolar sacs that are made up of the alveoli. Gas exchange takes place between the alveoli and the capillaries in the lungs.

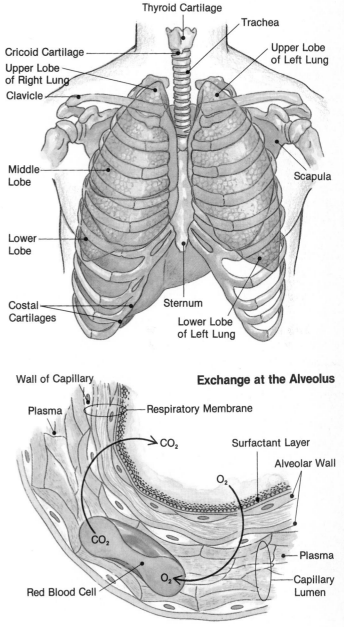

Thyroid Cartilage

Trachea

Cricoid Cartilage

Upper Lobe of Right Lung

Upper Lobe of Left Lung

Clavicle

Middle Lobe

Scapula

Lower Lobe

Costal Cartilages

Sternum

Lower Lobe of Left Lung

Wall of Capillary

Exchange at the Alveolus

Plasma

Respiratory Membrane

CO_2

Surfactant Layer

Alveolar Wall

O_2

CO_2

O_2

Plasma

Red Blood Cell

Capillary Lumen

FIGURE 12-1
The respiratory system.

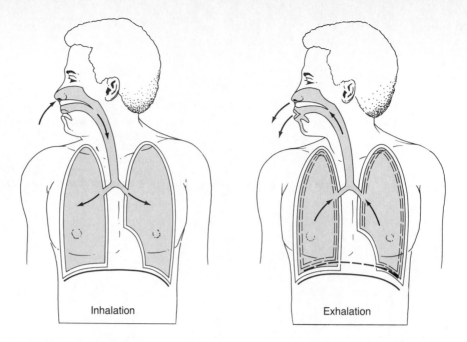

FIGURE 12-2
Inhaling and exhaling.

Inhalation

Exhalation

called the **epiglottis.** It covers the trachea when foods or fluids are swallowed. This prevents substances from entering the trachea and causing choking, obstruction, or aspiration into the air passages. **Aspiration** occurs when small pieces of food or fluid, mucus, or vomitus are taken into the air passages.

·The lungs almost stand on the **diaphragm.** The diaphragm is a muscular organ that separates the thoracic (chest) and abdominal cavities. The diaphragm flattens during inhalation, which increases the size of the chest cavity and allows the lungs to expand. The diaphragm expands on exhalation, reducing the size of the chest cavity.

RESPIRATORY EMERGENCIES

As a nursing assistant, you must be alert for signs of a respiratory emergency and take immediate action to report the emergency and start appropriate life-saving measures. The following conditions can signal a respiratory emergency:

- No chest movements or uneven chest movement.
- No exhange of air can be heard or felt at the mouth or nose.
- Breathing is very difficult (**dyspnea** means difficulty in breathing).
- The resident's skin becomes blue-gray or ashen (called **cyanosis**). The nailbeds and lips lose their normal pink or red color due to lack of oxygen in the circulatory system.
- The rate of breathing becomes too fast or too slow (below 8 or above 30 respirations/minute).
- Respirations become very shallow or noisy and periods of **apnea** (no breathing) occur.

These conditions require the immediate attention of a licensed nurse! Call for help and initiate mouth-to-mouth ventilation when it is determined a respiratory emergency exists by following the step-by-step procedures. In a facility setting, you will rarely need to use mouth-to-mouth ventilation. The facility's emergency equipment will contain disposable airways and a ventilator bag, usually called an **ambu bag.** Use of the airway takes away the need to put your mouth directly on the mouth of the resident. The ambu bag includes a mask that fits over the nose and mouth of the resident. Squeezing the bag forces air into the resident's lungs. The mask must be positioned to provide a tight seal and the resident's head must be positioned to allow the air to enter. The positioning is the same as for mouth-to-mouth ventilation.

MOUTH-TO-MOUTH VENTILATION

This procedure is very efficient in providing **artificial ventilation** (rescue breathing). It can be done by one person without any special equipment. This procedure would have to be modified if there were any indication the resident had sustained neck or spinal cord injuries.

1. *Open the airway* — by properly positioning the resident on his or her back using the head-tilt or chin-lift maneuver. Place one hand on the forehead and apply pressure to tilt the head back. Place the fingers of the other hand under the resident's chin and lift the chin forward with your fingers.

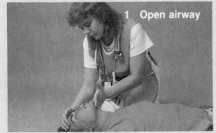

2. *Look, listen, and feel* — while maintaining the proper head tilt and determine whether the resident is breathing by: *Looking* for chest movements — are they present, are they even? *Listening* for air flowing into and out of resident's mouth and nose. Notice any unusual sounds (gurgling, snoring). *Feeling* for air exchange at the resident's mouth and nose. Take at least 3 to 5 seconds to accurately determine whether or not the resident is breathing.

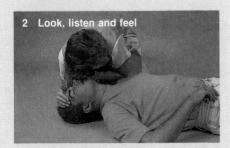

3. *Ventilate* — by maintaining the maximum head tilt and pinching the resident's nose closed with the thumb and forefinger of the same hand you are using to hold the resident's forehead. Open your mouth wide and take a deep breath in. Place your open mouth around the mouth of the resident, making a tight seal with your lips against the resident's face. Ventilate the resident by exhaling slowly into the resident's mouth until you can see the chest rise and feel resistance to the flow of your breath. The ventilation should take 1 to $1\frac{1}{2}$ seconds. If the first attempt fails, reposition the head and try again.

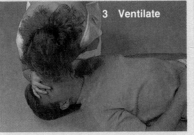

4. *Allow passive exhale* — by breaking contact with the resident's mouth and allowing air to flow from the lungs. Quickly take another deep breath and begin again until resident begins breathing independently (**spontaneous breathing**). Deliver repeated breaths to the adult at the rate of one breath every 5 seconds or 12 breaths per minute. Check to see if the resident has started breathing.

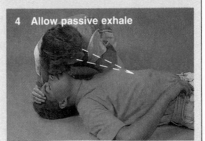

299

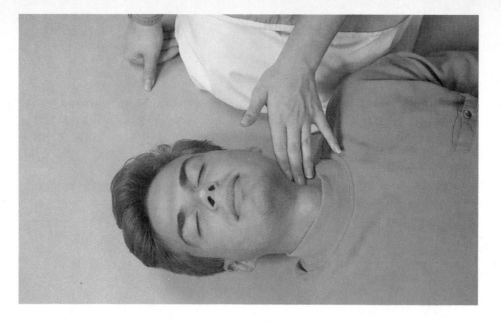

FIGURE 12-3
Signs of cardiac arrest: unresponsiveness, lack of breathing, lack of pulse.

If the resident does not begin breathing again, is unresponsive, and has no carotid pulse, **cardiac arrest** has occurred (Fig. 12-3). Cardiac arrest means the heart has stopped, and **cardiopulmonary resuciatation** (CPR) must be started immediately. *Cardio* refers to the heart and *pulmonary* refers to the lungs.

Cardiopulmonary resucitation is an emergency procedure used to restore circulation and oxygenation when heart, lung and/or certain brain functions have stopped (see Chapter 13). Check the carotid pulse by placing the index and middle fingers on the resident's trachea (windpipe), then slide your fingertips to the side of the neck nearest you, just under the jaw bone. Check the location of the carotid pulse on yourself so that you are familar with its location.

Remember the *signs of cardiac arrest.*

Note: When for any reason there is obstruction or injury to the mouth or oral cavity, it may be necessary to ventilate by using the mouth-to-nose procedure. Most of this procedure is the same as for mouth-to-mouth ventilation with the following exceptions:

1. Keep one hand on the resident's forehead to tilt the head back, and use the other hand to lift the resident's lower jaw and close the mouth. The nose is left open.
2. After taking a deep breath, seal your mouth around the resident's nose.
3. Ventilations are delivered through the resident's nose. Be certain that the resident's mouth is kept closed.
4. When allowing the resident to exhale, break contact with the nose and slightly open the mouth. Keep your hand on the resident's forehead to keep the airway open.

In some cases, blood or vomit may be present. The mouth-to-mask method, using the pocket face mask, is used to help prevent the spread of disease (Fig. 12-4). This technique cuts down on the effort required to keep the resident's airway open and allows you to provide breaths without having to make direct contact with the resident's mouth and nose. It is important to keep a good seal between the face mask and the resident's face. If the mask has a second entry for oxygen, you can at the same time breathe for the patient with air from your own lungs and oxygen from an oxygen source.*

*Adapted from material on page 92 in *First Responder*, 3rd Ed., by J.D. Bergeron, published by Prentice Hall, 1991.

FIGURE 12-4

The Pocket Face Mask and Rescue Breathing.

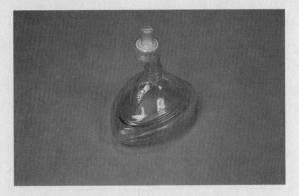

Pocket face mask with one-way valve.

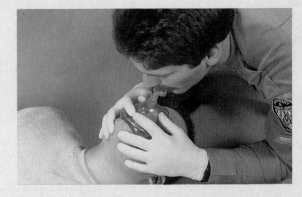

Providing breaths with a pocket face mask.

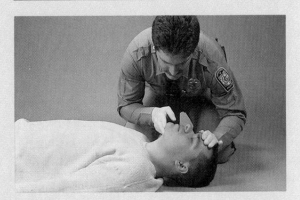

1 Open the airway.

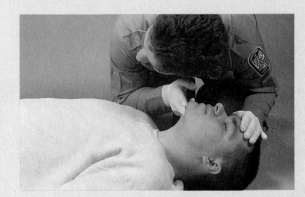

2 Look, listen, and feel for air exchange.

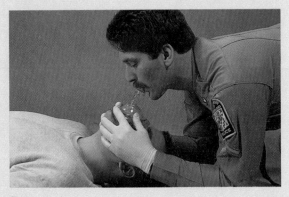

3 Breathe out into mask, watching for the chest to rise.

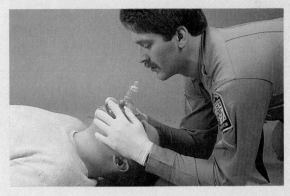

4 Allow passive respiration, watching for the chest to fall.

ONE BREATH EVERY 5 SECONDS EQUALS 12 BREATHS PER MINUTE.

You will know that you are performing these procedures correctly when you are able to:

- *Feel* resistance to your ventilations as the resident's lungs expand
- *See* the chest rise and fall
- *Hear/feel* air leaving the resident's airway as the chest falls

AIRWAY OBSTRUCTION

Another common respiratory emergency is "airway obstruction." Airway obstruction can occur under many different circumstances (Fig. 12-5):

- *Obstruction by the tongue* — the tongue falls back to block off the throat. This can occur when for any reason the resident's head flexes forward, as in the case of sudden unconsciousness or even when too large a pillow is placed under the head.
- *Tissue damage* — this occurs following accidents or injuries where the soft tissues of the neck and throat are crushed or punctured, resulting in swelling of these tissues and blockage of the airway.
- *Diseases* — some respiratory infections and chronic conditions (e.g., asthma) can cause tissue swelling and/or muscle spasms that will lead to airway obstruction.
- *Obstruction by foreign objects* — this type of obstruction, also called "mechanical obstruction," occurs when any object or substance blocks the airway. This could occur with food, toys, or dentures as well as blood or vomitus, which could pool in the back of the throat.

The most frequent cause of airway obstruction in adults is choking on meat or other large, poorly chewed pieces of food. Many elderly residents experience difficulty in swallowing due to aging and disease. If the airway is obstructed down in the lower airway passages, there is usually very little that can be done. However, upper airway obstructions can often be removed with a few simple procedures.

Signs of partial airway obstruction:

- Unusual breathing sounds
- Snoring, often caused by the tongue obstructing the back of the throat
- Gurgling, often caused by a foreign object or fluid in the airway
- Crowing, often caused by spasm of the larynx (voicebox), producing a high-pitched sound that is called **stridor**
- Wheezing, usually due to tissue swelling in the lower air passages (*Note:* Wheezing that is not severe does not generally result in airway obstruction.)

When there is only partial airway obstruction, the resident may be capable of either good or poor air exchange.

If a conscious resident appears to have a partial airway obstruction, have the resident cough. A strong forceful cough indicates that enough air is being exchanged. Encourage the resident to continue coughing in hopes that any foreign object will be dislodged and expelled. Do not interfere with resident's attempts to expel the foreign object.

If the resident cannot cough or the cough is very weak, begin to treat the resident as though *complete airway obstruction is present!*

FIGURE 12-5
Various types of airway obstruction.

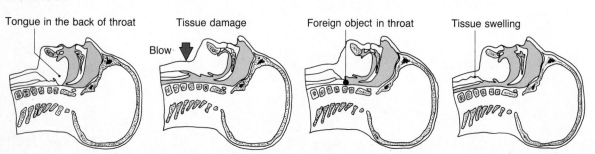

Tongue in the back of throat   Tissue damage   Foreign object in throat   Tissue swelling

Blow

Complete Airway Obstruction

Complete airway obstruction is recognized in a conscious resident when:

- A person is suddenly unable to speak or cough
- A person grasps his or her neck and opens the mouth in an effort to indicate an inability to breathe (Fig. 12-6)

Prompt action is required before the resident loses consciousness!

CORRECTING AIRWAY OBSTRUCTION

In recent years the procedure known as the Heimlich maneuver included the use of back blows when partial or complete airway obstruction was present. However, back blows are no longer recommended for children or adults with complete airway obstruction. This previously taught technique is recommended only for infants who can be placed in a head-down position when the back blows are delivered.

The following procedures are for use with adults. They are not recommended for infants, very small children, pregnant women, or for anyone who has had recent chest or abdominal surgery. Special procedures for infants, very small children, and pregnant women are available from the American Red Cross and the American Heart Association.

You must assess the total situation quickly and determine whether or not complete or partial airway obstruction is present. Follow the steps below for correcting airway obstruction.

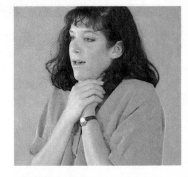

FIGURE 12-6
A person indicating an inability to breathe.

PROCEDURE

CORRECTING AIRWAY OBSTRUCTIONS

1. Determine if there is *complete obstruction* or partial obstruction that must be treated as complete obstruction. Be certain to ask the conscious resident "Are you choking?"; "Can you speak?" Look, listen, and feel for the signs of complete obstruction or poor exchange. Quickly tell the resident you are going to help.
2. Give six to ten abdominal thrusts (the application of these thrusts is known as the **Heimlich maneuver**) in rapid succession.
   - Position yourself behind the resident if the resident is standing or sitting.
   - Slide your arm under the resident's armpits, wrapping both of your arms around the waist.
   - Make a fist and place thumb side of this fist against the midline of the resident's abdomen, just above the navel. Keep your fist below the resident's rib cage, taking extra caution to avoid the area just below the breastbone **(sternum).**

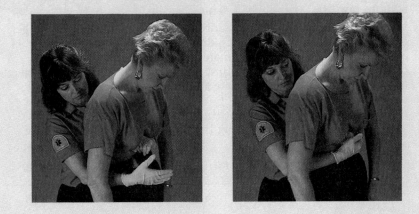

If the resident's brain cells do not receive oxygen, lethal changes can begin to occur within 4 to 6 minutes. It is very important to monitor the resident carefully during any of these procedures to determine if cardiac arrest has occurred. The checking of the carotid pulse is generally the most reliable indicator. If at any time during these procedures it is determined that cardiac arrest has occurred, you would need to begin cardiopulmonary resuscitation (CPR) immediately (see Chapter 13).

AGE-RELATED CHANGES

Respiratory problems are among the more common and life-threatening problems the aged face. Various types of influenza and pneumonia are the fourth-leading cause of death in the aged, and emphysema, bronchitis, and asthma rank eighth. Respiratory disease can be very debilitating, preventing many people from leading a full and active life. There are a number of age-related changes that affect the respiratory system:

- The rib cage becomes more rigid as the cartilage between the ribs becomes calcified (hardened). This prevents full expansion of the chest and lungs during inspiration.
- Postural changes occur, which produce a stooped effect that also limits expansion of the chest.
- The muscles of the abdomen become weaker, affecting the movement of the diaphragm.
- The lungs themselves lose some of their elasticity.

All of these changes lead to decreased exchange of oxygen and carbon dioxide. Older residents without respiratory diseases are usually able to meet ordinary respiratory demands despite these changes. However, the elderly adapt less efficiently if they have to cope with stressful circumstances or vigorous physical activity. The older adult has a decreased resistance to respiratory infections. Once a respiratory problem develops, they are slower to recover and require aggressive treatment.

SECTION 2 THE RESIDENT WITH RESPIRATORY DISEASE

OBJECTIVES/WHAT YOU WILL LEARN

When you have completed this section, you will be able to:
- Identify the single most important factor contributing to respiratory disease
- Explain why residents confined to bed are at risk for pneumonia
- Describe two nursing measures to prevent pneumonia
- Identify correctly statements related to providing oxygen therapy

DISEASES OF THE RESPIRATORY SYSTEM

Smoking is the most important factor contributing to respiratory disease in all ages (Fig. 12-7). Many older adults started smoking in the years before the health hazards associated with smoking were recognized. Smoking is the

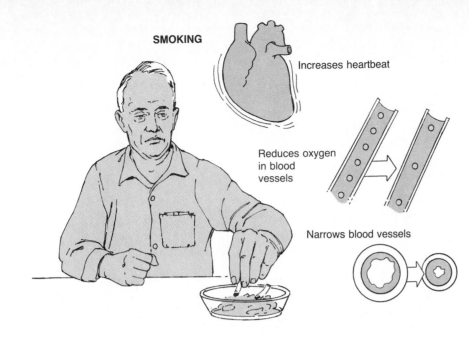

SMOKING

Increases heartbeat

Reduces oxygen in blood vessels

Narrows blood vessels

FIGURE 12-7
Some of the destructive results of smoking.

major cause of chronic bronchitis. Smokers are twice as likely to develop lung cancer as nonsmokers. Research statistics show a direct parallel between the increase in cigarette smoking and an increase in lung cancer rates.

Cessation of smoking is associated with a rapid decline in incidence, reaching the level of a nonsmoker within 13 years. For this reason, it is important that the elderly population be made aware of the dangers of cigarette smoking and the benefits of quitting at any age.

Smoking habits are not easy to change. Many local health departments, the American Heart Association, the Lung Association, and the Respiratory Diseases Association will provide specific information on various antismoking programs. As a nursing assistant, you can help residents become aware of these programs.

Common respiratory diseases of the elderly are:

- Pneumonia
- Emphysema
- Asthma
- Tuberculosis

PNEUMONIA

Pneumonia is an acute inflammation or infection of the lung. Until the discovery of antibiotics, most elderly people who developed pneumonia died. Pneumonia can be caused by either bacteria or viruses. The microorganisms that cause pneumonia are always present in the upper respiratory tract and are not disease producing unless resistance is severely lowered. Age and immobility are contributory factors. When a resident is in a reclining position, the chest does not expand completely and fluids and mucus "pool" in the lungs, causing congestion (Fig. 12-8). Many bedridden residents are too weak to cough up these pooled secretions, which provide a good medium for bacterial growth, resulting in infection.

Signs and symptoms associated with pneumonia include:

- Cough
- Fever
- Rapid, labored, or shallow respirations
- Noisy respiration such as wheezing, gurgling, and rattling
- Confusion, which can occur as a result of decreased oxygen

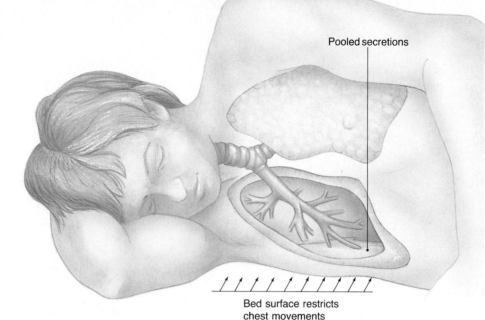

Pooled secretions

Bed surface restricts
chest movements

FIGURE 12-8
When a person is in a
reclining position, fluids
pool in the lungs.

- Restlessness, which can occur as a result of decreased oxygen
- Complaints of pain in the chest

EMPHYSEMA

Emphysema is a disease where tiny bronchioles become plugged with mucus. The lungs become less elastic and air inhaled is trapped in the lungs, making breathing difficult, especially during exhalation. Chronic emphysema takes the lives of over 10,000 Americans each year, and the death rate is increasing sharply. Many times emphysema results after prolonged respiratory problems such as bronchitis, asthma, tuberculosis, or prolonged irritation from pollutants. Individuals who smoke are at high risk for development of emphysema. The disease can be extremely debilitating. Some residents require continuous oxygen and must severely limit their activity. Others are able to pace their activities according to their tolerance.

Emphysema is a diagnosis established by the physician based on pulmonary (lung) function tests and X-ray. Residents with emphysema generally exhibit the following signs and symptoms:

- Persistent cough (moist coughing and wheezing)
- Fatigue
- Loss of appetite
- Weight loss
- Anxiety (due to difficulty breathing)
- Coughing up thick secretions, especially in the morning
- Resident sits leaning forward with shoulders hunched to facilitate breathing
- Breathing with "pursed lips"

ASTHMA

Asthma is another common respiratory disease that affects the elderly. Some elderly have been affected with asthma all their lives; others develop asthma during their later years. Asthma is a disease of the bronchi, characterized by difficulty breathing, wheezing, and a sense of tightness or constriction in the chest due to spasm of the muscles (Fig. 12-9). This causes narrowing of the air passages.

Asthma is often the result of an allergic reaction. The person has developed a sensitivity to a particular substance and, when exposed, the body reacts, sometimes in a life-threatening manner. More than half the cases of asthma are related to allergies. For this reason, it is essential that residents are protected from being exposed to substances to which they are allergic.

The resident's medical record will contain a notation related to allergies. The diet card will identify any foods to which the resident is allergic. Some residents are allergic to certain kinds of tape, soap, medications, animals, fabrics, and pillow fillings. You must be aware of residents' allergies.

Some types of asthma are related to the resident's emotional state. Nervous tension, stress, and emotional upsets all can bring on an asthma attack or make an attack worse. You can help protect the resident from sources of emotional excitement and provide a quiet, relaxed atmosphere.

There are specific drugs and special medicated inhalers used to treat the resident with asthma. Observing for the symptoms of an asthma attack and reporting these observations promptly to the charge nurse are very important. Frequently, if medication is administered in the initial phase of the attack, the severity of the reaction is reduced.

Emphysema, asthma, and chronic bronchitis are often referred to as **chronic obstructive pulmonary disease** (COPD). You may see this term used on a health-care plan identifying problems related to these diseases.

TUBERCULOSIS

Tuberculosis is an infectious disease that commonly attacks the lungs. It is a communicable disease usually spread by contact with the sputum of an infected person. It can also be spread by coughing, sneezing, or speaking.

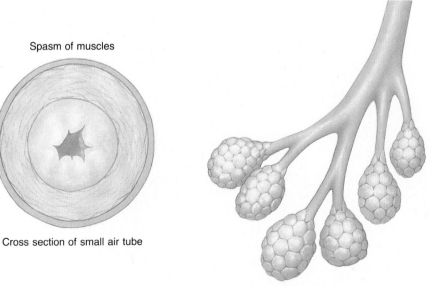

FIGURE 12-9
Bronchial asthma.

Spasm of muscles

Cross section of small air tube

Unfortunately, the incidence of tuberculosis is increasing in the elderly, especially in hospital settings. They may have had it in the past, and as they become debilitated, the disease reactivates.

Symptoms of tuberculosis are:

- Loss of appetite
- Weakness
- Night sweats
- Weight loss
- Fever (not always)

All residents are screened for tuberculosis on admission, usually by a chest X-ray or skin test. Employees are also screened for the presence of tuberculosis when they are hired and annually thereafter. There are excellent drugs that can control the disease and make the resident noncontagious after a short period of time. Reporting signs and symptoms of tuberculosis is important for your own protection as well as for the protection of other employees and residents.

Respiratory disease imposes drastic restrictions in lifestyle and activity for many residents. Having difficulty breathing is one of the most anxiety-producing conditions anyone can experience. There is a feeling of panic when breathing is impaired for any reason. A number of nursing procedures are related to care of the resident with respiratory disease. Study your facility procedures carefully so that you can react quickly and efficiently.

OXYGEN THERAPY

Every cell requires oxygen. There is a balance required between the supply and the body's demand. If the demand is greater than the supply, additional oxygen may be administered. The physician will specify the method, rate, and length of time for oxygen therapy. Some residents with respiratory disease may not be able to tolerate too much oxygen. *Therefore, you should not adjust oxygen flow rates. This is the responsibility of the licensed nurse.*

Nasal cannulas, or tubes, are used to give oxygen to a resident (Fig. 12-10). The cannulas are inserted into the resident's nostrils. The **cannula,** which is made of plastic, is a half-circle of tubing with two openings in the center. It fits about $\frac{1}{2}$ inch into the resident's nostrils. Nasal cannulas are held in place by an elastic headband secured around the resident's head and are connected to the source of oxygen by a length of plastic tubing.

FIGURE 12-10
A nasal cannula.

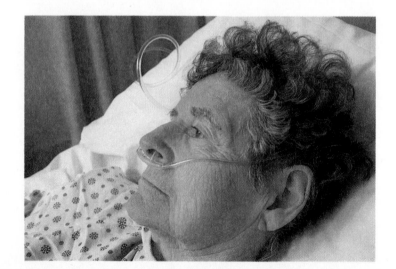

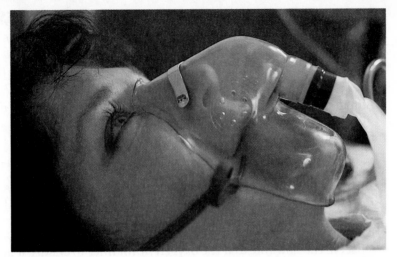

FIGURE 12-11
A face mask.

A plastic face mask may be used when the resident breathes through the mouth or requires a higher concentration of oxygen (Fig. 12-11). The mask is placed over the mouth and nose and is fitted to the nose with the metal nosepiece. The mask is held in place by an elastic headband secured around the resident's head and connected to the source of oxygen by a length of plastic tubing. Residents who require long-term oxygen therapy generally prefer the nasal cannula to the face mask as they feel less confined.

Oxygen can be supplied through a portable oxygen cylinder, through a wall outlet at the resident's bedside from a central oxygen system, or through a portable machine referred to as an oxygen concentrater (Fig. 12-12). Oxygen is administered by passing it through water to reduce its drying effect. The water container is called a **humidifier.** The humidifier should never be allowed to run dry. Report any problems to the licensed nurse.

Oxygen is essential to life; however, it must be considered a potential hazard when stored because it supports combustion. Review Chapter 2 dealing with oxygen safety. Remember, a "No Smoking" sign must be posted in the resident's room and on the door when oxygen is in use.

The licensed nurse is responsible for administration of oxygen to residents according to the physician's order and will set the flow rate as indicated. However, the nursing assistant should understand how to read the flow meter and oxygen gauge as well as how to observe the resident and equipment.

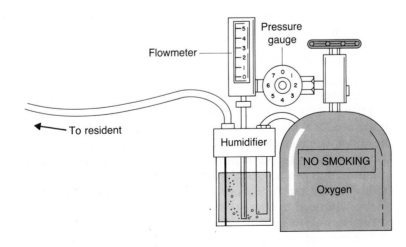

FIGURE 12-12
An oxygen concentrator.

have very thin walls, which are one cell thick. They allow exchange of oxygen, carbon dioxide, and other substances through their thin walls. Capillaries nourish all body cells.

- **Veins** are the blood vessels that always carry oxygen-poor blood back to the heart, lungs, and kidneys (with the exception of the pulmonary vein).

- **Venules** are the very tiny veins of the body. They carry blood from the capillaries to the large veins of the body.

- **Lymph vessels** are tiny capillary-like structures that collect lymph (tissue fluids) from the tissue spaces (areas between the cells). The lymph vessels follow the veins of the body and eventually empty into the large veins. Lymph is a colorless fluid with a salty taste circulating through the system. It is 95 percent water. Lymph is called tissue fluid when it is surrounding the cells. It is called lymph when it is drained from the tissues and collected by the lymph vessels. Along the course of the lymph vessels are lymph nodes. The main lymph nodes are in the neck, under the arms, and in the groin. These nodes often become enlarged when infection or disease occurs.

THE HEART

The heart receives blood through the veins and pumps it out through the arteries to all cells of the body. As blood circulates through the blood vessels, a force called **blood pressure** is created. Blood pressure is the measurable force of the blood against the walls of a blood vessel.

The **heart** is a cone-shaped muscle about the size of a fist. It is located a little to the left of the midline of the chest (Fig. 13-3). This efficient pump beats 100,000 times a day to circulate the blood through approximately 100,000 miles of blood vessels. The heart is divided into right and left halves by a tissue called the **septum.** Each half consists of two chambers — a **right atrium** and **right ventricle** and a **left atrium** and **left ventricle.** The heart is composed of cardiac muscle, and the ventricles have thick muscular walls.

The heart has a specialized "conduction system" that is responsible for the iniation of the heartbeat. The cardiac muscle is capable of continuous rhythmic contraction. There is a place in the right atrium called the **pacemaker** that transmits an electrical impulse through the atrium to another specialized area, which sends impulses into the ventricles. This causes them to contract. An **electrocardiogram** (EKG) records the heart's electrical conduction system on a graph for analysis by the physician. Through the EKG, disturbances in the normal conduction system can be identified.

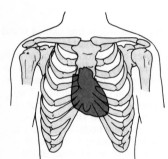

FIGURE 13-3
The position of the heart in the chest cavity.

BLOOD FLOW THROUGH THE HEART

Blood flows through the heart in one direction because of four heart valves that prevent backflow. Knowing how the blood flows through the heart and lungs will help you understand some of the changes that occur when heart disease is present (Fig. 13-4). The right atrium (2) receives unoxygenated (oxygen-poor) blood through the largest veins in the body, the superior and inferior venae cavae (1) (3). Blood passes from the right atrium (2) through a valve **(tricuspid)** (4) into the right ventricle (5). The right ventricle (5) contracts (squeezes) and pumps blood up through another valve **(pulmonic)** (6) into the pulmonary artery (7). The blood passes through the pulmonary artery (right and left) (7) to the lungs, where waste products in the blood and carbon dioxide are disposed of and oxygen is taken into the blood.

This oxygenated (oxygen-rich) blood returns to the left of the heart through the pulmonary veins (8) into the left atrium (9). The blood drains from the left atrium (9) through a valve (mitral) (10) into the left ventricle (11). The left

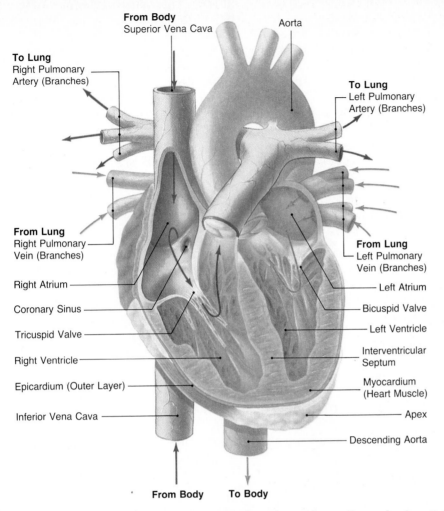

From Body
Superior Vena Cava

Aorta

To Lung
Right Pulmonary
Artery (Branches)

To Lung
Left Pulmonary
Artery (Branches)

From Lung
Right Pulmonary
Vein (Branches)

From Lung
Left Pulmonary
Vein (Branches)

Right Atrium

Left Atrium

Coronary Sinus

Bicuspid Valve

Tricuspid Valve

Left Ventricle

Right Ventricle

Interventricular
Septum

Epicardium (Outer Layer)

Myocardium
(Heart Muscle)

Inferior Vena Cava

Apex

Descending Aorta

From Body   **To Body**

The heart is a hollow, muscular organ that pumps 450 million pints of blood in the average lifetime. Its superior chambers, the atria, receive blood. Both atria fill and then contract at the same time. The inferior chambers are the ventricles. They pump blood out of the heart. Both ventricles fill and then contract at the same time. When the atria are relaxing, the ventricles are contracting.

The right side of the heart receives blood from the body and sends it to the lungs (pulmonic circulation). The heart's left side receives oxygenated blood from the lungs and sends it out to the body (systemic circulation).

The heartbeat originates at the sinoatrial node (pacemaker) and spreads across the atria to stimulate contraction. After a slight delay, the impulse is sent from the atrioventricular node, down the bundles of His, and out across the ventricles. This stimulates the ventricles to contract while the atria are relaxing.

The heart muscle (myocardium) receives its blood supply by way of the right and left coronary arteries. These vessels are the first branches of the aorta.

FIGURE 13-4
Blood flow through the heart.

ventricle (11) contracts and pumps the blood up through another valve (aortic) (12) into the **aorta** (13), the largest artery in the body. The aorta branches into smaller arteries leading to all areas of the body, which in turn branch into **arterioles** (Fig. 13-5).

The arterioles deliver blood to the tiniest blood vessels of the body, including capillaries. The capillaries surround all the cells in the body. They deliver nutrients and oxygen to the cells and remove waste products. They in turn pass the blood into the large veins so that the waste products can be disposed of through the lungs, the kidneys, and the sweat glands. The heart itself receives its oxygenated blood from the coronary arteries, the first branches from the aorta.

AGE-RELATED CHANGES

There are numerous age-related changes to the cardiovascular system. Some are not serious, while others can lead to acute illness. The heart muscle may become enlarged in the older adult with **hypertension** (high blood pressure). When hypertension is present, the heart muscle has to work harder to circulate the blood through vessels that are more rigid and less elastic. When you increase the work of a muscle, it becomes larger. When you decrease the work of a muscle, it becomes smaller. In some older adults, when physical activity has been drastically reduced, the heart muscle can decrease in size.

The heart rate in the older adult is decreased, and the amount of blood pumped out into the circulatory system with each heart contraction is generally

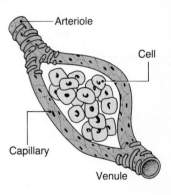

Arteriole

Cell

Capillary

Venule

FIGURE 13-5
An arteriole.

lessened (called decreased cardiac output). It is estimated that cardiac output decreases as much as 40 percent between the ages of 25 and 65. This explains why older people tire more easily and have less reserve energy.

Other age-related changes occur in the blood vessels themselves. They become thickened and less elastic in many instances. These changes are not usually great enough to produce disease, other than slight increases in blood pressure or minor changes in heart sounds due to thickening in the heart valves. When these and other changes progress to the point that cardiac function or circulatory function is impaired, heart disease is present. Understanding the changes experienced during the aging process, as well as some of the common forms of heart disease, will assist you in providing better nursing care.

CARDIAC EMERGENCIES

All the functions of the cardiovascular system depend on the heart pumping the blood in a constant, one-directional flow. When, for any reason, this process is interrupted, a serious cardiac emergency exists. There is an important relationship between breathing, circulation, and certain brain activity.

- If breathing stops, the blood being circulated to the brain will not contain enough oxygen, and the brain will send a signal to the heart, and it will soon stop pumping.
- When the heart stops pumping, breathing stops almost instantly.
- If the centers in the brain that control breathing and cardiac function are damaged, heart and lung action will soon stop.

The activities of the heart, lungs, and brain are interdependent (Fig. 13-6). If one fails, they all will fail.

Whenever you read about basic life support, you will see references made to the ABCs of emergency care. ABC stands for:

A = airway   B = breathing   C = circulation

FIGURE 13-6
Interdependence of the activities of the heart, lungs, and brain.

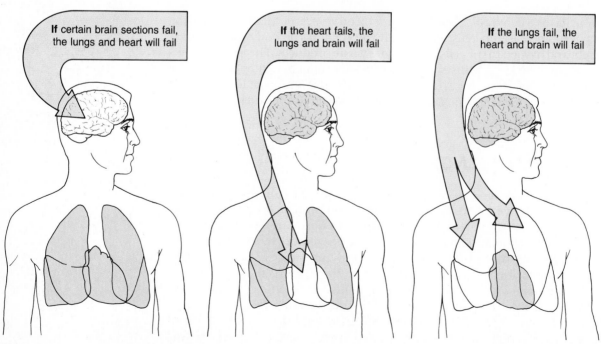

If certain brain sections fail, the lungs and heart will fail

If the heart fails, the lungs and brain will fail

If the lungs fail, the heart and brain will fail

CARDIOPULMONARY RESUSCITATION

In Chapter 12 you learned how to maintain an open airway and how to perform rescue breathing. When performing CPR, you must continue to keep an open airway and breathe for the victim. Your breaths provide oxygen for the blood. In addition, you must circulate the oxygenated blood to the vital organs of the body. During CPR the increased pressure in the chest cavity forces the blood into circulation (Fig. 13-7).

It is important to remember that when someone stops breathing and the heart stops pumping, **clinical death** results. Within just 4 to 6 minutes, lethal changes begin to take place in the brain, and generally within 10 minutes **biological death** will occur as the brain and other body cells start to die. For these reasons, quick action to start CPR on someone who is in cardiac arrest is essential. *Start CPR immediately* even if you could worsen existing injuries, for without CPR the victim will quickly go from clinical death to biological death.

The following procedure is a step-by-step outline for performing one-rescuer CPR. The procedures covered here follow the recommendations of the American Heart Association (AHA). Your instructor will inform you of any recent changes made by the AHA. This procedure should be learned exactly as presented. Extensive research by the AHA has determined that the procedures presented here are the most efficient in saving lives of victims in cardiac arrest.

Note: There are slightly different techniques to be used on infants and small children under the age of 8. For an average-sized child 8 years and older, the adult techniques presented here can be used. The variations to be used on infants and small children are not presented in this book; however, specific information is available through the American Red Cross and the American Heart Association.

ONE-RESCUER CPR

Because CPR is a lifesaving procedure, it is essential that the rescuer understand exactly how to perform these procedures correctly. Therefore, it is recommended that these procedures be taught by an instructor certified by the American Heart Association and/or the American Red Cross.

FIGURE 13-7
The mechanics of CPR.

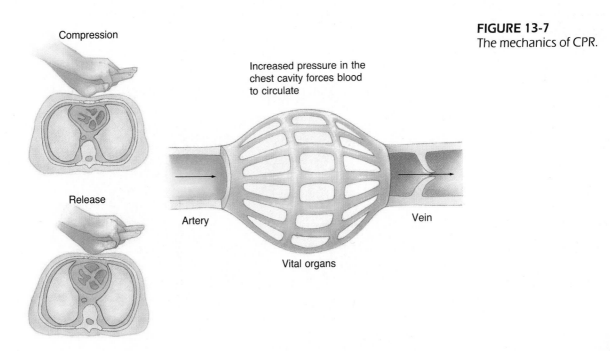

Compression

Release

Increased pressure in the chest cavity forces blood to circulate

Artery

Vein

Vital organs

1. *Establish unresponsiveness.* Gently shake the victim and ask, "Are you okay?" If the victim is unresponsive, immediately *call for help.*

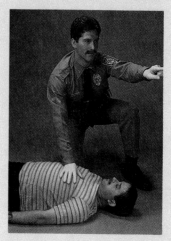

2. *Properly position the victim and yourself.* Place the victim on a flat surface face up. Kneel beside at chest level with your knees pointing in toward the patient's chest.

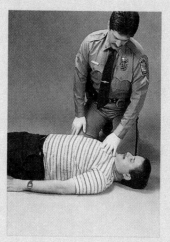

3. *Establish an open airway.* Use the head-tilt, chin-lift method to ensure an open airway.

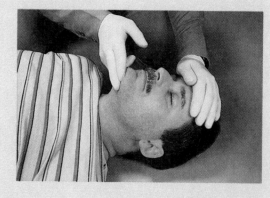

4. *Check for breathing — look, listen, and feel* for air exchange. This should take 3 to 5 seconds.

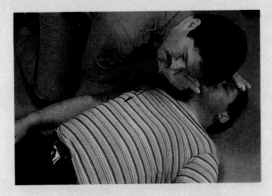

5. *Provide two adequate breaths.* Use the procedure outlined for mouth-to-mouth ventilation in Section 1 of Chapter 12, presented on pages 299–301.

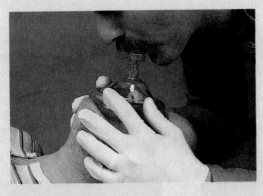

6. If necessary, *clear the airway.* Use the techniques of manual thrusts, finger sweeps, and ventilations described in Chapter 12, pages 303–306.

7. *Establish cardiac arrest.* Check for circulation by feeling for a carotid pulse. This should take 5 to 10 seconds. If a carotid pulse is present but no breathing is present, give one breath every 5 seconds. If there is no carotid pulse, start CPR.

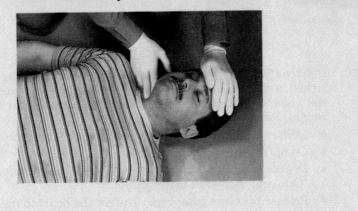

TWO-RESCUER CPR

The procedure for two-rescuer CPR varies slightly in that one rescuer delivers the ventilations and the second person delivers chest compressions (Fig. 13-8). In two-rescuer CPR:

- Compressions are five every 3 to 4 seconds.
- Provide one ventilation every five compressions, or 12 per minute.
- The person giving ventilations checks the carotid pulse.
- The person doing compressions counts out loud the one to five cycles.
- Check for carotid pulse every few minutes.

Because these are lifesaving procedures, it is essential that you learn them by memory in order to be prepared at all times to provide the *ABCs of emergency care!*

SECTION 2 THE RESIDENT WITH HEART DISEASE

OBJECTIVES/WHAT YOU WILL LEARN

When you have completed this section, you will be able to:
- Identify three types of heart disease and signs and symptoms associated with each
- Describe nursing measures needed when a resident takes nitroglycerin
- Apply antiembolism stockings
- Identify three important measures associated with providing care to the resident with an amputation
- List three guidelines for providing care to the resident with heart disease

TYPES OF HEART DISEASE

Heart disease is the number one cause of death in the United States. Although heart disease is associated with all ages, as age increases so does the incidence of heart disease. Approximately 18 percent of those over 65 years of age must limit their daily activities due to various heart conditions. There is a great deal of interest and public education concerning ways to prevent heart disease. Maintaining a proper diet, getting regular exercise, keeping weight within normal limits for height and build, along with regular physical examinations are the more important preventative measures that people can take to guard against heart disease.

New techniques for the treatment of various types of heart disease along with a health-conscious society are major factors in the reduction of deaths due to heart disease in recent years. It is helpful to understand which heart diseases are most common and how you can assist residents with heart disease to lead healthy, productive lives.

Cardiovascular insufficiency is a form of heart disease in which there is decreased blood supply to the major organs of the body. The most important cause of cardiovascular insufficiency is associated with arteriosclerosis or atherosclerosis.

FIGURE 13-8

Two-Rescuer CPR

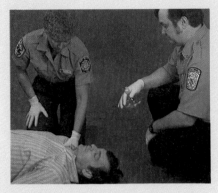

1 Determine unresponsiveness. Reposition resident.

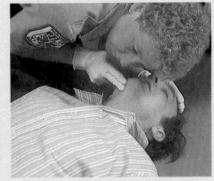

2 Open the airway and look, listen, and feel (3-5 sec.)

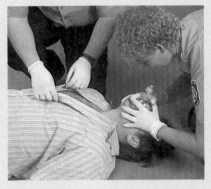

3 Ventilate twice (1-1.5 sec/ ventilation)

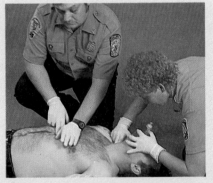

4 Determine pulselessness. Locate CPR compression site.

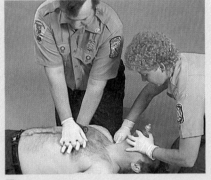

5 Say "no pulse." Begin compressions.

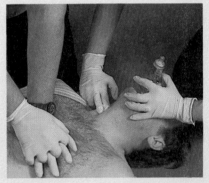

6 Check compression effectiveness. Deliver five compressions in 3-4 seconds. (rate = 80-100/minute)

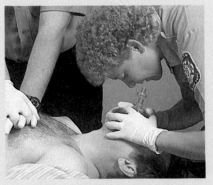

7 Ventilate once. (1-1.5 sec./ ventilation) Stop for ventilation

Continue with one ventilation every five compressions.

8 Continue with one ventilation every five compressions.

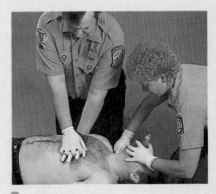

9 After ten cycles, reassess breathing and pulse. No pulse—ventilate and say "continue CPR." Pulse—say "stop CPR."

NOTE: Assess for spontaneous breathing and at the end of the first minute, and then every few minutes thereafter.

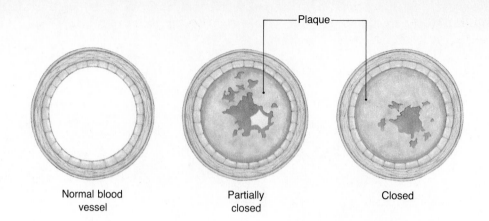

FIGURE 13-9
Artherosclerosis.

Plaque

Normal blood
vessel

Partially
closed

Closed

Arteriosclerosis is a thickening and loss of elasticity in the arteries of the body (often referred to as a *hardening of the arteries*). **Atherosclerosis** is a form of arteriosclerosis in which the arteries become clogged or blocked with various substances, such as **plaque** and deposits of calcium and/or fat (Fig. 13-9).

Arteriosclerosis is the major cause of heart disease and cerebral vascular accident (CVA or stroke). It is estimated that 1 million deaths occur in the United States each year that are directly related to arteriosclerosis or atherosclerosis. Both conditions result in an inadequate blood supply to the heart muscle and other vital organs, such as the brain, kidneys, lungs, stomach, and intestine. The heart muscle receives its blood supply from the coronary arteries, which branch off the aorta (Fig. 13-10).

Deaths from heart disease are decreasing due to earlier diagnosis and effective surgical and nonsurgical techniques designed to improve blood flow throughout the heart muscle by restoring circulation through the coronary arteries. **Cardiac bypass surgery** is becoming more and more common. The surgeon removes a blood vessel from the patient's leg and replaces a portion of the coronary blood vessel that is clogged or blocked, thereby restoring cardiac circulation. The patient is placed on special equipment to maintain circulation

FIGURE 13-10
The coronary arteries.

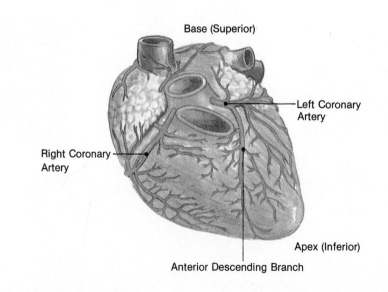

Base (Superior)

Left Coronary
Artery

Right Coronary
Artery

Apex (Inferior)

Anterior Descending Branch

while surgery is performed on the heart itself. This type of surgery has proven to be very successful.

Another procedure called **cardiac angioplasty** is being used to open clogged coronary arteries. A special pressurized balloon is threaded through the clogged portion of the artery and pressure is used to open the artery.

When the heart muscle does not receive an adequate blood supply, parts of the heart muscle die **(infarct).** This is called a **myocardial infarction,** often referred to as an MI, or a heart attack. Heart attack can also occur when the conduction system of the heart fails.

PACEMAKERS

Many people have **pacemakers** (Fig. 13-11) implanted to stimulate the heart to beat properly. The heart rate is controlled by a specialized node in the heart. When this node does not function normally, the heart rate can decrease severely or become very irregular. An electronic pacemaker may be implanted in the chest wall to correct this. This device substitutes for the nonfunctioning conduction system of the heart.

There are different types of pacemakers:

- *Fixed rate:* the rate is fixed between 60 to 70 beats per minute. This is only used if the heart is totally dependent on the implanted electrical device for stimulation.
- *Demand pacemaker:* the rate is not preset, and it provides electrical stimulation to produce a beat only when the heart beat falls below a predetermined rate.

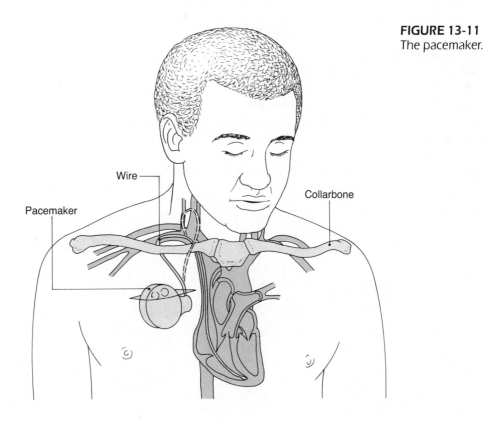

FIGURE 13-11
The pacemaker.

- Electrical appliances should be used cautiously.
- Microwave ovens should not be used within 10 feet of residents with pacemakers.
- If the resident has hiccoughs, report this immediately, as this could indicate the pacemaker is not in its proper place.
- If the resident's pulse is below the preset rate of the pacemaker, report it immediately.
- Report pain or discoloration of the skin around the implanted pacemaker.
- Report any complaints of dizziness, edema (swelling), shortness of breath, or irregular heart beat immediately.

There are new methods of testing the pacemaker by using telephone telemetry. A call is made to the determined source, and the pacemaker can be checked. This is generally done on a monthly basis by the licensed nurse.

SIGNS AND SYMPTOMS OF HEART ATTACK AND HYPERTENSION

You should be aware of the symptoms of heart attack:

- Chest pain — described as a heavy, squeezing, or crushing feeling in the chest
- Pain in the left arm and neck
- Irregular, weak, or thready pulse
- Faintness, dizziness
- Difficulty breathing, shortness of breath
- Shocklike symptoms — pale, cold, clammy skin, weakness, decreased blood pressure

Some residents frequently experience chest pain. **Angina pectoris** is a term used to describe acute chest pain caused by decreased blood supply to the heart.

Residents who have been diagnosed with angina frequently have a medication called *nitroglycerin* prescribed by the physician. This medication is one of the very few that the physician will allow residents to keep at the bedside. These tiny white pills, which are placed under the tongue to dissolve, act rapidly to increase the blood flow to the heart. Find out which residents have nitroglycerin prescribed and assist a resident as instructed in taking this medication. You must always report and record any time you observe or assist a resident in taking nitroglycerin. The charge nurse will need to evaluate the resident's condition and measure vital signs.

Hypertension is a natural partner of arteriosclerosis. When the blood vessels become rigid, less elastic, or partially blocked, the heart has to work harder to propel the blood through the vessels. The increased resistance of the vessels raises the blood pressure. Hypertension often leads to heart failure. Hypertension exerts excessive pressure of the blood against the arterial walls.

Generally, a person is considered to be hypertensive if systolic pressure is consistently above 160 mm and diastolic pressure is over 90 mm. Hypertension is very common in the older adult. Signs and symptoms of acute hypertension are:

- Feeling faint or dizzy
- Headache
- Difficulty with vision or speech
- Nosebleed
- Flushed red face
- Sudden changes in behavior, orientation

SIGNS AND SYMPTOMS OF CONGESTIVE HEART FAILURE

Congestive heart failure is an abnormal condition characterized by circulatory congestion caused by cardiac disorders. Signs and symptoms of congestive heart failure are:

- Congestion in the lungs
- Difficulty breathing
- Restlessness, anxiety
- Edema of legs, feet, hands, face
- Weight gain
- Weakness, fatigue
- Dizziness, confusion
- Chest pain

Congestive heart failure is treated by prescribed medications, treatments, and skilled nursing care. Commonly used medications are digitalis preparations and diuretics. Digitalis preparations slow the heart rate and increase the force of the contraction. Diuretics decrease the work load of the heart by ridding the body of excess fluids. Because these fluids are eliminated through the urinary system, a resident receiving diuretics will urinate frequently. With less fluid to move through the blood vessels and a slower, stronger heart beat, the heart works more effectively. The licensed nurse administers these drugs. However, you should know if the resident is being given these medications in order to observe and report special problems. Other treatments for congestive heart failure include periods of prolonged rest and oxygen therapy.

SIGNS AND SYMPTOMS OF PERIPHERAL VASCULAR DISEASE

Residents with heart disease very often experience poor circulation, called **peripheral vascular disease,** especially of the lower extremities (legs and feet). Due to changes in the blood vessels resulting from arteriosclerosis, blood supply to the area decreases, causing tissue death. Signs and symptoms of peripheral vascular disease are:

- Edema or swelling of extremities — hands, fingers, legs, feet, toes
- Changes in skin temperature — infection produces red, warm skin and poor circulation produces cold, pale, or bluish skin
- Shiny, dry, flaky skin
- Pain
- Absence of pulse in legs and feet

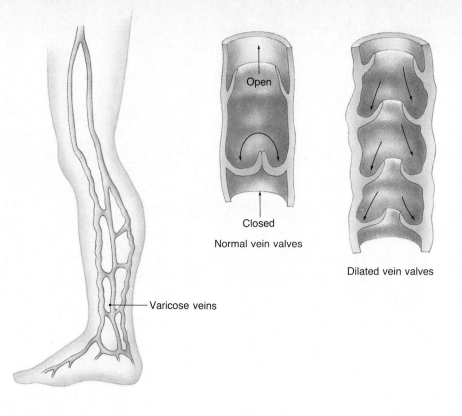

FIGURE 13-12
Varicose veins.

Open wounds or sores on the legs are referred to as **stasis ulcers.** *Stasis* means a stoppage of flow. Stasis ulcers are caused by a stoppage of blood flow. Residents with heart disease and diabetes are particularly likely to develop stasis ulcers.

Varicose veins are another type of vascular disease (Fig. 13-12). These swollen (distended) veins are especially prominent in the legs. Varicose veins can be caused by lack of exercise and prolonged standing as well as loss of elasticity associated with aging. The resident will experience dull pain and cramping of the legs. Pain is relieved by elevation of the limb and rest. Elastic stockings are used to reduce the pooling of blood in these distended veins and to reduce the possibility of a blood clot formation. A blood clot (called a **thrombus**) is more likely to form in the veins than in arteries because the blood flow is slower. If a blood clot breaks loose from the wall of a vessel and moves within the bloodstream, it is called an **embolus.** If an embolus enters a major organ such as brain, heart, kidney, or lungs, death is likely. Elastic stockings (Ace wraps, "Ted" stockings, or "antiembolism stockings") may be applied to compress and smooth out the distended walls of the veins. The blood moves through them without pooling. These stockings also help blood return to the heart more efficiently, reducing the workload of the heart. On some occasions they may be used to provide support and comfort in the event of a sprain or strain at a joint.

APPLYING ANTIEMBOLISM STOCKINGS AND ELASTIC BANDAGES

Antiembolism stockings can be knee length or full length (Fig. 13-13). You should always apply antiembolism stockings with the resident in bed. The legs should be elevated briefly prior to application. This helps drain the limb of blood, increasing the efficiency of the stocking when applied. Gather the stocking up and slip over the toe and heel, taking care to smooth out wrinkles. Gently stretch the stocking over the ankle and leg. The stocking should fit snugly. A

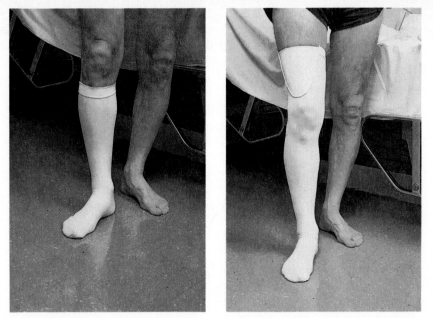

FIGURE 13-13
Antiembolism stockings.

stocking that is loose is ineffective. One so tight as to impair circulation is dangerous. Elastic stockings must be removed and reapplied at least once every day or more frequently if the physician orders it. Some physicians will order "out of bed only with antiembolism stockings."

Elastic bandages (often referred as "Ace wraps") are long strips of elasticized cotton. They are wound into rolls and secured with a metal clip or a strip of Velcro. They are used for the same purpose as antiembolism stockings or to provide support or to hold a dressing in place. The antiembolism stocking is much more effective because it is not apt to slip and wrinkle and cannot be wrapped in such a way as to impair circulation. If you are instructed to apply elastic bandages, several precautions must be kept in mind:

- Never wrap a limb so tightly that you impair circulation. You must check toes or fingers to ensure adequate circulation.
- Never wrap in a way that pinches or applies undue pressure as this can cause tissue injury or skin breakdown.
- Check the resident often since elastic bandages slide as the resident moves and can become dislodged or "bunch up," causing pressure and discomfort.
- Never tie an elastic bandage. The wrap should be smooth and even. Ask your charge nurse for assistance when you are unsure on how to wrap an elastic bandage.

Probably the most important nursing function related to peripheral vascular disease is observation for changes. If circulation is severely impaired, skin breakdown will occur, and **gangrene,** a disease associated with dead tissue, develops. Gangrenous extremities almost always require amputation.

CARING FOR THE RESIDENT WITH AN AMPUTATION

Amputation (cutting off) of any body part is traumatic, both physically and psychologically. The change in body image requires a great adjustment. Each person has an image or a mental picture of how their body looks. We think of ourself as fat or thin, tall or short, young or old, attractive or unattractive. We visualize ourselves with all of our body parts present and working properly. When there is an image change, such as an amputation, it can take a long time to adjust and form a new body image. When a body part is removed, most individuals also experience feelings of increased dependence and decreased value. The person loses both the part and the function performed by that part, resulting in a need to depend on others.

Emotional or psychological support includes:

- Listening to the resident
- Giving the resident opportunities to make decisions about his care
- Encouraging maximum independence
- Having a matter-of-fact attitude about the amputation

Usually, by the time the new amputee has arrived in an LTC facility, the surgical wound is almost healed. There may still be some sutures in place covered with a dressing. Nursing measures should include:

- Promote healing of the wound
- Prevent infection
- Prevent contractures
- Decrease swelling in the "stump" (remaining part of the amputated limb)
- Protect the stump from injury

The nursing assistant should report any sores, bleeding, or drainage from the wound. The resident should be positioned to prevent contractures. If the amputation is below the knee (BK), the knee joint should be kept in extension (straight out) as much as possible. If the amputation is above the knee (AK), the hip should be regularly extended by positioning the resident onto his abdomen (proning) every day, as tolerated. Swelling is usually controlled by wrapping the stump with an elastic wrap or by using a "stump sox," a cone-shaped elastic stocking that fits snugly over a stump.

Since most residents who have amputations also have poor circulation, you must be on guard against bumping or injuring the tender stump. They may not even be aware that an injury has occurred.

Rarely is the elderly debilitated resident fitted with an artificial limb. Frequently, there is a lack of motivation to complete the strenuous rehabilitation as well as a lack of strength and energy. The cost is high, and the chance of success is often poor. Since crutches are difficult to use, requiring considerable strength and coordination, the elderly debilitated amputee is usually confined to a wheelchair.

Some amputees experience pain in the amputated limb. These pains are called *phantom limb pains*. Although the limb is gone, the resident actually feels pain in the absent part. The pain is not only real but can be quite severe. Report any complaints of pain to the charge nurse immediately. The nursing care you give and the emotional or psychological support you provide can greatly affect the adjustment of the resident who has had an amputation.

NURSING CARE OF THE RESIDENT WITH HEART DISEASE

The nursing care of residents with any kind of heart disease or circulatory impairment is primarily devoted to decreasing the amount of work the heart has to do and to observing and reporting changes in condition. The following guidelines should be followed when providing care to residents with heart disease.

Plan and organize care to assist the resident in balancing activity with rest (Fig. 13-14).

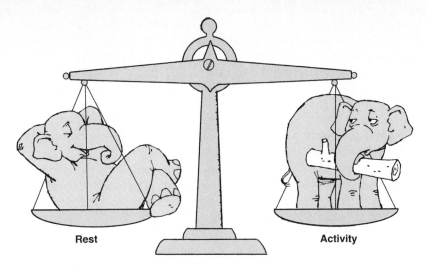

FIGURE 13-14
Activity and rest should be kept in balance.

Rest

Activity

The activity of the resident with heart disease must be limited to what he or she is able to tolerate. If the resident's activity causes chest pain or difficulty breathing, the pace must be slowed. Rest periods should be planned throughout the day, and activities should be scheduled around the rest periods. Too often, the needs of residents for adequate rest are placed in a secondary position to facility routines and schedules. The nursing assistant must plan rest periods for all residents and especially those with heart disease.

When a resident is acutely ill, even a bed bath can be exhausting. Be observant; listen to the resident. Remember, rest needs to be both physical and emotional. The resident with heart disease and hypertension needs an environment that is nonanxiety producing. Anger, frustration, and emotional upsets all increase the work of the heart and raise blood pressure.

You can help promote rest and reduce anxiety by assisting residents as needed. Many residents with heart disease have difficulty breathing and require special positioning to help them breathe easier. Some will need to sleep in a semisitting position supported with pillows.

Take time to evaluate how the resident rests best. This is particularly important to the totally dependent resident who is unable to communicate his or her needs. Residents with edema also require special positioning. Edema interferes with circulation, which leads to skin breakdown. When the resident has edema of the feet and legs, you should keep them elevated as much as possible to reduce the edema. Elevating a limb improves the flow of blood back to the heart.

In order to decrease the workload of the heart, the resident needs to be at a weight that is appropriate for his or her body height and build. Many times the physician will order a calorie-restricted diet. The resident may need a good deal of support, encouragement, and teaching in order to follow the diet.

Assist the resident to follow the diet ordered by the physician.

Most residents with heart disease have a problem with fluid retention. Fluid retention causes the heart to work harder and produces edema. An important factor related to fluid retention is sodium intake. Sodium is contained in **sodium chloride** (table salt). Sodium causes tissues to hold onto water. If the average adult did not add salt to food, they would lose approximately 10 pounds of fluid in a year. There are many foods that are naturally high in sodium, such as baking soda (and items made with baking soda — bread, cake, etc.). Milk, cheese, ham, bacon, cold cuts, and soft drinks are all foods high in sodium content. The physician will order a sodium-restricted diet for many residents with heart disease. Salt restriction is not easy to live with. Residents complain the food is bland and tasteless. When the physician's orders permit, a salt substitute can be used, but the taste is still poorly accepted by most residents. You will need to watch the food intake closely and report any departure from the physician's order to your charge nurse. Helping the resident and family understand the reasons for dietary restrictions or modifications helps them to follow the physician's orders.

Be alert for signs and symptoms of heart disease or changes in the resident's condition.

When you recognize the signs and symptoms of various forms of heart disease, you are able to notice subtle changes and report them immediately. Medications and treatments can then be started before an emergency arises. Develop good observational skills and be accurate! Take vital signs carefully. Pay attention to the rate, rhythm, and strength of the pulse. Observe and report sudden changes in behavior, orientation, sleeping and eating patterns. Pay particular attention to circulatory changes such as the presence of edema.

Never assume that symptoms are due to "old age." Most symptoms are related to disease processes and need attention and treatment. Too often those who provide care attribute all problems to "aging" and thereby neglect to evaluate and provide care that really needs to be given.

CHAPTER 14

The Endocrine System

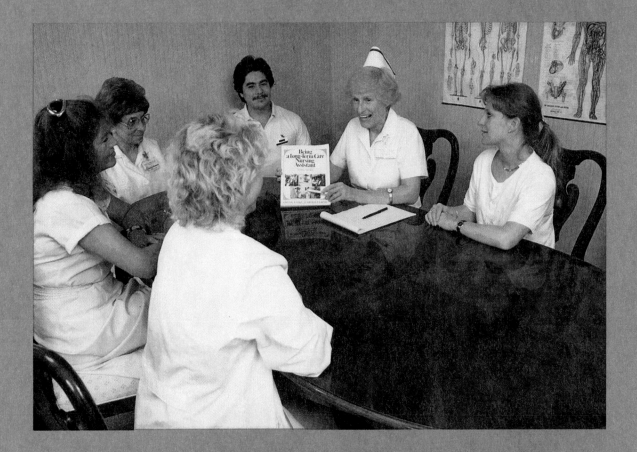

OBJECTIVES/WHAT YOU WILL LEARN

When you have completed this section, you will be able to:
- ■ Identify the endocrine glands
- ■ Match the functions of the glands with their names
- ■ Identify and describe the most common endocrine disease

The endocrine system (Fig. 14-1) is composed of:

- ● Endocrine glands
  - —pituitary   — adrenal
  - — thyroid   — pancreas
  - — parathyroid   — ovaries
  - — thymus   — testes
- ● Exocrine glands
  - — sweat glands of the skin
  - — salivary glands of the mouth
  - — other glands that secrete digestive juices

FIGURE 14-1
The endocrine system.

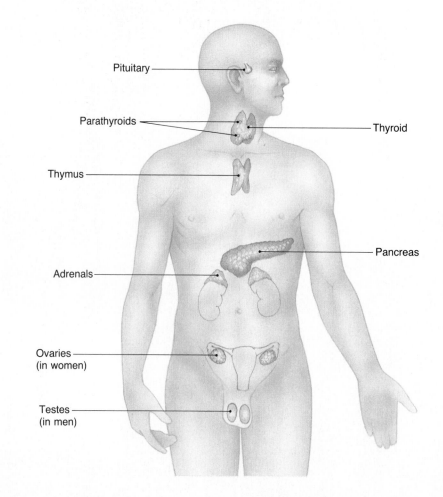

The functions of the endocrine system are to:

- Secrete hormones to regulate body functions related to growth and development
- Regulate body functions of metabolism and reproduction

The endocrine glands of the body secrete fluids called **hormones** (hormone is a Latin term meaning to arouse or set in motion).

- The **pituitary gland** is considered the "master gland" of the body. The hormones secreted regulate metabolism (the work of the cell). The hormones secreted by the pituitary gland affect other endocrine glands, stimulating them to secrete their hormones. *[handwritten: — controls hormone production of other glands.]*
- The **thyroid gland** is the largest of the endocrine glands. It produces hormones that regulate growth and the metabolic rate. Hormones secreted by the thyroid are mainly responsible for the individual's energy level. They influence skeletal growth, sexual development, as well as skin texture and hair luster. *[handwritten: — produce tyroxine. must have iodine to produce adeq. tyroxine]*
- The **parathyroid glands** are two pairs of small glands located within a capsule of the thyroid gland (one on each side of the thyroid gland). They produce a hormone that together with the thyroid regulates the level of calcium and phosphorus in the body. *[handwritten: — produces parathormone]*
- The **thymus gland** is a two-lobed ductless gland, larger in childhood than in adulthood. It has the structure of a lymph node. The exact function is not understood, but it is believed to play a role in the immune system of the body.
- The **pancreas** is the large gland located below and behind the liver and stomach. It is both an endocrine and exocrine gland. The endocrine portion secretes two very important hormones, insulin and glucagon. Insulin decreases the level of sugar in the blood. Disturbances of the insulin-producing gland lead to the disease known as *diabetes mellitus.* Glucagon increases the level of sugar in the blood.
- The **adrenal glands** are two small glands located on the top of each kidney. They are important in the metabolism of proteins, fat, and carbohydrates. They influence the levels of sodium and potassium in body fluids and are important in fluid and electrolyte balance. They produce hormones that help the body react and adapt to stress.
- The **ovaries** are the primary female reproductive organs and have two basic functions (see Chapter 15):
  — **Ovulation**, the process by which an ovum (egg) is discharged from an ovary at regular intervals
  — Production of the hormones estrogen and progesterone. These two hormones are essential in the reproductive processes and also influence a woman's feminine physical characteristics.
- The **testes** are the primary male reproductive organs and have two basic functions:
  — Production of sperm, which are ejaculated during sexual intercourse.
  — Production of the hormone testosterone, which is responsible for the masculine physical characteristics and which stimulates the production of sperm.

The hormones secreted by the endocrine system interact with the nervous system to organize and control many activities of the body. These glands are ductless, which means they empty hormones directly into the bloodstream. This makes secretions immediately available to cells in all parts of the body.

The hormones secreted by the exocrine glands are secreted through ducts into a body cavity or to the surface of the body. **Exocrine** means secreting externally. These glands do not secrete directly into the bloodstream.

Functions of the exocrine glands are varied.

- The **sweat glands** are located over the surface of the skin, with approximately 2 million in the body. The largest sweat glands are in the axilla (underarms) and groin. Sweating produces an evaporative cooling of the body. Some waste products are excreted as sweat.
- The **salivary glands** secrete saliva from various areas of the mouth. Saliva is necessary to moisten the mouth and to lubricate the food, making it easier to chew and swallow. Saliva contains enzymes essential to begin the process of food breakdown. The salivary glands produce approximately 3 pints of saliva each day.
- Other exocrine glands are the **mammary glands,** located in the breast in females, the **bulbo-urethral glands,** located near the prostate in males, and various intestinal glands associated with the digestive processes.

There are a number of diseases associated with malfunctions of the endocrine system. Such diseases are usually a result of overproduction or underproduction of a hormone. Not many disorders of aging are related directly to malfunctions of the endocrine glands. An older person can develop malfunctioning glandular problems just as a young person can. Some age-related changes do occur naturally—a gradual decrease in thyroid, parathyroid, and adrenal hormone secretions are examples of this.

The most common endocrine disease is diabetes mellitus. Diabetes is not just a disease of the elderly; it affects people of all ages.

There are four groups of people who are most susceptible:

- Those who are obese or who have a history of obesity (80% of all diabetics)
- Those over 40
- Women
- Those who have a history of diabetes in their family

In people over 65, diabetes is the eighth leading cause of death. There are over 3 million people in the United States suffering from diabetes. Understanding the nature of diabetes and how to provide nursing care to the resident with diabetes is a very important responsibility.

SECTION 2 CARE OF THE RESIDENT WITH DIABETES MELLITUS

OBJECTIVES/WHAT YOU WILL LEARN

When you have completed this section, you will be able to:
- Describe diabetes mellitus
- Define four terms related to diabetes mellitus
- List four common complications associated with diabetes mellitus
- Describe nursing actions that prevent complications of diabetes
- Demonstrate the proper technique for testing the urine for sugar and acetone
- Explain why you should report what is *not* eaten by the resident who takes insulin

Diabetes mellitus is a disorder of carbohydrate metabolism in which the ability to break down and use carbohydrates is lost due to disturbances in insulin production. Diabetes affects almost all the body systems and is a complex disease process. If insulin protection is too low or absent, the carbohydrates eaten cannot be utilized to nourish the cells of the body. Cells must be nourished in order to live!

Normal Carbohydrate Metabolism (Fig. 14-2)

- Carbohydrate types of food are eaten.
- The food is digested in the stomach.
- The food is converted to a simple sugar (glucose), which is an essential nutrient of the cell.
- The glucose enters the bloodstream for distribution to the millions of cells in the body.
- **Insulin** is secreted into the bloodstream. It is the "key" that opens the door to allow the right amount of glucose to leave the bloodstream.
- Glucose leaves the bloodstream and provides nourishment to the cells.
- Cells metabolize glucose and give off waste products, which are excreted through the kidneys, lungs, and skin.

Remember, if nutrients (glucose) cannot get to the cells, they are undernourished and may deteriorate or die no matter how much a person consumes.

Diabetic Carbohydrate Metabolism (Fig. 14-3)

- Carbohydrate types of foods are eaten.
- The food is digested in the stomach.
- The food is converted to a simple sugar (**glucose**), which is an essential nutrient of the cell during digestion.
- The glucose enters the bloodstream for distribution to the millions of cells in the body.

FIGURE 14-2
Normal carbohydrate metabolism.

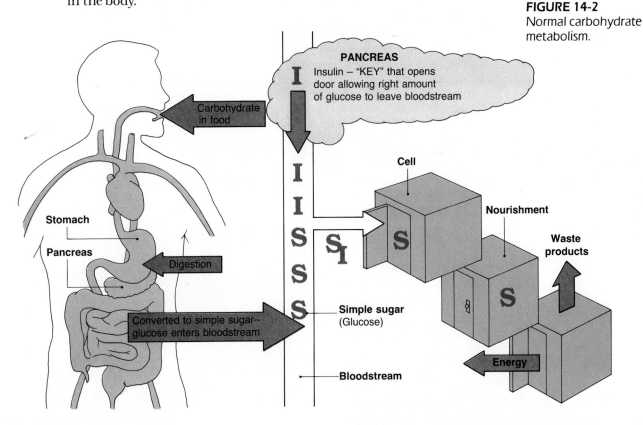

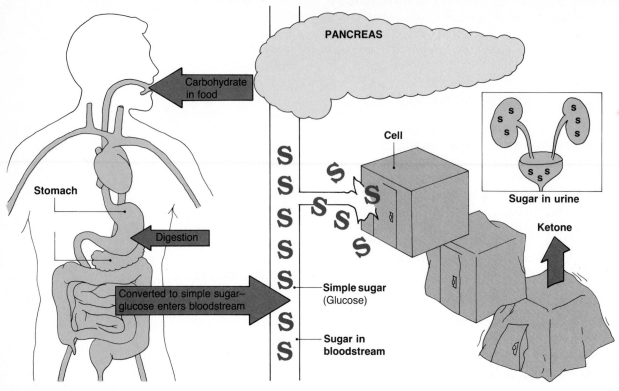

PANCREAS

Stomach

Carbohydrate
in food

Digestion

Converted to simple sugar–
glucose enters bloodstream

Cell

S S S S S S S S

Simple sugar
(Glucose)

Sugar in
bloodstream

Sugar in urine

Ketone

FIGURE 14-3
Diabetic carbohydrate
metabolism.

- There is no insulin or too little insulin, so there is no "key." The door remains locked, and glucose accumulates in the bloodstream (called **hyperglycemia**).
- The kidneys spill some of this excess glucose into the urine (called **glycosuria**).
- The cells are starving. They have no nourishment, so the body begins to use fats for nourishment. When fats are metabolized abnormally, there is a by-product created called **acetone.** Acetone is a type of ketone. Some ketones may be excreted in the urine (called **ketonuria**). When the acetone ketone buildup is excessive, the body is unable to excrete these toxic substances safely, and they can reach dangerous levels. The condition is called **acidosis.** Severe acidosis leads to coma and death.

Markedly elevated blood sugar and acidosis are the basis of the diagnosis of **diabetic coma.** Diabetic coma is a life-threatening problem that requires immediate diagnosis and treatment. For these reasons you will need to be familiar with signs and symptoms of diabetic coma. They are:

- Gradual onset
- Fruity odor to breath
- Skin hot and dry, face may be flushed
- Deep, labored breathing
- Loss of consciousness
- Nausea
- Glycosuria (sugar in urine)
- Hyperglycemia (high blood sugar)
- Drowsiness and lethargy

The treatment of most diabetes mellitus victims includes administration of insulin. Insulin is a hormone given by injection. Insulin cannot be taken by mouth because it is destroyed by the digestive enzymes. Residents who have no insulin production must take insulin in order to live. Residents who have some production may take oral drugs to stimulate the pancreas to secrete more insulin, or they may be able to control the disease by diet alone.

Just taking insulin injections is not enough. The resident must take the right amount of insulin, which is determined by the physician.

Establishing the correct dosage is often very difficult. Residents who are not easily controlled are referred to as "brittle" diabetics. For some residents, one daily dose of insulin is adequate, but in other cases insulin will be administered later in the day as well, based on the results of urine or blood testing.

One of the most common and serious complications associated with diabetes is **diabetic shock** or **insulin shock.** When insulin shock occurs:

1. Insulin is administered. Different types of insulin have their peak effect at different times—some are relatively fast acting; others are slow.
2. Carbohydrate types of foods are eaten.
3. The food is digested in the stomach.
4. The food is converted to simple sugar (glucose), which is an essential nutrient of the cell during digestion.
5. The glucose enters the bloodstream for distribution to all the cells of the body.
6. If the resident has received *too much insulin or failed to eat enough food,* too much glucose leaves the blood. The central nervous system must have a certain blood sugar level to function normally. Too low a blood sugar is called **hypoglycemia.**
7. Severe hypoglycemia leads to coma and death.

Signs and symptoms of insulin shock or diabetic shock:

- Sudden onset
- Perspiration, skin pale, cold, and clammy
- Shallow breathing
- Hunger
- Mental confusion, strange behavior
- Nervousness
- Double vision
- Loss of consciousness
- Low blood sugar (hypoglycemia)

It is often difficult even for the experienced licensed nurse to differentiate between diabetic coma and insulin or diabetic shock. Therefore, it is very important to recognize the little changes and report them before loss of consciousness occurs. If severe, *both diabetic coma and insulin shock can result in irreversible brain damage.*

Hypoglycemia (too *little* sugar) and hyperglycemia (too *much* sugar) are serious emergency conditions related to diabetes. However, there are many long-term complications that must be recognized in residents with diabetes. Residents with diabetes are at high risk to develop arteriosclerosis, heart disease, and stroke due to poor fat metabolism. Peripheral vascular disease is very common, resulting in poor circulation to the legs and feet. The poor circulation and elevated blood sugar make the diabetic very susceptible to infection. Once infection or injury occurs, the diabetic has decreased ability to heal or recover. For this reason, many amputations of the lower extremities become necessary due to ulceration and gangrene associated with the resident's diabetic condition.

Impaired vision and blindness are common complications of diabetes. The capillaries that supply blood to the retina of the eye develop weakened areas (**aneurysms**) and rupture, leading to detachment of the retina and blindness. In most cases diabetes can be controlled, although there is no known cure at the present time. The treatment and control of diabetes is a team effort that involves the physician, the licensed nurse, the nursing assistant, and the resident (Fig. 14-4).

The physician will order a calorie-restricted diet designed to limit the amount of carbohydrates consumed. The resident, the licensed nurse, and the nursing assistant must monitor the resident's intake carefully to ensure that the amount of carbohydrates consumed does not exceed that ordered by the physician. To provide the resident with the right amount of insulin, the physician will order the dosage based on blood tests done in the laboratory and blood and urine testing done in the facility. You must carefully follow the procedures for testing urine for sugar and acetone as well as record and report the results accurately! The nursing assistant will also need to record and report accurately what the diabetic resident *does not consume* with each meal.

Remember, insulin shock can occur when either *too much insulin is given or too little food is consumed.* If the resident refuses a meal and has taken insulin, there is a danger of insulin shock.

- Physical activity of the resident must be coordinated with the carbohydrates consumed and the insulin given. The licensed nurse and nursing assistant must observe and report changes in physical activity to the physician so that dosages of insulin can be adjusted accordingly. Generally, whenever exercise or heavy activity is planned, the diabetic must either increase carbohydrates or cut down on the insulin.
- Complications such as injury or infection must be prevented. Special skin care is essential. Any break in the skin can lead to severe infection. A small cut or laceration of the legs or feet can, and often does, lead to amputation of the limb. Diabetic residents require special foot care.
- Never attempt to trim the toenails of the diabetic resident. This is done by the podiatrist or licensed nurse only.
- Never cut corns or callouses.
- Note and report any signs of irritation.
- Make sure that the resident's feet are protected with well-fitting shoes and stockings.
- Make sure that there is never any restriction of circulation from elastic hose, garters, or bed covers.
- Protect the resident from overexposure to heat or cold.
- Report any complaints of pain, redness, discoloration, or changes in skin temperature to your charge nurse immediately!

FIGURE 14-4
Understanding diabetes.

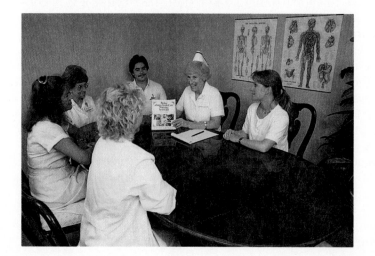

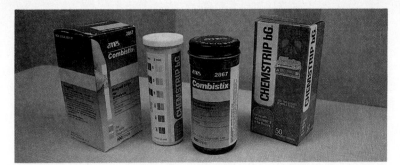

FIGURE 14-5
A number of preparations are available for diabetic testing.

Another important nursing function is testing urine for sugar and acetone (Fig. 14-5). Study carefully the procedures for testing urine. Testing urine is an efficient, easy method of checking the resident's metabolism of carbohydrates. When performing any test of urine, remember the UNIVERSAL PRECAUTIONS and wear gloves.

The Clinitest and Clinistix test determine the amount of glucose (sugar) in the urine. The Acetest or Ketostix reagent strip determines the amount of acetone or ketones in the urine. These tests are ordered by the physician and are generally done four times a day: one-half hour before breakfast, lunch, supper, and at bedtime. In residents whose diabetes is under control, the tests may be ordered less often.

For each test you will be using either a reagent strip or a reagent tablet. A **reagent** is a substance used in a chemical reaction to determine the presence of another substance. The names for these tablets or strips vary greatly according to geographical area and the company that makes them. When testing for sugar (doing the Clinitest), you will use Clinitest tablets, Tes-tape, Clinistix, or Uristix. When testing for acetone (doing the Acetest), you will use Ketostix, Tes-tape, Acetone Tablets, Uristix, or Labstix. Instructions for these tests are on their containers.

All tablets and strips used for these tests are *poisonous.* Always place equipment in a safe place where it is not accessible to residents. You will need to handle the equipment carefully because heat is generated during the Clinitest, and the bottom of the glass tube gets hot.

A fresh fractional urine specimen is needed for each testing. Since the sugar test and the acetone test are done at the same time, only one specimen is needed. The word *fresh* is used to refer to urine that has accumulated recently in the urinary bladder. To obtain fresh urine, it is necessary to discard the first urine voided in the AM because this urine has remained in the urinary bladder for an unknown length of time. One-half hour after discarding the urine, collect a fresh urine specimen for the test. This will be urine recently accumulated in the urinary bladder. The word *fractional* is used to refer to a small portion of urine voided. Only a very small amount of urine is needed for these tests.

Remember, testing urine for sugar and acetone accurately is vital to the resident's care. If you have questions regarding a reading or obtaining a specimen, ask your charge nurse for assistance.

Many facilities are now checking the blood in addition to or in place of checking the urine of diabetic residents. There are kits used by the licensed nurse that are called Glucoscan, Glucometer, or Acucheck, for example. The kits contain a sharp object, called a **lancet,** to prick the skin of a fingertip or earlobe to obtain a small sample of blood. A drop of blood is then placed on a treated strip. The glucose content of the blood is read by a device in the kit, which displays the results on a calibrated dial.

Measuring the blood sugar is believed to be more accurate and meaningful than testing urine. In many cases, urine testing has been eliminated for the diabetic resident. Make sure that you follow the instructions of the licensed nurse. Providing care to the resident with diabetes requires knowledge and skill in order to prevent life-threatening complications.

CHAPTER 15

The Reproductive System and Human Sexuality

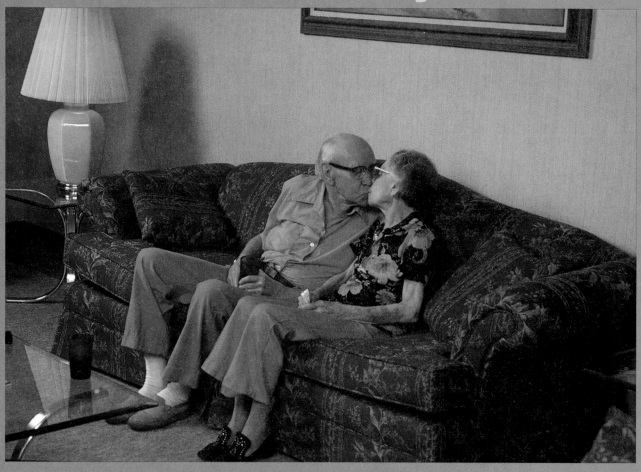

OBJECTIVES/WHAT YOU WILL LEARN

When you have completed this section, you will be able to:
- List the two basic functions of the male and female reproductive systems
- Name the primary sex hormones in the male and the female
- List four common symptoms associated with prostatic hypertrophy
- List two age-related changes that may affect the reproductive organs of the elderly female resident
- Give a vaginal douche

THE MALE REPRODUCTIVE SYSTEM

The reproductive system in the male (Fig. 15-1) is composed of:

- Testes
- Scrotum
- Penis
- Seminal vesicle
- Prostate gland

Functions of the male reproductive system are to:

- Reproduce an organism like itself
- Achieve sexual pleasure and release

In the male, the primary reproductive organs are the **testes.** The testes produce **sperm** (reproductive cells released upon ejaculation). The two testicles lie in a sac called the **scrotum** (outside the body and posterior to the penis). The **penis** is the primary male sex organ. The penis is capable of enlargement and erection upon stimulation. It is an important organ for sexual arousal in the male. The hormone **testosterone** influences both sexual activity and reproduction.

During intercourse, sperm travel up the vas deferens to enter the urethra. The sperm mix with secretions from other glands in the male reproductive system, seminal vesicles, prostate gland, and Cowper's gland. These glands contribute water, nutrients, and vitamins that, when added to sperm, make up **semen.** This is the fluid that is *ejaculated* (expelled) at the time the male experiences orgasm.

The **urethra** is the only duct in the penis. It expels urine and ejaculates semen. During the process of intercourse, the internal sphincter of the male's urinary bladder closes tightly so that urine is not mixed with semen.

AGE-RELATED CHANGES IN MEN

Probably the most significant age-related change that affects the male reproductive system is enlargement of the prostate. A majority of all elderly men develop some degree of **benign prostatic hypertrophy** (noncancerous enlargement of the prostate gland). The **prostate gland** encircles the urethra like a donut and is a firm, muscular gland. When it becomes enlarged, it squeezes against the urethra, causing painful urination, hesitancy, decreased force of

The reproductive system consists of the organs, glands, and supportive structures that are involved with human sexuality and procreation. In the male, spermatozoa and the hormone testosterone are produced in the testes. The female produces ova (eggs) and the hormones estrogen and progesterone in her ovaries. The union of ovum and sperm produce a single cell called a zygote. Through growth, cell division, and cellular differentiation (the formation of specialized cells) the new individual develops and matures.

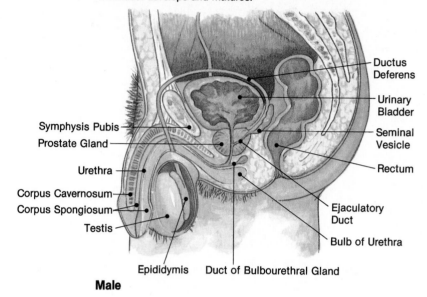

Male

FIGURE 15-1
The male reproductive system.

FIGURE 15-2
The female reproductive system.

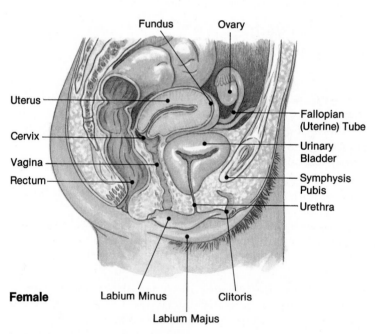

Female

Labium Minus (singular), Labia Minora (plural)
Labium Majus (singular), Labia Majora (plural)

the urinary stream, and frequency of urination, which usually results in **nocturia** (the need to get up at night to urinate).

If the condition persists and goes untreated, dribbling, poor urinary control, bleeding, obstruction, and kidney damage may occur. Some men are embarrassed and do not seek medical attention until the condition is advanced. There are a number of treatments that can help resolve the problem.

One of the most common is **trans-urethral surgery.** This type of surgery involves removing some of the prostate tissue. It is compared to "coring an apple" because the part of the prostate surrounding the urethra is removed. This surgery does not cause **impotence** (loss of sexual function).

Tumors of the penis, testes, and scrotum also occur but not more often than in younger males. Any lesion, growth, or lump should be reported at once so that proper medical examination can be scheduled.

Older men, in general, do experience a slowing down process of sexual desire and function that results in needing more time to achieve an erection. Usually, the erection is not as firm as it was in younger years, but the erection lasts longer.

THE FEMALE REPRODUCTIVE SYSTEM

The reproductive system of the female (Fig. 15-2) is composed of:

- Ovaries
- Clitoris
- Fallopian tubes
- Uterus
- Vagina

Functions of the female reproductive system are to:

- Reproduce an organism like itself
- Achieve sexual pleasure and release

In the female, the primary reproductive organs are the two **ovaries.** The main function of the ovary is to produce **ova** (eggs). These specialized cells are able to unite with the sperm cell released from the male during intercourse. This fertilized ovum grows for a period of 40 weeks into a human being.

The primary sex hormone in the female is **estrogen,** which enters the bloodstream during ovulation. **Ovulation** is a cyclical process that occurs monthly. An ovum is released from one ovary into the fallopian tube, where it may or may not be fertilized before it moves to the **uterus** (womb). This occurs once each month, usually 14 days prior to the first day of the next menstrual period. It is during this time that a woman is **fertile** (able to become pregnant). The estrogen released during ovulation causes a buildup in the lining of the uterus, preparing it for pregnancy. If pregnancy does not occur, menstruation starts. The hormones from the pituitary gland are involved in the development of the ovum and in maintaining pregnancy.

Menstruation is simply the monthly release of blood and the lining of the uterus. This bloody discharge flows out of the vagina generally for between four and seven days.

The human female has three openings in the perineal area: the urethra, the vagina, and the anus (Fig. 15-3). The **clitoris** is the primary female sex organ. It is capable of enlargement and erection upon stimulation. It is an important organ related to sexual satisfaction in the female.

AGE-RELATED CHANGES IN WOMEN

There are a number of age-related changes that affect the female reproductive system. Many of these problems could be managed more easily if regular physical examinations were done.

One of the most significant age-related changes in the female is the ending of menstruation, or **menopause.** The menopause, which usually occurs from age 42 to 50, ends the reproductive ability and results in decreased hormone

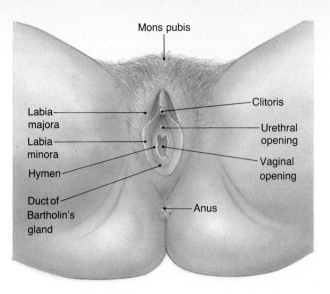

Mons pubis

Labia majora

Labia minora

Hymen

Duct of Bartholin's gland

Clitoris

Urethral opening

Vaginal opening

Anus

FIGURE 15-3
External female genitalia.

production. This decrease in estrogen is thought to contribute to the other changes described here.

The vulva of the elderly female loses hair and the labia (fatty tissue) have a flat and folded appearance. These changes cause the vulva to be more sensitive and susceptible to infection called **vulvitis.** For this reason great care must be taken to ensure that the perineal area is kept clean and free from irritation. When irritation occurs, the resident can scratch and cause more irritation and inflammation. Good personal hygiene, adequate hydration, and good nutrition will help eliminate this problem.

Vaginitis is an inflammation of the tissue of the vagina, which is a common problem due to loss of elasticity of the vaginal tissue and decreased secretions. These changes make the elderly female resident particularly susceptible to irritation and infection. Because of the decrease in secretions, some women experience painful intercourse. This can be remedied by use of water-soluble lubricants. Sometimes the physician will order special vaginal creams or suppositories, and sometimes a vaginal douche or vaginal irrigation is ordered.

The introduction of a solution into the vaginal canal with an immediate return of the solution by gravity is called a **vaginal irrigation** or **douche.** This irrigation is generally ordered to clean the vaginal canal or to relieve inflammation. If this procedure is overused, it will wash away the natural protective secretions, leaving the area more susceptible to irritation and infection. In an LTC facility a vaginal douche would be administered only when ordered by the physician. In some facilities the licensed nurse may administer the douche.

PROCEDURE

THE VAGINAL DOUCHE

1. Assemble your equipment:
   - Disposable douche kit—irrigating container, tubing clamp, douche nozzle
   - Solution
   - Bedpan and cover
   - Disposable bed protector
   - Disposable gloves
2. Wash your hands.
3. Identify the resident.

4. Provide privacy.
5. Explain the procedure to the resident.
6. Put on gloves.
7. Offer the bedpan—explain the results of the douche will be better if the bladder is empty.
8. Remove bedpan and measure urinary output if the resident is on intake and output.
9. Empty and rinse the bedpan and change gloves.
10. Place a disposable bed protector under the resident's buttocks.
11. Raise the bed to its highest horizontal position.
12. Open the douche kit, clamp the tubing, and pour the solution into the irrigating douche container.
13. Pour the cleansing solution over the cotton balls.
14. Place the bedpan under the resident's buttocks.
15. Cleanse the vulva using the saturated cotton balls. Separate the folds of the labia (lips) and wipe with cotton ball from front to back on one side. Discard cotton ball in bedpan. Wipe the other side with a cotton ball, again from front to back, and discard the cotton ball into the bedpan. Wipe down the middle from front to back with a cotton ball and discard.
16. Open the clamp to expel air. Allow the solution to flow over the vulva—do not touch the nozzle to the vulva.
17. With solution flowing, insert the douche nozzle tip into the vagina 2 to 3 inches with a gentle upward, then downward, and backward movement.
18. Allow the solution to flow, holding the douche container no more than 12 inches above the vulva or 18 inches above the mattress.
19. Rotate the nozzle until all the solution has been given.
20. Clamp the tubing and remove the nozzle gently. Wrap in tissue to prevent contamination and place the tubing inside the douche container for disposal.
21. Assist the resident in sitting upright on the bedpan. This will help drain the solution from the vagina.
22. Assist the resident to dry the perineal area as necessary with tissue and discard into the bedpan.
23. Remove the bedpan—place on chair.
24. Remove the bed protector.
25. Lower the bed.
26. Empty the bedpan, clean, rinse, and return to bedside cabinet.
27. Discard used equipment appropriately.
28. Remove gloves.
29. Make the resident comfortable.
30. Wash your hands.
31. Assist the resident to wash her hands.
32. Wash your hands.
33. Report and record any unusual observations.

The uterus, fallopian tubes, and ovaries are connected to each other by ligaments that normally hold each in their proper place. Sometimes these ligaments are stretched during childbirth and cause the uterus to **prolapse** (fall down into the vagina). This can cause problems in urination and also makes good hygiene more difficult. Sometimes surgery is done to repair the ligaments, or in other cases the uterus is surgically removed (called **hysterectomy**). A hysterectomy is usually necessary when tumors are present or when persistent bleeding occurs.

Because many people are embarrassed to discuss problems related to their reproductive organs, simple problems often develop into more serious ones. Observe carefully for abnormalities or complaints and report them promptly.

SECTION 2 HUMAN SEXUALITY

OBJECTIVES/WHAT YOU WILL LEARN

When you have completed this section, you will be able to:
- Define the term *sexuality*
- List two common myths associated with sex and the elderly
- Describe three ways you can acknowledge the resident's sexuality as you provide care

In addition to physical problems, there are age-related sexual concerns that require a sensitive, informed approach by the health-care team. Residents of LTC facilities have sexual feelings and needs that are frequently ignored due to reluctance to deal with this very natural and normal aspect of life.

In years past health-care professionals have often overlooked the sexual rights and needs of residents. Discussion and education regarding sex have been avoided and discouraged. The reluctance to deal openly and intelligently with our own as well as our residents' sexuality has led to ignorance, prejudice, and misinformation.

Sexuality is defined as the quality of being male or female. Sexuality includes the warm, loving, caring feelings shared between people. Sexuality is not age limited. We are sexual beings during our entire lifespan. Individuals who have over their lifetime established patterns of sexual behavior will generally continue these patterns into old age.

When the topic of sex and the elderly is presented, many social prejudices appear. For example, when a 70-year-old man shows a healthy interest in sex, he may be regarded as a "dirty old man," while the 35-year-old man is considered a "swinger" or "playboy." It is acceptable for young women to be concerned with fashion, sexy lingerie, and makeup, but eyebrows are raised if a grandmother shows interest! The aging process does not take away one's sexuality or one's need for meaningful relationships (Fig. 15-4).

SEX AND THE ELDERLY

Common myths associated with sex and the elderly are:

- Older women have lost all interest in sex.
- Older men are not capable of sexual intercourse.
- Older people don't need sexual satisfaction or pleasure.
- Older people don't care how they look and are not concerned about being attractive to the opposite sex.

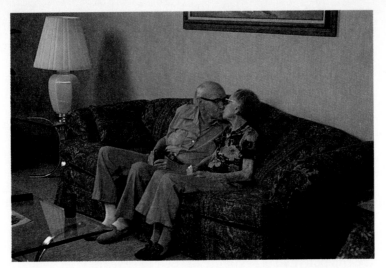

FIGURE 15-4
Sexuality is a part of our entire life span.

These misconceptions are often imposed on the elderly to the point that they either give up warm, meaningful sexual experiences or they harbor feelings of guilt and shame about having them. They are often deprived of the joy and comfort of feeling important and wanted by someone else.

One of the common reasons residents may not experience sexual fulfillment is the lack of an appropriate partner. They may have lost a spouse through death or divorce and feel that sex without marriage is immoral. For this reason, some may meet their needs for release of tension and sexual satisfaction through **masturbation.** Masturbation is sexual self-stimulation. Contrary to myths surrounding it, masturbation is a normal means of sexual satisfaction that does not harm the individual. You may observe one of your residents in the act of masturbation. If so, provide privacy by drawing the curtain or closing the door. It is never appropriate to ridicule or embarrass the resident. Some disoriented residents or those with dementia may masturbate without seeming to know what they are doing. In that case, be sure to take them to a private place and emphasize that what they are doing is not appropriate in public. Emphasize the inappropriateness of the place, not the activity itself.

Some residents may express their sexual frustration by reaching out to you. They may pat you or grab you where you don't wish to be touched. Handle the situation calmly and without anger. Simply state, "I don't like it when you do that," or "I don't like it when you touch me there." Show the resident affection in ways that you feel are appropriate. If your efforts to stop the inappropriate touching are not successful, ask the charge nurse if you can have a conference on how to handle the behavior. You may also obtain the help of the social worker or other members of the health-care team.

There are a number of ways that members of the health-care team can acknowledge the sexuality of each individual. Helping residents understand the effects of aging on sexual function is a beginning. A willingness on the part of the nurse to discuss sex openly demonstrates concern, acceptance, and respect for the resident's sexuality. Be observant and report special concerns to the charge nurse so that positive steps can be taken to deal with the resident's sexual needs.

You can recognize and accept the resident's sexuality as you provide care by following these guidelines:

Assist as necessary with personal hygiene.
Allow the residents to choose attractive clothing, cosmetics, and hairstyles. Help them to prepare for special occasions or outings.

- Assist them to maintain their sexual identity by dressing them in appropriate masculine or feminine attire.
- Always consider the resident's feelings and need for privacy. Take care not to expose residents unnecessarily. Close privacy curtains and doors.
- Help them establish a positive self-image. Never discuss their incontinence or episodes of confusion in the presence of others. Treat them as valued members of society.
- Show understanding and acceptance when they show interest and affection for each other.
- Residents should never be made to feel foolish or guilty for their expressions of love or sexuality.
- Consider the individual's right to privacy by allowing residents time alone, knocking before entering, and—when requested—assisting residents to find areas where privacy can be assured.

The nursing assistant has an important role in helping the residents realize the full potential of sexuality in their later years.

CHAPTER 16

Developmental Disabilities

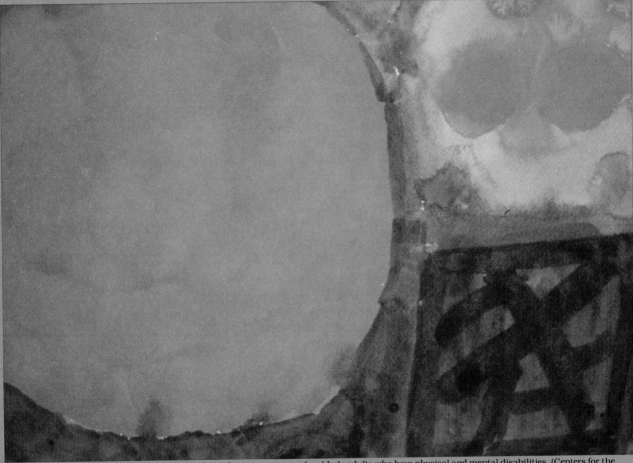

Opportunities for self-expression are available through an art program for elderly adults who have physical and mental disabilities. (Centers for the Handicapped, Inc., Silver Spring, MD.)

SECTION 1 INTRODUCTION TO DEVELOPMENTAL DISABILITIES

OBJECTIVES/WHAT YOU WILL LEARN

When you have completed this section, you will be able to:

- Define the term *developmental disability*
- List three causes of developmental disability
- Define the term *mental retardation*
- Describe what is meant by the concept of normalization, giving examples of a normalized environment
- Define the terms *age appropriate, developmental model, least restrictive alternative,* and *active treatment.*

Certain long-term care facilities are established for the care of the developmentally disabled. Nursing assistants play a vital role in these facilities. The nursing assistant functions as both a teacher and a caregiver. You may be called a trainer, a developmental aide, or a direct care staff member. Special knowledge and skills are required. In addition to the many nursing skills you have learned, you will need behavior management, teaching, and data collection skills.

The term **developmental disability** (DD) is a legal definition mandated by Congress in 1970 and revised in 1978. *Developmental disability* means a severe, chronic disability of a person that:

1. Is attributable to a mental or physical impairment or combination of mental and physical impairments
2. Is manifested (shown) before the person attains age 22
3. Is likely to continue indefinitely (chronic)
4. Results in substantial functional limitation in three or more of the following areas of major life activity:
   — self-care (activities of daily living)
   — receptive and expressive language (understanding others and making self understood)
   — learning (ability to acquire new skills and new knowledge)
   — mobility (ability to move from place to place without assistance)
   — self-direction (ability to make decisions about one's own life)
   — capacity for independent living
   — economic self-sufficiency (ability to support oneself)
5. Reflects the person's need for a combination and sequence of special, interdisciplinary, or generic care, treatment, or other services that are of lifelong or extended duration and are individually planned and coordinated

Four categories or diagnoses account for the majority of the individuals who are developmentally disabled. They are mental retardation, cerebral palsy, epilepsy, and autism. The new definition does, however, include accident victims and those who sustained brain damage due to illness.

MENTAL RETARDATION

More than 6 million people are believed to be mentally retarded. More than 100,000 babies born each year are likely to join this number. One out of every ten Americans has a mentally retarded person in the family.

Mental retardation is defined as "significantly subaverage general intellectual functioning existing along with deficits in adaptive behavior and manifested during the developmental period."* Although this definition sounds complex, it becomes clear when broken into parts. *General intellectual functioning* refers to the IQ (intelligence quotient) or score obtained on a standard test. The average IQ is 100. Significantly below average is considered to be an IQ of 70 or below. About 3 percent of the population would be classified as mentally retarded based on IQ alone.

Deficits in adaptive behavior are limitations in the person's ability to learn, to be independent, and to be socially responsible (Fig. 16-1). The person is evaluated based on what is considered normal or average for his or her age and cultural group. The *developmental period* is the period of time between conception and the eighteenth birthday.

Causes of mental retardation are usually divided into three categories: prenatal, perinatal, and postnatal. **Prenatal** causes are those that are hereditary or occur during the pregnancy of the mother. Examples of hereditary causes include Down's syndrome and Tay-Sachs disease. An example of retardation caused by an event during pregnancy would be an instance when the mother abuses drugs or alcohol during the pregnancy, and the baby is born mentally retarded. **Perinatal** causes are those that occur during the birth process. There may be a problem that cuts off the supply of oxygen to the baby, such as an umbilical cord around the neck or physical injury to the brain from difficulty going through the birth canal. **Postnatal** causes include any event that occurs after the birth, including illness, accidents, or physical abuse.

Mental retardation is divided into levels based on IQ scores:

Level	IQ Range
Mild mental retardation	50–55 to approximately 70
Moderate mental retardation	35–40 to 50–55
Severe mental retardation	20–25 to 35–40
Profound mental retardation	Below 20 or 25

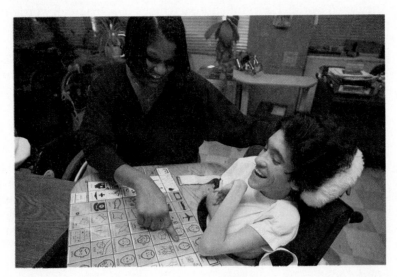

FIGURE 16-1
Communicating with a mentally retarded person.

*From: Grossman, H., ed., *Manual of Terminology and Classification in Mental Retardation*. Washington, D.C.: American Association on Mental Deficiency, 1973.

Most of the mentally retarded persons you will care for in a facility for the developmentally disabled will be either severely or profoundly retarded. The *profoundly retarded* person rarely is able to speak. Often this person will have sensory, skeletal, and other physical abnormalities. Most are either bedfast or chairfast. Fifty percent live in institutions. Research shows that they are placed in institutions earlier, are least often visited by family and friends, and die at the youngest age. One study showed that the average age of death of the profoundly retarded is 38. The major cause of death is pneumonia.

The *severely retarded* person will generally have some useful speech by adolescence. The severely retarded have fewer multiple physical handicaps, and their life span is longer than the profoundly retarded.

CEREBRAL PALSY

Cerebral palsy is a developmental disability caused by damage to the brain that results in the person having difficulty controlling the muscles of the body. Because the muscles often include those used in speech, a capable individual can be hidden within a body that cannot be controlled or understood. About 750,000 people in the United States have cerebral palsy. The causes of cerebral palsy are similar to the causes of mental retardation. They occur during pregnancy or birth and may be due to prematurity, lack of oxygen, or injury to the head. Many persons with cerebral palsy live active, successful lives in the community. Examples include a successful rock singer and a well-known comedienne. The person with cerebral palsy who is living in a facility for the developmentally disabled will probably have severe or multiple handicaps and may also be mentally retarded. Never assume, however, that someone with cerebral palsy is mentally retarded. Cerebral palsied persons are unique individuals who should not be labeled, categorized, or treated as part of a group.

AUTISM

Autism affects about 60,000 children under 18 years of age in the United States. Boys are affected three to four times as often as girls. Although very little is known about the cause of autism, it is thought to be a disability that results from a lack of organization in the functioning of the brain. Autistic children appear to be aloof and withdrawn from contact with others. They seem to live in their own world. The name *autism* comes from a Greek word *autos*, meaning self. The autistic person seems to respond in unpredictable ways to things he sees and hears. Some never develop speech. Some seem unaware of pain. Although some may become friendly and cheerful, many have severe behavior problems that include violence toward themselves, others, or their immediate environment.

EPILEPSY

Epilepsy is a condition or disorder in the electrical functioning of the brain that results in various kinds of seizures. Epilepsy does not cause mental retardation nor is everyone with epilepsy mentally retarded. In fact, the vast majority of those with epilepsy are *not* retarded. (Chapter 11, "*The Nervous System*," includes information on seizures and epilepsy; review that information now.) Epilepsy is, however, often present along with mental retardation and cerebral palsy because it may be caused by the same event that caused the other conditions.

NORMALIZATION

A facility providing care to the developmentally disabled adopts guiding principles or a philosophy of care that establishes not only how care will be given, but also the kind of environment in which it will be given. The most basic concept is called "normalization." **Normalization** means creating an atmosphere that is as close as possible to the atmosphere provided those citizens who are not mentally retarded (Fig. 16-2). It means offering the same opportunities and kind of treatment. Principles of normalization require that positive attributes or qualities of the individual be emphasized while negative qualities are eliminated. For example, if a developmentally disabled resident or client has a physical abnormality such as crossed eyes that would make the client appear unusual or abnormal, the crossed eyes should be corrected with surgery or special glasses. Great care should be taken in the grooming and dressing of your clients so that any negative physical traits are either disguised or offset by attractive, age-appropriate clothing and good grooming (based on chronological age, not mental or developmental age). With older clients, make special effort to select an appropriate hairstyle as well as clothing. For example, an older woman might look absurd in a ponytail with childlike bows or barrettes. There are, however, ways to pull the hair back that are more adult. A child's ponytail is placed high on the back of the head while an adult's is secured lower, at the back of the neck.

In order to create a normalized environment, it is essential that every staff member hold a particular belief: that all human beings are worthy of being treated with dignity and respect. If you believe that you are somehow "better" than those you serve, you will have difficulty treating your clients or residents as they deserve to be cared for.

Some of the ways you will know normalization when you see it are:

- Staff members treat people under their supervision with dignity and respect.
- Staff members do not exert undue power over the resident.
- Staff play the role of an associate or assistant, not a parent.
- Residents are encouraged to do all they can for themselves.
- Residents' rooms contain many personal items.
- Residents are encouraged to have personal belongings that are age appropriate.

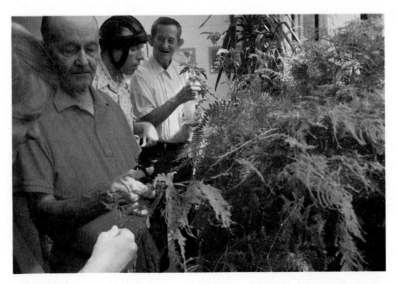

FIGURE 16-2
Normalization activities.

- Residents' clothing is individualized and age appropriate (not "uniform").
- Privacy is available for all residents. This means both visual privacy and privacy of information about the resident.
- Residents are encouraged to make choices about their lives (when to get up, when to go to bed, how to spend leisure time, what to wear, etc.)
- Residents are encouraged to become involved in the community. They are taught skills that will allow them to function successfully away from the facility. For example, if possible they should learn to use the telephone, take a bus, manage money, shop, and so on.

If you are now working in a facility for the developmentally disabled, use the list to see how your facility measures up when it comes to the principle of normalization. If you are seeking employment in this rewarding field, ask questions and observe for these concepts in action.

THE DEVELOPMENTAL MODEL

Another important factor for those working in this setting is a belief in the developmental model. The developmental model is based on the philosophy that all human beings have potential. Human beings thrive only to the extent that they are allowed and encouraged to change and to develop. The change and growth you see can seem very small, but to the resident it may be enormous. Your role will be to help each resident achieve as much growth as possible for that person.

LEAST-RESTRICTIVE ALTERNATIVE

Another guiding principle is that of choosing the least-restrictive alternative. Whenever there is a choice to be made in method of treatment or selection of activities or living arrangements, the goal is to choose the option that least limits the freedom and independence of the individual resident. In terms of medical care, this means that the physician orders the lowest dosage of a drug that will effectively manage the problem, or it means that instead of using a medication for a behavior problem, behavior management is attempted first. The least-restrictive alternative principle is also shown when residents are taught skills that allow greater independence and the ability to live in an environment where they can experience greater freedom and a more "normal" living situation.

PROGRAMMING

Each facility for the developmentally disabled has a program or program plan that describes in writing how the principles of normalization, least-restrictive alternative, and the developmental model will be made a reality. You might think of the program as parallel to a curriculum in a school. In fact, that's a good way to think of a DD facility. It is like a boarding school in that it serves as both home and school. The main purpose of the school is to teach skills that maximize or accentuate the positive aspects of each individual client and eliminate the negative aspects. The curriculum is designed to provide individual educational plans, which are called **IPP**s or individual program plans. A team of skilled professionals develop the individualized plan based on assessment of each client's abilities. The team includes the client, the parents of the client (if appropriate and possible), any agency that monitors the client's care, professionals including a registered nurse, physical therapist, speech therapist, psychologist, social worker, occupational therapist, special education teacher, and the program director of the facility. This team is referred to as the **ID team** or interdisciplinary team. The team is headed by a person called the **QMRP** or qualified mental retardation professional. The QMRP may have education and training in any of the professional disciplines mentioned above. For example, the QMRP might be a psychologist, physical therapist, nurse, and so on. This person must have knowledge and experience beyond the basic training in their particular field or discipline. Most often they must be approved by a state agency to serve as the QMRP.

Your role is to assist in carrying out the IPP as you work with the client individually and in small groups (Fig. 16-3). Clients are usually grouped according to ability, common interests, and common learning activities. In order to carry out the IPP, it is essential that you know what the objectives or goals and activities are for each client in your assigned group. At first, you may have to memorize the goals and plans. Normally these written plans are readily available to you in the classroom where you carry out your activities.

The program plan includes descriptions of all the activities involved in assisting each client to reach her or his individual goals. Activities may be grouped under categories such as functional life skills, fine motor skills, gross motor skills, and sensory-motor skills.

- **Functional life skills** are the skills necessary to allow the person to function as independently as possible. These may be ADL skills for some or activities such as making change or using the telephone.
- **Fine motor skills** require use of the fine muscles such as those of the hands. Fine motor skills would include such tasks as buttoning, writing, and feeding oneself.
- **Gross motor activities** involve the use of the larger muscles of the body. For example, physical fitness exercises or activities such as walking, swimming, or dancing are gross motor activities.
- **Sensory-motor activities** are designed to improve the thinking of the client by improving the information coming into the brain through all the senses, including sight, sound, smell, and touch. For example, in order to develop understanding of what "round" means, the resident might feel a ball, watch it roll and bounce, and even listen to a sound it makes. The concept of round would be important to learning about money (coins are round) or to learning certain types of jobs.

LEAST RESTRICTIVE ENVIRONMENT

Whatever the category of skills in the program, the goal is to provide skills that will allow the client or resident to live in the *least restrictive environment* possible. This means that of all the choices available for the living arrangements, the

FIGURE 16-3 (a) Learning to weigh oneself; (b) learning to self-administer insulin.

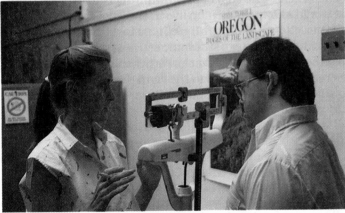
(a)

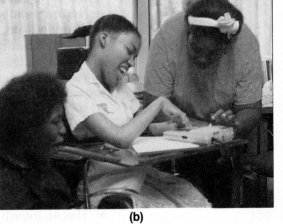
(b)

CHAPTER 17

The Restorative Nursing Assistant

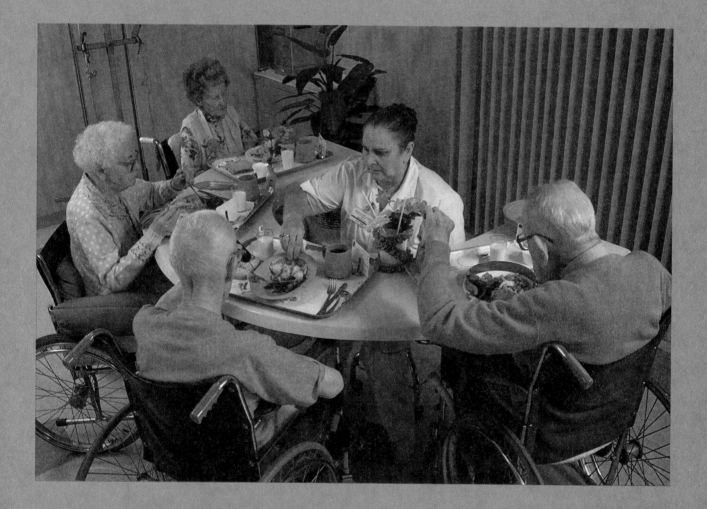

Section 1 Role and Responsibilities of the Restorative Nursing Assistant

OBJECTIVES/WHAT YOU WILL LEARN

When you have completed this section, you will be able to:

■ Explain why health promotion and prevention of disease are essential to any LTC facility's restorative program

■ Describe the overall philosophy of the restorative nursing program

■ Identify the basic job differences between a nursing assistant and a restorative nursing assistant

■ Correctly select from a given list those tasks that would be performed by a restorative nursing assistant

■ Write a restorative weekly summary using measurable behavioral terms from the information provided

HEALTH PROMOTION

There is a great need for LTC facilities to focus their efforts toward health promotion and prevention of disease and disability in addition to the treatment of existing and chronic illnesses. Health-promotion activities are programs designed to encourage good health practices. Components might include:

- Exercise
- Good nutrition
- Antismoking
- Discouraging substance abuse
- Health screening
- Immunization
- Socialization

Many of these programs can be offered in the LTC facility through in-house activity, social service, and nursing staff participation as well as through community agencies. When providing care and services to the elderly, prevention of disease and disability must be one of the primary goals!

RESTORATIVE NURSING PROGRAM

In most LTC facilities, there are one or more nursing assistants assigned as restorative nursing assistants (RNAs). These nursing assistants are usually certified nursing assistants who have received additional training in rehabilitation and restorative programs. This training is most often provided by licensed nurses, physical therapists, occupational therapists, and speech therapists.

In other LTC facilities, each nursing assistant will perform specific restorative services as part of her daily routine of providing care. Even when the restorative nursing program is delegated to RNAs, the rehabilitative care cannot be isolated and designated as the responsibility of a few. It is the responsibility of the *entire* health care team to continue to focus and direct their care toward maximum rehabilitation of the resident (Fig. 17-1). The National Council on Rehabilitation defines **rehabilitation:** "Rehabilitation means the restoration of the individual to the fullest physical, mental, social, vocational, and economic capacity of which he is capable."

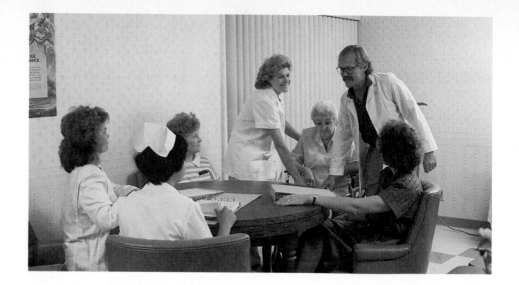

FIGURE 17-1
The rehabilitation team.

Throughout the book the importance of preventing disease and deformity as well as maintaining abilities and restoring lost functions has been stressed. It is important to remember that rehabilitation programs should never be limited to physical disabilities or conditions alone. The resident's psychological and social needs must also be included for any program to be successful. These concepts combined are the essential elements of any rehabilitation program.

Nursing assistants selected to work in the restorative nursing program must have a positive attitude about the potential for restoring and retraining residents in basic activities of daily living. This positive attitude should be based on knowledge as well as specialized skills.

The RNA will use all of the restorative skills expected of any nursing assistant but will also learn additional techniques related to activities of daily living in order to teach and motivate residents to do as much as they are physically capable of doing by themselves.

JOB DESCRIPTION — RESTORATIVE NURSING ASSISTANT (RNA)

In order to help you understand the responsibilities of the RNA, a sample job description is included for your review. The role of the RNA differs from the nursing assistant in several important ways, but *teaching* the resident to become as independent as possible is one of the most important.

Nursing service:	Restorative Nursing Assistant
Position summary:	The RNA is responsible to provide direct resident restorative care and training under the supervision of the Director of Nursing. The Director of Physical, Occupational, and Speech Therapies will provide additional training and will coordinate ongoing restorative programs for residents when professional therapies are discontinued.
	The RNA will follow facility's established policies and procedures and will assume other nursing assistant duties as assigned.
Responsible to:	Nursing Supervisor
Workers supervised:	None

	(Unless there are several RNAs where one person has been designated as team leader)
Interrelationships:	Director of Nursing
	Nursing Supervisor
	Charge Nurses
	Therapy Personnel
	ALL Health-Care Team Members
	Families
	Consultant Personnel
Education:	High School Diploma Desirable
Training experience:	Certified nursing assistant or equivalent experience/training plus documented inservice with therapy personnel at least quarterly.
Personal:	Presents neat, well-groomed appearance and has good physical health and stamina. Demonstrates emotional stability as well as an enthusiastic attitude toward restorative programs.

1. Follows established performance standards and performs duties per nursing service and restorative policies and procedures.

2. Requests clarification and/or training for policies and procedures that are not clearly understood.

3. Assists, as requested, new employees during orientation with implementation of facility's policies and procedures.

4. Provides direct restorative care as assigned, completing work accurately, safely, and in a timely manner.

5. Identifies special resident needs or problems and reports them to appropriate nursing and/or therapy staff.

6. Assists other nursing personnel with difficult or special assignments as necessary.

7. Identifies safety hazards and emergency situations and initiates corrective action immediately.

8. Provides care to residents without violating patient rights.

9. Participates in facility educational programs as required and/or assigned, orientation, inservice, precertification training, as well as quarterly therapy inservices.

10. Attends all classes as assigned and completes assignments on time.

11. Consistently demonstrates an attitude of cooperation and enthusiasm toward residents and other facility personnel.

12. Assumes personal responsibility for following facility procedures related to control of equipment and supplies.

13. Assumes accountability for compliance to federal, state, and local regulations related to restorative nursing care.

14. Reports to appropriate nursing personnel any incidents, problems, or failures of other personnel to adhere to facility policies and procedures.

15. Accurately documents incidents and/or unusual occurrences per facility policy and procedures.

16. Demonstrates consistent ability to work cooperatively with residents, members of the health-care team, families, and consultant personnel.

17. Participates in interdisciplinary care planning conferences and rehabilitation conferences as necessary.

18. Participates in the development of an individualized plan of restorative

care for assigned residents and implements restorative plan of care consistently.

19. Documents the specific restorative care, service, treatment, or program provided daily and documents residents' response or lack of response to care weekly.

20. Documents residents' progress or lack of progress to care plan restorative goals in behavioral, measurable terms.

21. Demonstrates concern for all residents by rendering immediate assistance to any resident in need.

22. Greets residents and their families by name and is consistently courteous and thoughtful.

23. Controls angry feelings and only expresses anger in appropriate areas.

24. Works wherever assigned to meet resident care needs.

25. Works as scheduled and is consistently dependable.

26. Comes to work on time and is consistently punctual.

27. Follows facility policies related to absences and notification of appropriate personnel.

28. Follows facility dress code and adheres to good personal grooming and personal hygiene standards.

29. Performs assigned restorative nursing tasks competently on a consistent basis.

30. Develops good interpersonal relationships with residents and utilizes acquired teaching skills to help resident become as independent as functionally possible.

RESTORATIVE NURSING TASKS

Review the specific text related to the tasks listed below and be sure you are prepared to perform these tasks competently. If you need assistance, seek help!

Specific tasks performed by the restorative nursing assistant include:

- Range of motion (passive and active), beginning on page 197
- Transfer training/development, pages 190–193
- Achieving balance — sitting, standing, walking
- Ambulation development -— increasing strength and stamina, pages 205–8
- Special positioning techniques, pages 208–14
- Special procedures to prevent contractures, foot drop, external rotation, skin breakdown, and other complications of immobility
- Indication for and use of assistive devices/adaptive equipment
- Weighing and measuring height, pages 101–6
- Giving whirlpool treatments/baths, pages 381–82
- Behavior management and reinforcement, pages 365–69 and 382
- Communication development/reinforcement, pages 382–83
- Providing assistance/training in activities of daily living
  — Self-feeding, pages 384–85
  — Bowel/bladder retraining and/or management, page 244 and page 386
  — Self-grooming, pages 386–87
  — Self-dressing, pages 387–88

The physician, licensed nurses, and various therapists will assess the resident's special needs and develop a plan of care that should be followed in order to prevent further disease or deformity. The specific restorative care to be provided is communicated to the resident's physician and a physician's order is given. When you understand that providing restorative care according to the physician's orders is as important as giving the resident the right medication and diet, you will begin to see what an important responsibility RNA assumes.

The restorative nursing plan will be found on the resident's care plan along with all the other care that is to be provided for the resident. It is helpful for the nursing assistant to understand specifically the goals established for the resident so that all care provided is goal directed. Take time to review the goals and approaches for the resident for whom you will provide restorative nursing care.

DOCUMENTATION BY THE RNA

All of the principles of observation and charting previously studied are applicable to the RNA. Accurate documentation is very important due to the fact that the RNA is the only nonprofessional staff member who documents progress or lack of progress to established resident goals in the resident's health record. The RNA will chart care given or attendance at special retraining programs each day by initialing in the appropriate place. Daily programs may require specific narrative charting describing what was done for the resident and the resident's response to the care provided. Notes that would be useful in writing the weekly summary should be kept daily. At a minimum, the resident's progress or lack of progress toward specific goals should be summarized weekly. This weekly summary should be specific, clearly reflecting resident's progress toward goals in behavioral and measurable terms:

Correct: Resident able to stand at bedside with assistance of one for 3 minutes. Balance and strength improving as minimum steadying support is now necessary.
Incorrect: Resident is doing better.
Correct: Resident feeding self using spoon 50 percent of the time versus only 25 percent of the time last week. Requires fewer reminders to use spoon than last week.
Incorrect: Resident using her spoon more, is doing better.

There may be times when residents fail to cooperate with the RNA by refusing to participate in a program or any specific care ordered. When this occurs, it is essential that you:

- Notify the charge nurse of the resident's refusal.
- Chart the resident's refusal as well as the stated reason for refusal: "I'm too tired to walk today"; "My son is coming today, I want to get ready for him early."

SECTION 2 TEACHING THE RESIDENT

OBJECTIVES/WHAT YOU WILL LEARN

When you have completed this section, you will be able to:
- Describe the best learning environment for the resident
- List four principles of adult learning

- Interview a resident and determine the nursing actions most helpful during her or his rehabilitation
- Select from a list those statements that would positively reinforce the resident's behavior
- Describe how depression interferes with residents' rehabilitation progress.

Teaching is defined as "to cause to learn by example or experience." The teacher *must* be able to answer these questions before starting any teaching program:

- What do I want to achieve?
- How do I proceed to achieve it?
- How do I know when I've achieved it?

These questions need to be answered by the professional medical staff during the interdisciplinary conferences for each resident who needs a restorative teaching program.

- What do we hope the resident will be able to do as a result of the teaching program? This is the goal.
- What should we do to help the resident achieve the desired goal? This is the approach.
- How will we measure the resident's progress or lack of progress toward the goal? This involves observation and charting.

It is important to understand that when we establish goals and proceed with a resident teaching program there may be a big difference between what *we* have decided *we* would like the resident to do and what he or she may be willing to do. It is always best when the resident is involved in the goal-setting process because if the resident is not motivated to achieve the goal, the task becomes much more difficult and often impossible to achieve.

We all had our first learning experiences as infants and children when we were totally dependent on others for our care. As we grew older, our parents gave up some of their control and allowed us to assume responsibility for our own learning.

When adults face the task of relearning a lost skill or function, they resent being placed in a dependent role again. Often this resentment is expressed in anger, frustration, and/or withdrawal and depression.

Many residents who need specialized restorative nursing care and retraining will be in some stage of depression. It is a natural reaction to experience grief and anger when functional losses occur. The resident may believe there is "no use in trying" and indicate an attitude of "giving up." Social withdrawal as well as episodes of crying or irritable and demanding behavior are not uncommon. One of the major reasons for depression is related to dependence and the loss of control the resident feels. Sometimes well-meaning nurses tend to make the situation worse by treating residents as if they are helpless, which seems to the resident synonymous with worthless. Therefore, it is always appropriate to assist the resident to do as much as possible for himself, even if he is slow and inefficient.

It is always important to explain to the resident what you are going to do for and with him. It is not helpful to be unrealistic or to give the resident false hope.

Providing supportive encouragement and giving praise when small successes are achieved will help reinforce the resident's sense of hope. Putting emphasis on the resident's abilities rather than disabilities is an essential part of rehabilitation.

Even though residents may be physically dependent, we should *never* treat them or talk to them as if they were children. When an adult is forced to resume the dependent learner role, learning is impaired. There are some basic principles of adult learning that you must understand in order to help your residents learn most efficiently.

- Adults expect to be treated with respect.
- They need to understand specifically what they are going to do (the goal).
- They need to understand what they will have to do as well as how you are going to help them (the approach).
- They need to feel accepted and free to express their frustrations, feelings, or ideas.
- Adults learn more quickly from the shared experiences or successes of others.
- They should have their learning tasks start at their present level of function.
- They need to have learned skills put into immediate use — do not delay practicing after a new skill is learned.
- Some residents have to *unlearn* some things that are inconsistent with new ideas or techniques. (Sometimes the licensed nurse may need to explain why a particular approach is being used that may be different from what the resident had previously learned.)
- They need reinforcement, praise, and encouragement for even the smallest successes or progress.
- They will learn better and faster if you help them understand that they are making progress. Comments such as "last week you were only able to walk to the bathroom and now you can go to the dining room and back" help the resident clearly recognize the progress she has made, and this positive reinforcement helps motivate her to continue.

The physical therapist, occupational therapist, or speech therapist will generally do the initial "teaching" or retraining during the rehabilitation program. Once the resident has reached certain therapeutic goals, the therapist will assign continued restorative care to the RNA under the supervision of the licensed nurse. The RNA will be responsible to continue the therapy by practicing and supervising the resident as he or she performs the skill or task.

A useful technique to assist residents in performing the skills or tasks is prompting. **Prompting** is a verbal reminder of what to do next — a verbal clue: for example, to remind the resident to look up while walking by saying, "Chin up, Mr. Jones." Keeping the clue simple and encouraging all who provide care to use the same clue consistently helps reinforce the desired actions. The prompting clues should be included in the approach portion of the care plan.

The environment in which anyone learns has a direct relationship to how well they learn. Generally an area that is free from distractions where privacy can be maintained is desirable. The resident should be comfortable and at "his best." Most people are at their best when they are not overly tired or anxious.

A positive environment that invites open discussion between the resident and the RNA will help the resident to feel accepted, worthwhile, and comfortable. This type of environment facilitates learning and therefore progress toward reaching the rehabilitation goals.

OBJECTIVES/WHAT YOU WILL LEARN

When you have completed this section, you will be able to:
- Demonstrate teaching a resident to perform range-of-motion exercises independently
- Demonstrate teaching a resident to transfer independently
- Select from a given list those statements that are true regarding achieving balance and increasing strength for ambulation
- Demonstrate special positioning techniques to prevent pressure, contractures, and foot drop
- Demonstrate the correct procedure for giving a whirlpool bath
- Describe why performing ADLs independently is an important goal for most residents whose functional abilities have been lost or are impaired

RESTORATIVE NURSING PROCEDURES/GOALS

Range-of-Motion Exercises (ROM)

The restorative goal is to preserve the resident's present range, thereby preventing further deterioration, and when possible teach the resident to assist and eventually do ROM independently. The resident may require both active and passive ROM with varying degrees of assistance from the RNA. The physical therapist will provide the RNA with specific instructions if resistive types of exercises are to be used with residents.

Transfer Training

The restorative goal could be to achieve independence in transferring from wheelchair to various objects or to transfer with minimal assistance.

Achieving Balance in Standing, Sitting, or Walking

The restorative goals could be to achieve balance in standing, sitting, and walking through increasing strength and practice with the RNA (Fig. 17-2).

FIGURE 17-2
Ambulating the resident.

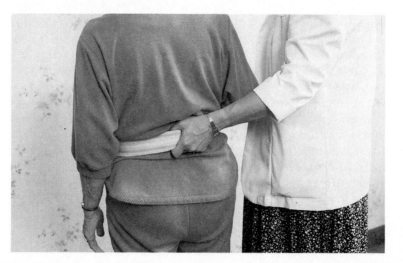

Ambulation Development

The restorative goals could be achieving independence in ambulation, independent ambulation with the use of assistive devices, or increasing ambulation strength and endurance through practice with RNA. Remember to use the safety belt while assisting residents to ambulate.

Use of Special Assistive Devices

The RNA should be very familiar with how assistive devices can increase independence for residents. The occupational or physical therapist will provide the RNA with additional training in the use of assistive devices. The RNA should observe and monitor the use of these devices with all residents as well as make recommendations to the charge nurse whenever a resident seems to need additional assistive equipment. It is very important that these assistive devices are properly measured and fitted for the resident. The occupational or physical therapist will make necessary recommendations regarding specific equipment. The restorative goals would almost always relate to the resident being able to function independently or with less assistance.

The following are basic guidelines for measuring, fitting, and adjusting assistive devices used in ambulation:

- *Walkers* — When the resident is standing erect with hands resting on the hand grips (Fig. 17-3), the walker should be at the height of the greater trochanter (straight across from the pubic bone; review the location on the skeletal diagram, page 176). There should be approximately 20 degrees flexion at the elbows when the walker is moved forward. The resident should be able to stand erect when moving the walker forward.

- *Crutches* — should be measured from the axilla (arm pit) to the floor and then add 2 to 4 inches. You should be able to insert two to three fingers between the axillary pad on the crutch and the axilla when the crutches are forward 4 inches and 6 inches out to the side. The hand-grip level should be adjusted to allow 20- to 30-degree flexion of the elbow when moving forward.

- *Canes* — The highest part of the cane should be at the height of the greater trochanter when the cane is at the side. The shoulders should not be elevated or depressed when walking with the cane; they should be level. There should be 20- to 30-degree flexion of the elbow upon movement forward.

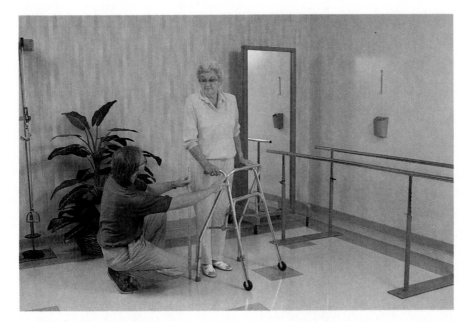

FIGURE 17-3
The walker should be at the proper height.

The following guidelines should be followed when assisting a resident to relearn how to walk using a walker:

- *Pick-up walker* (Fig. 17-4) — used in non-weight-bearing with progression to full-weight-bearing gait. It is better than crutches for most elderly residents as they feel more secure, and the walker requires less strength and coordination than crutches.
- *Four-wheeled walker* — used to take pressure off the lower back when only moderate or minimal balance impairment exists. It may be used when the resident's upper body strength is poor and she or he is unable to physically pick up and move a walker. It is frequently used when the resident is very close to full weight bearing.
- *Semiwheel walker* (Fig. 17-5) — This is the same as a pick-up walker but used when the resident lacks enough strength or endurance.

Essential steps to follow when walking a resident with a walker:

- Verify the physician's or physical therapist's order
- Instruct/inform the resident about the procedure
- Check joint range of motion and muscle strength
- Check standing balance
- Measure and adjust height of walker properly
- Instruct resident regarding standing and balancing before taking any steps
- While assisting ambulation with a walker, stand behind the resident and slightly to one side with one hand grasping the safety belt and the other hand ready to grasp the resident's shoulder.
  Note: The gait to be taught will be determined by the physical therapist, based on the disability and its severity. The physical therapist should instruct and initially observe as you assist residents with gait retraining to ensure that proper technique is used. Be sure to follow the therapist's directions.
- For non-weight-bearing gait: Stand with weight on uninvolved extremity assisted by walker and use of both upper extremities. Move walker forward and shift weight to upper extremities. Have resident hop forward with uninvolved extremity. Many elderly residents are unable to hop and will use a forward shuffling motion. This is acceptable as long as there is no weight placed on the involved extremity.

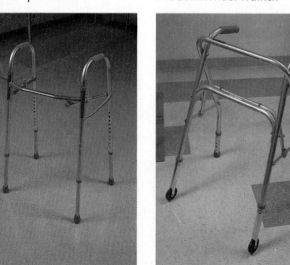

FIGURE 17-4
The pick-up walker.

FIGURE 17-5
The semiwheel walker.

- For the partial-weight-bearing gait: Stand with weight on the uninvolved lower extremity, resting involved extremity on the floor but applying no pressure by supporting the body with the upper extremities on the walker. Move the walker forward, keeping the weight on the upper extremities. Step forward with involved lower extremity, allowing partial weight bearing as ordered by the physician or therapist. Then bring uninvolved lower extremity forward. (Repeat)
- For full-weight-bearing gait: Stand with weight evenly distributed or balanced on both lower extremities, resting hands on walker. Move walker forward, and shift weight to upper extremities. Step forward with involved extremity, and then bring uninvolved extremity forward.

Special Positioning/Preventative Techniques

The restorative goals could be to prevent development of pressure areas or contractures, to use protective devices to position residents so range of motion is not impaired, to prevent foot drop, and to position residents to promote comfort and reduce pain.

Weighing, Measuring, and Reporting Changes

The RNA is commonly assigned to weigh and measure height of residents on admission as well as on a monthly basis. Because monitoring the resident's weight is an important nursing responsibility, it is often assigned to one person who has demonstrated competence in weighing and measuring residents and who is familiar with balancing the scales when necessary.

The RNA should understand the importance of weighing residents under the same conditions and at approximately the same time of day. Most facilities have the RNA report the monthly weights to the charge nurse for evaluation and recording in the resident's health record. The licensed nurse is responsible for notifying the physician, dietitian, or family of significant fluctuations in the resident's weight.

Giving Whirlpool Baths

The RNA works closely with licensed nursing personnel and the physical therapist when the physician orders whirlpool baths. Specific types of whirlpool therapy may be ordered to achieve a desired effect. Restorative goals could be:

- To stimulate circulation to a particular limb or area
- To cleanse a wound through circulation of water and antiseptic additives ordered by the physician
- To loosen and remove dead, necrotic tissue through the agitation of water against the area
- To relieve tension and discomfort as a relaxation technique

In some facilities, a mechanical lift will be used to place the resident in the whirlpool tub (Fig. 17-6). Water temperature should be the same as for a regular bath, 105 ° F. The physician may order a specific type of antiseptic solution to be added to the bath. The RNA should follow the directions of the licensed nurse or the physical therapist when adding solutions to the whirlpool.

Review the procedures for giving baths (pp. 153–158) and make sure to take all safety precautions. The whirlpool bath differs in that the water is agitated through a mechanical device. As with any equipment, it is essential that you understand the exact procedure to be followed for the equipment you are using. Follow manufacture's guidelines and clarify any questions or concerns. Special infection control procedures must be followed to properly clean and sanitize the whirlpool between residents. Due to the fact that open wounds are

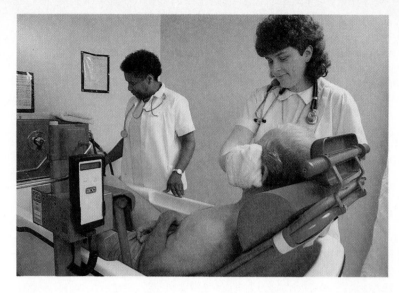

FIGURE 17-6
Giving a whirlpool bath.

treated with whirlpool therapy and there is a potential for cross-infection, the policies for cleaning and disinfection of the whirlpool must be followed strictly.

Behavior Management

The restorative goals of any behavior management program are directed toward changing behavior and replacing undesirable behavior with desirable or more acceptable behavior. The multidisciplinary health-care team will develop a plan of care designed to change or modify behavior. It may be the responsibility of the RNA to monitor the implementation of the plan along with the licensed nurse. Sometimes it takes several kinds of approaches to the problem before behavior changes.

The following is an example of what a behavior management care plan might include:

Problem: Resident yells "help me" continuously.

Approach: Identify times when yelling behavior is increased or decreased. Identify any possible "triggering" factors that initiate the yelling behavior.
Identify any factors that decrease yelling behavior. Have staff spend time with resident when he is not yelling. Implement factors identified that decrease yelling behavior. When resident is yelling, decrease communication to essential needs only.

Goal: Yelling behavior will decrease from continuous yelling to extend to periods of 30 minutes without yelling by date ____.

Throughout the book are many references to appropriate ways to deal with residents who have behavior problems. Be sure you review and understand the basic principles outlined. See the behavior management section in Chapter 16, pages 365–69.

Communication Development   *Study.*

Assisting residents who have difficulty speaking, expressing themselves, and making their needs known is one of the most challenging tasks of any nursing assistant. Probably the most important nursing skill that can be developed is *patience!* There is nothing more frustrating to residents or staff than the inability to communicate; taking time to listen as well as making every attempt to understand that meaning is essential to the emotional well-being of the resident.

The speech therapist will generally work with residents who have speech problems and will make specific recommendations to the staff regarding appropriate ways to communicate with the resident. Understanding the different types of speech problems outlined in Chapter 11 will assist you in working more effectively with these residents.

Frequently, the RNA will take the restorative program over from the speech therapist at the appropriate time. The speech therapist will instruct the RNA in exactly how to practice various speech patterns with the resident and how best to communicate with the resident. The communication development program will be outlined in the resident's plan of care so that all who provide care can consistently use the same approach with the resident. When communication can be reestablished for a resident, you will find this event one of the most rewarding experiences in providing nursing care.

ACTIVITIES OF DAILY LIVING

For those who are well and have no functional impairments, performing activities of daily living is almost automatic. However, when these basic functions are lost, it is frustrating and devastating to residents. The loss of control and then dependence on others is both frightening and humiliating. Because ADLs are so basic to our independent lifestyle, these are often the first problems to be addressed in therapy with the impaired resident.

Each resident should be evaluated to determine if he or she could benefit from the ADL program. The evaluation may be done with the physical and/or occupational therapists. Often a form is completed and placed in the resident's chart. The evaluation includes how much assistance is needed to perform each of the ADL skills.

Commonly used terms are: *supervision, standby assistance,* and *minimal, moderate,* and *maximum assistance.* Supervision refers to the need to have a staff member present to provide encouragement and verbal guidance. Standby assist means that a staff member is present to observe and be readily available if help is needed. Minimum assistance usually means that the resident performs about 75 percent of the task and the nursing assistant performs the remaining 25 percent. Moderate assist means that the resident performs about half or 50 percent and the nursing assistant performs the other 50 percent. Maximum assist usually refers to the resident performing 25 percent and the nursing assistant performing 75 percent of the task.

Figure 17-7 is an example of an evaluation that might be used to select candidates for an ADL program and to help set individual goals and approaches.

ADL EVALUATION

Name_____ Date of Birth_____
Date of Admission_____ Physician_____
Diagnosis_____
_____

MENTAL STATUS	yes	no
Able to make needs known		
Able to follow one- and two-step commands		
Can attend for at least 5 to 10 minutes		

HEARING
Normal _____
Wears prosthesis _____
Hard of hearing _____
Able to hear best in   Right_____ Left_____ ear.

VISION
Normal _____
Wears glasses _____
Blind _____

FIGURE 17-7
Sample evaluation form to select candidates for an ADL program.

RANGE OF MOTION	Able R L	Partially Able R L	Unable R L
Reach hands above head			
Cross arm across chest			
Reach down toward floor			
Bend knees			
Straighten legs			
Move leg away from the body			

Right-handed _____ Left-handed _____ Able to use nondominant hand

Tremor	mild	moderate	severe
Contractures	mild	moderate	severe

Specify joints involved_____

Pinch	good	fair	poor
Grasp	good	fair	poor

BALANCE/MOBILITY

Sitting	good	fair	poor
Standing balance	good	fair	poor
Transfers	light	moderate	severe
Mobility	fully ambulatory	amb. with equip.	nonambulatory
Sitting tolerance			_____ minutes.

DRESSING	SUPERVISE	STANDBY	MIN.	MOD.	MAX.	UNABLE
Put on shirt						
Line up buttons						
Button/fasten						
Unbutton/remove						
Get undergarments						
Pull pants over feet						
Stand to pull up						
Put on socks/shoes						
Tie/fasten shoes						
BATHING						
Wash face						
Wash upper body						
Wash perineal area						
Wash legs/feet						
GROOMING						
Brush teeth/dentures						
Brush/comb hair						
Shave						
Apply deodorant						
Apply makeup						

FIGURE 17-7
(cont.)

RESTORATIVE EATING OR SELF-FEEDING PROGRAMS

The restorative eating program is one of the most important responsibilities of the RNA. The major purpose of the program is to assist residents to attain their highest level of independence in eating (Fig. 17-8). Each resident should be evaluated by the occupational therapist prior to entry into the program. The resident must have some restorative potential for retraining. The resident who requires feeding and has little restorative potential should be identified and grouped with other residents with similar needs. You need to think of "feeding and restorative eating" differently.

Residents who are assigned to this program should be those who *do not* have swallowing difficulties but who have difficulty in eating independently. Residents with swallowing problems or other eating difficulties are at high risk for aspiration, and they require special therapeutic assessment as well as a specific plan of care that should be developed by the licensed nurse or the occupational therapist. Special feeding techniques to be used for residents with swallowing difficulties should be reviewed and practiced under the direction of the occupational or speech therapist.

Candidates for the program include those who have recently lost some of their self-feeding skills, who have physical disabilities that would benefit from learning to use adaptive equipment, or who have recently completed an occupational therapy program and need more practice. Some programs also include residents who take a long time to eat (more than 45 minutes) or who have been refusing to eat.

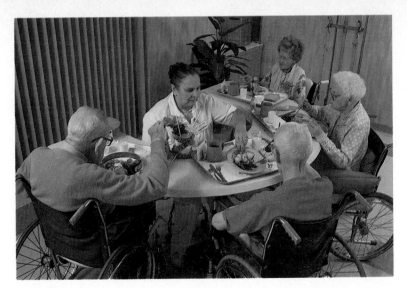

FIGURE 17-8
Assisting residents to attain their highest level of independence in eating.

Residents participating in the restorative eating program may be able to feed themselves but have other eating behaviors that are not socially acceptable such as food stealing, throwing food, making noises, or using hands to eat inappropriately. The format/structure of a dining program should include the following:

- Class size should be small with no more than four to six residents assigned for each RNA. (Class size should take into consideration the amount of assistance each participating resident needs.)
- The room for the program should be attractive, well-ventilated, with good lighting, and free from distractions. Making the environment as inviting as possible with tablecloths, flowers, and the like sets the stage for a positive dining experience.
- Residents participating in the dining program should be grouped together according to their functional abilities. When high-level functioning residents are placed with low-level functioning residents, they regress. If more than one seating is not possible, segregate seating by placing the groups at different tables.
- Each resident who participates in the program should have program goals as well as the appropriate actions and approaches identified on the care plan. This is usually coordinated by the occupational therapist and the licensed nurse. The RNA should follow the plan and report changes in condition or progress to the charge nurse immediately.
- Make sure that any necessary adaptive equipment that has been recommended for the resident is available at each meal. (The occupational therapist is generally responsible for recommending the type of adaptive equipment most appropriate for the resident.)
- Residents must be clean, dry, and properly positioned for mealtime.

RESTORATIVE EATING CARE PLAN ENTRIES

The multidisciplinary team will assess the resident and develop specific care plan goals based on each resident's identified needs. Sample care plan entries are shown below.

Problem: J. Jones uses her fingers for all foods and does not use appropriate utensils.

Approach: Hand spoon to Mrs. Jones when she is given her food. If she begins to use fingers, place your hand across the hand gently and

say, "No Mrs. Jones, use your spoon," and hand her the spoon
again. Repeat this process as often as necessary during a meal
period. Praise when using spoon.

Goal: Mrs. Jones will use a spoon rather than fingers to eat by date
_____.

Problem: Mr. Smith gets up and leaves table many times during meal
period.

Approach: Sit Mr. Smith at table when tray is ready to be served. Set up tray
for meal and get him started. When he starts to get up, place
hand on shoulder and encourage him to finish minimum of 50
percent before getting up. After getting up, return him to table
and repeat until 100 percent has been consumed. Praise for
staying seated.

Goal: Mr. Smith will consume 100 percent of food getting up only one
time by date _____.

Problem: Mr. Hall has left-sided paresis and is unable to use left hand to
stabilize dish while eating.

Approach: Use adaptive dish with suction cup to stabilize on table. Use plate
with an inner lip to make scooping food onto spoon or fork
easier. Praise successful attempts.

Goal: D. Hall will feed self 50 percent of meal using suction dish with
inner lip by date _____.

Residents who fail to make progress toward established goals need to be
reevaluated by either the licensed nurse or occupational therapist. Report lack
of progress immediately.

BOWEL/BLADDER RETRAINING PROGRAMS

Bowel and bladder retraining programs cannot be delegated to the RNA alone
because a successful program must involve all those who provide care to the
resident. However, once a plan has been developed, the RNA may be assigned to
assume responsibility for:

- Monitoring its implementation
- Teaching other nursing assistants basic elements of the program
- Monitoring daily documentation of nursing assistants
- Monitoring completion of accurate intake/output records

The key to a successful retraining program is consistency. The staff must
follow the plan developed and chart residents' progress or lack of progress each
day. If a plan is not working, report this information to the licensed nurse, who
can reassess and change the plan if necessary.

SELF-GROOMING PROGRAMS

The development of a self-grooming program can be fun, and residents generally respond positively to programs designed to improve their appearance (Fig.
17-9). Sometimes it is easier to motivate them toward improved self-grooming
than it is toward improved personal hygiene, which always needs to be
included with any self-grooming program. Because self-grooming tasks are
usually performed along with the AM care or the bath/shower, group classes
are not as appropriate as an individualized approach.

The RNA along with the licensed nurse and the occupational therapist can
develop a plan for self-grooming after assessment of the resident's functional

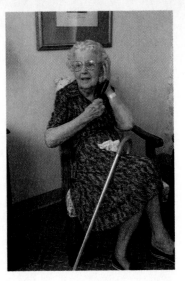

FIGURE 17-9
Self-grooming is an important step toward independence.

abilities. The RNA as well as the assigned nursing assistants will be responsible for the implementation of the plan. Documenting the resident's progress or lack of progress each week in the weekly summary is essential. The RNA frequently becomes the "coordinator" of the self-grooming program, working with the assigned nursing assistants to see that the plan is implemented consistently. Remember, the primary purpose of the program is to teach the resident to perform self-grooming and personal hygiene tasks as independently as possible.

Appearance is generally important to all of us; however, if residents do not have access to mirrors, they may not be as motivated to improve their appearance. Having hand mirrors and wall mirrors in residents' rooms has a positive impact on their willingness to work at improving their appearance.

Teaching residents to brush their teeth again, to shave, and comb their hair is not difficult if you are able to carry out these basic procedures competently for a dependent resident. Review these procedures and make the necessary adaptations to allow the resident to perform independently if possible or with minimal assistance. Remember, regaining skills takes time and patience in addition to accepting the reality that the end result may not be as good as if the task were performed by someone else. Some residents particularly enjoy having makeup applied for them or having someone give them a manicure. Reward residents who are working toward self-grooming goals with these "extras" when possible.

SELF-DRESSING PROGRAMS

Again the RNA along with the licensed nurse and the occupational therapist will need to assess the resident's special needs in order to set up a plan of care. The plan must be very specific because the assigned nursing assistant will most often be responsible for implementing the plan. The RNA can review the plan as well as special dressing techniques with the nursing assistant and monitor the resident's progress several times a week in order to document in the weekly summary specifically what progress has been made.

Relearning to dress oneself takes time! At first, it may take a resident up to one hour to complete the task. Later, after much practice, dressing may be completed in fifteen minutes. Your patience in allowing as much time as needed makes the difference between a resident who is frustrated by what he can't do and the resident who is proud of what he can do!

Remember the goal is to teach the resident to dress independently if possible. If the resident needs to use assistive devices to reach the goal, be sure they are available consistently. If you have any questions regarding the need for or use of special assistive devices, talk with the occupational therapist.

Physical fitness and group exercise programs are among the most well-received restorative nursing programs offered. Groups of residents with similar abilities can be brought together to perform exercises. In a group they encourage one another and work harder to keep up with the group. Music is used to create an atmosphere of fun and energy. The program usually includes active range of motion beginning with the head and working down to range each of the joints about three times. Sometimes the exercise is provided by kicking and tossing a beach ball or by using a parachute to wave up and down. There are also simple dance records such as "the Hokey Poky" that provide fun and exercise. The exercise program is an opportunity for almost every resident to participate regardless of mental status, ability to communicate, or ability to perform ADL skills. Residents feel good about themselves when they participate in an exercise program.

The restorative nursing program must be a total program that involves all who provide care. When a program can be developed that directly involves each nursing assistant providing the above-mentioned kinds of care every day, the facility can be proud of its commitment to restorative and rehabilitative philosophies.

■ Glossary

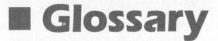

A

abdominal respiration breathing using mostly the abdominal muscles

abduction to move an arm or leg away from the center of the body

accuracy factual or being correct

acetone byproduct of the metabolism of fat; a type of ketone

acidosis a dangerous condition related to diabetes when toxic substances build up in the body

acquired immune deficiency syndrome (AIDS) a terminal condition in which the body's immune system is damaged by attack from a virus

active done by the resident independently

active treatment program plan including interdisciplinary evaluation and an individual plan of care with measurable goals and an integrated program of activities

activities of daily living (ADL) activities or tasks needed for daily living, such as eating, grooming, dressing, bathing, washing, and toileting

adduction to move an arm or leg toward the center of the body

adrenal glands two small glands located on top of each kidney; produce hormones that help the body react and adapt to stress

adult day care center provides meals and activities for the elderly who cannot or do not want to be alone during the day

advocates persons who represent residents or clients and act to protect their interests

age appropriate appropriate to the chronological age of a person

AIDS (acquired immune deficiency syndrome) a condition in which the body's immune system is damaged by attack from a virus (HIV)

alignment to put in a straight line

alimentary tract route taken by food as it passes from the mouth to the anus

alopecia loss of scalp and body hair

alveoli tiny air sacs in the lungs where oxygen enters the blood

Alzheimer's disease incurable disease affecting the brain that occurs predominantly in older adults and affects memory, thinking, and judgment

AM care assisting the resident with toileting needs, washing face, hands, providing oral hygiene and preparing the resident for breakfast

ambu bag a ventilator bag

ambulation walking or moving about in an upright position

ambulation device any apparatus to assist with walking; includes braces, canes, crutches, and walkers

amino acids the units of structure in proteins

amputation cutting off a body part, usually an arm or leg

anatomical position term of reference used when a person is standing facing you, with palms out and feet together

anatomy study of body parts, how the body is made, and what it is made of

anemia insufficient supply of red blood cells

aneurysm bulging out of the wall of an artery creating a weakened area subject to rupture

angina pectoris acute chest pain caused by decreased blood supply to the heart

ankylosed condition where joints become very stiff, unmovable and frozen

aorta largest artery in the body

apathy lack of feeling or interest in things

aphasia loss of language or communication ability

apical pulse heartbeat measured at the apex of the heart

apnea absence of breathing

appendages attachments of the skin

appendix small projection of tissue located where the small and large intestines meet

ARC (AIDS-related complex) non-life-threatening illnesses caused by a decreased immune response due to AIDS infection

arteries blood vessels that carry blood away from the heart

arterioles tiny arteries that carry blood from the large arteries to the capillaries

arteriosclerosis thickening and loss of elasticity in the arteries

artificial ventilation rescue breathing

aseptic   free of microorganisms

aspiration   inhaling food or fluid into the lungs

assault   threat or unsuccessful attempt to commit bodily harm

asthma   a disease of the bronchi characterized by difficulty breathing, wheezing, and a sense of tightness or constriction in the chest due to spasm of the muscles

atherosclerosis   clogging of the arteries with plaque and deposits of calcium or fat

atrophy   decreasing of muscle mass; wasting of muscle tissue

autism   a disability related to lack of organization in the functioning of the brain

autoclaving   sterilizing using superheated steam under pressure

autonomic dysreflexia   in spinal cord-injured victims, a life-threatening condition that is caused by stimuli from the skin, the bowel, and the bladder

autonomic nervous system   part of the nervous system that controls organs not under voluntary control

axillary   in the armpit

B

backward chaining   teaching the last step in a skill first, then the next to last, and so on

bacterium   singular of bacteria, a type of microorganism

base of support   foundation of an object or person

battery   assault that is carried out, resulting in harm to another person

behaving courteously   putting the needs of others before your own

behavior   action that can be observed and measured

behavior modification   a process of changing behavior patterns by eliminating useless behaviors and teaching or reinforcing useful ones

behavior shaping   process of creating a new set of behaviors

benign prostatic hypertrophy   noncancerous enlargement of the prostate gland

bereave   to be left desolate by death

bile   substance stored in the gallbladder that aids in the digestion of fats

biological death   occurs when vital activity in the cells of the body stops

blood pressure   measurable force of the blood against the walls of a blood vessel

blood pressure cuff   common name for a sphygmomanometer

body mechanics   special ways of standing and moving one's body

Bowman's capsule   part of the kidney containing the glomerules

brain syndrome   signs or symptoms that indicate the presence of brain disease

bridging   technique used to support areas above and below a designated area

bronchi   two main branches of the windpipe

bulb   portion of the thermometer which is placed in direct contact with the resident's body

bulbo-urethral glands   exocrine glands located near the prostate in males

bursa   small fluid-filled sac that allows one bone to move easily over another bone

bursitis   inflammation of the fluid-filled sacs between bones causing pain on movement

C

calculi   stones in the kidney or bladder

calibrated   marked with graduations, as on a thermometer or graduate

cancer   form of cellular disorder in which the normal mechanisms of the cell (that control rate of growth, cell division, and movement) are disrupted

cannulas   tubes used to give oxygen

capillaries   smallest blood vessels in the circulatory system; they nourish all body cells

carcinogen   substance known to cause cancer

carcinoma   a form of cancer found most often in the skin and the lining of hollow organisms and passageways

cardiac angioplasty   procedure used to open clogged coronary arteries

cardiac arrest   when the heart stops beating

cardiac bypass surgery   procedure in which a blood vessel is removed from the leg to replace a portion of a coronary blood vessel that is clogged or blocked

cardiac muscle tissue   type of muscle in the heart that controls the heartbeat

cardiovascular insufficiency   type of heart disease in which there is decreased blood supply to the major organs of the body

caring   compassion; understanding fears, problems, and distress of another

cartilage   tough gristle-like substance that forms a pad at the end of or between bones

cataract   condition in which the lens becomes cloudy to the point of complete blindness

catastrophic reactions   sudden changes from baseline behavior that are socially unacceptable

cell   fundamental building block of all living organisms

cell membrane   rim or edge of the cell

Celsius (C)   measurement of temperature in which 0 degrees is the freezing point and 100 degrees is the boiling point for water

center of gravity   place where the bulk or mass of an vv object is centered

central line   catheter placed into the atrium of the heart

cerebellum   part of the brain that coordinates voluntary movement

cerebral palsy   a developmental disability caused by damage to the brain

cerebral vascular accident (CVA)   stroke

cerebrum part of the brain responsible for thinking, learning, and memory

chart written health or medical record, which is a legal document

chemotherapy use of drugs or medications to treat disease

chromosomes threadlike structures that carry genetic material

chronic obstructive pulmonary disease (COPD) emphysema, asthma, and chronic bronchitis, and problems related to these diseases

cilia small hair-like projections of the respiratory passages

cirrhosis inflammation of a tissue or organ, particularly the liver

clean uncontaminated; free from known pathogenic organisms

clinical death when breathing stops and heart stops

clitoris primary female sex organ

clonic phase stage of a convulsion in which the muscles jerk or spasm

closed urinary drainage system method of collecting urine that prevents contamination as it is uninterrupted

code of ethics rules of conduct for a particular group

colostomy opening into the colon

communicable conditions diseases and infections that spread from one person to another

communication involves a sender, a message, and a receiver; it may take place in speaking or writing, or without words through facial expressions, tone of voice, gestures, body position, and movement

complete airway obstruction blocking of the airway so that no air passes through

confidentiality not revealing private information to others

congestive heart failure inability of the heart to pump out all the blood returned to it from the veins

constipation buildup of fecal material in the large intestine

contaminated not sterile; in contact with micro-organisms

continuity doing the same thing in the same way

contracture shortening of the muscles from inactivity

control stopping or limiting of growth

convulsions jerking of the muscles as they contract and relax

counter-traction exertion of pull in the opposite direction of traction

cranium bones of the head

crede pressing on the area of the abdomen over the bladder to push the urine out

cross-infection acquiring an infection from someone else

culture specimen of body tissue or fluids kept under special laboratory conditions to detect the presence of microorganisms

cure correction or removal of a problem

cyanosis blue or gray color of the skin, lips, and nailbeds, indicating lack of oxygen

cytoplasm material surrounding the nucleus of a cell

D

debridement removal of dead or unhealthy tissue

decubitus ulcers tissue breakdown resulting from pressure or reduced blood flow (often called pressure sores or bed sores)

defamation of character making false or damaging statements about another person which injure his or her reputation

defecation process of eliminating waste material from the bowel

dehydration condition in which fluid output is greater than fluid intake

dementia deprived of reason; mentally deteriorated

dermis second layer of skin

developmental disability a chronic condition related to or needing treatment similar to mental retardation

diabetes mellitus disease in which the pancreas secretes insufficient amounts of insulin

diabetic coma high blood sugar with presence of ketones in the urine

diabetic shock very low blood sugar with symptoms of shock

dialysis use of a machine that performs the base functions of the kidney

diaphragm muscular organ that separates the chest and abdominal cavities

diarrhea semi-fluid feces

diastolic pressure pressure when the heart is relaxed (the lowest pressure)

diencephalon area of the brain where control is exercised over body activities such as regulation of body temperature and the endocrine glands

dirty contaminated, used, or exposed to disease-producing organisms

disabled limitation in the ability to function normally

discharge long-time absence or permanent exit from an acute care hospital

disinfection process of killing most microorganisms

dislocation disruption of the normal alignment of bones where they form a joint

dorsiflexion to flex the ankle (away from the sole of the foot)

douche introduction of a cleansing solution into the vaginal canal with immediate return by gravity

dry application application where no water touches the skin

duodenum first loop of the small intestine and most major area of digestion

dyspnea difficult or labored breathing

E

edema   swelling of joints, tissue or organs

ejaculated   released at the time the male experiences orgasm

elder abuse   abuse of an elderly person

electrocardiogram (EKG)   tracing of the heart's electrical conduction system

embolus   a blood clot that moves within the blood stream

emesis   vomiting

emotional lability   overreaction of the emotions to a stimulus, e.g., crying or laughing inappropriately

empathy   ability to put yourself in another's place and to see things as they see them

emphysema   disease in which tiny bronchioles become plugged with mucus, making breathing difficult, especially during exhalation

encephalitis   inflammation of the brain

enema   introduction of fluid into the rectum and colon

enemas until clear   there is no solid fecal material present when the solution is expelled

environmental control   means of providing a safe environment that is as free as possible of pathogenic organisms

enzymes   digestive secretions

epidermis   outer layer of the skin

epiglottis   cartilage which covers the opening of the trachea when foods and fluids are swallowed

epilepsy   a disorder in the electrical functioning of the brain resulting in seizures

erythema   redness of the skin

eschar   a slough produced after an injury (often called a scab)

estrogen   primary female sex hormone

euphoric   experiencing an exaggerated feeling of well-being

exacerbation   return or increase of symptoms

exocrine   secreting externally

extension   to straighten an arm or leg

F

fading   a technique in behavior management where the amount of guidance is decreased

Fahrenheit (F)   measurement of temperature in which 32 degrees is the freezing point and 212 degrees is the boiling point for water

fallopian tubes   tubes from the ovary to the uterus through which the ovum passes

false imprisonment   keeping or restraining a person without proper consent

fecal impaction   serious and painful condition in which feces remain in the S-shaped area of the colon and rectum, where they may block the intestinal passage

feces   solid human waste

fertile   able to become pregnant

fine motor skills   skills which require use of fine muscles such as those of the hands for writing, buttoning, eating

finger probes   manual removal of a foreign body by using the index finger

flaccid   limp

flexion   to bend a joint (elbow, wrist, knee)

fluid balance   the individual takes in and eliminates about the same amount of fluid

fluid intake   total amount of fluid taken into the body over a given amount of time

fluid output   total amount of fluid eliminated from the body in a given amount of time

focal or Jacksonian seizure   type of seizure that affects only part of the body

follicles   roots of the hair

force (pulse)   strength or power described as weak or bounding

force fluids   encourage fluid intake

formed elements   those parts of the blood that are not fluid, e.g., red blood cells and platelets

forward chaining   complex skills broken down into specific steps and taught in the order in which they would normally be completed

fracture   breaking or cracking of a bone

frequency   the need to urinate often

functional life skills   skills necessary to allow an individual to function as independently as possible

G

gait belt   a belt placed around a patient's waist that allows better control over the center of gravity

gallstones   cholesterol crystals that settle out of the bile stored in the gallbladder

gangrene   a disease where tissue dies and amputation is often necessary

gastritis   inflammation of the stomach caused by many different factors

gatch   handle or crank used to raise and lower the bed, head of bed, or foot of bed

genuineness   being yourself

glaucoma   increased pressure within the eye that can lead to blindness due to pressure on the optic nerve

glomerulus   a network of capillaries in the kidney that filters the blood

glucose   simple sugar to which food is converted

glycosuria   sugar in the urine

graduated guidance   a technique of behavior management where the amount of assistance or prompting that is necessary is gradually decreased

grand mal seizure   type of seizure involving loss of consciousness and convulsions

gravity   attraction that the earth has for an object on or near its surface

grief process   emotions experienced by people following a loss

gross motor activities involves use of the large muscles such as those used in walking, dancing, and swimming

gross negligence person responsible shows so little care that it appears that he or she is indifferent to the welfare of others

H

Harris flush return flow enema; irrigation of the rectum

health care plan written guidelines for providing care

hearing aid a mechanical device used to make certain sounds louder

heart muscle that pumps blood through the vessels

Heimlich maneuver application of abdominal thrusts during airway obstruction

hemiplegia paralysis of one side of the body

hemispheres halves

hemorrhage bleeding

hemorrhoids enlarged blood-filled vessels that surround the rectal area

home health care agencies businesses that provide health services to clients in the home

homeostasis the body's attempt to keep its internal environment stable and in balance

hormone fluid secreted by an endocrine gland

hospice a facility that provides care to residents who have limited life expectancy

humidifier water container through which oxygen is passed to reduce its drying effect

hyperactive extremely, abnormally active

hyperextension to move beyond the normal extension

hyperglycemia high blood sugar

hypertension high blood pressure

hypoglycemia low blood sugar

hypotension low blood pressure

hypothalamus gland in the brain that controls body temperature and the function of the endocrine glands

hysterectomy surgical removal of the uterus

I

ID the interdisciplinary team which works with the developmentally disabled client

ileostomy opening into the ileum

imbalance lack of equality

immobilized unable to move

implement to carry out or accomplish a given plan

impotence inability to engage in sexual intercourse

incidence number of occurrences

incident report written description of an accident involving resident, visitor, or staff member

incontinent no control over bowel and bladder function

individualized health-care plan plan of care tailored to reflect the individuality of each resident

indwelling catheter tube inserted through the urethra into the bladder to drain urine into a collection bag

infarct death of part of the heart muscle

infection invasion of the body by a disease-producing organism

infectious objects objects that have come in contact with a person who has an infection or communicable disease

infectious waste disposable items used by residents and any body discharges

inferior toward the feet

inflammation tissue reaction to disease or injury characterized by heat, redness, pain and swelling

insulin hormone secreted by the pancreas

insulin shock low blood sugar, usually from too much insulin or not enough food intake

intramuscularly injection into muscle

intravenously injection into the vein

invasion of privacy when personal information is exposed publicly, violating an individual's right to privacy

IPPs the individual program plans used with developmentally disabled clients

I.Q. intelligence quotient or score obtained on a standard test

irregular respiration a change in the depth of breathing and an unsteady rate of rise and fall of the chest

isolation to separate or set apart

isolation techniques safety measure to prevent spread of communicable conditions

J

jaundice a yellow coloring of skin and the white portion of the eye caused by the substance bilirubin, which is secreted by the liver

job description describes the duties of a particular job category

K

ketonuria presence of ketones in the urine

kyphasis hunchback or forward curving of the spine

L

labored respirations difficult breathing that may include gurgling, rattling, or wheezing sounds

lancet sharp object used to prick the skin of a fingertip or earlobe to obtain a small sample of blood

larynx voice box

laxative medication that loosens the bowel contents and encourages evacuation

legal according to the laws of the community, state, or nation

level of injury in spinal cord injury, the location of injury in relationship to the vertebrae that surround the cord

libel a written type of defamation of character

ligaments tough, white, fibrous cords that connect bone to bone

log-rolling a technique of turning a patient

LTC abbreviation for long-term care

lymph fluid which surrounds the body cells

lymph vessels tiny capillary-like structures that collect lymph

M

mammary glands glandular tissue of the breast

manual thrusts series of rapid thrusts to the upper abdomen or chest that force air from the lungs

masturbation sexual self-stimulation apart from intercourse

medulla vital center in the brain that controls breathing, swallowing, and heartbeat

meningitis inflammation of membranes surrounding the brain

menopause the period of time when menstruation stops, ending reproductive ability and resulting in decreased hormone production

menstruation monthly shedding of the lining of the uterus

mental retardation a significantly subaverage general intellectual functioning existing with deficits in adaptive behavior

metabolism complex processes of the living cells where oxygen is used and carbon dioxide is given off (called the work of the cell)

metastasize spread to other parts of the body

microorganisms tiny living things seen only with a microscope

midbrain part of the brain through which nerve impulses pass

midstream clean-catch urine specimen type of urine specimen obtained under clean conditions by collecting urine while it is being eliminated from the body

modeling a technique of behavior management where the client is shown how to perform a task

moist application application where water touches the skin

multidisciplinary team professionals with different educational backgrounds who work together

multiple sclerosis chronic degenerative disease of the nervous system

muscular dystrophy a group of related muscle diseases that are progressively crippling due to weakness and atrophy of muscles

myelin an insulating material that surrounds the nerve fibers

myocardial infarction heart attack in which part of the heart muscle dies

N

nasal cannulas tubes inserted into the nostrils to supply oxygen

nasogastric tube tube inserted through the nose and into the stomach

negligence failure to act as an average nursing assistant would act under the same circumstances

nephrons microscopic filtering units of the kidney

neurons specialized cells of the nervous system

nitroglycerin medication which, when placed under the tongue to dissolve, will act rapidly to increase blood flow to the heart

nocturia waking at night to urinate

nonpathogenic not capable of producing disease

nonprofit operated without profit or gain

normalization creating an atmosphere that is as close to normal as possible

NPO consuming nothing by mouth

nucleus part of the cell which directs growth of the cell and cell division

nursing care Kardex "nursing assistant information" record, which may be handwritten or printed from a computer

nutrition science of food and its actions or relationship to health

O

objective observations facts observed and not distorted by personal feelings

observation recognizing and noticing a fact or occurrence

obstruction blocking of the airway

occupied bed one with the resident in it

olfaction sense of smell

ombudsman an impartial person who investigates complaints and acts as an advocate for residents and/or families

opportunistic infection occurs when organisms take advantage of a diseased immune system

oral in the mouth

oral hygiene care of the mouth, teeth, gums, and tongue

organ body part where two or more tissues work together to perform a particular function

organism any living thing

orientation ability to accurately describe person, place, and time

osteoarthritis disease characterized by deterioration of joint cartilage and formation of new bone at joint surfaces

osteocytes living cells of the bone

osteoporosis disease characterized by porous or chalk-like bones which fracture very easily

ostomy surgical opening made on the surface of the abdomen to release waste from the body

otologist a specialist in hearing

ova eggs

ovaries primary female reproductive organs

ovulation process in which an ovum is discharged from an ovary at regular intervals

P

pacemaker part of the conduction system of the heart which creates the stimulus for the heart to beat

palliation to relieve symptoms

pancreas large gland located in the abdomen; secretes insulin and glucagon

paralysis loss of voluntary movement

paraplegic person with paralysis of the lower limbs

parasympathetic nervous system part of the autonomic nervous system that conserves energy

parathyroid glands two pairs of glands located within the thyroid that produce a hormone to help regulate the level of calcium and phosphorus in the body

parenterally through a tube inserted into a vein or into the atrium of the heart

partial airway obstruction incomplete blocking of the airway, allowing some air to pass through

partial bath bathing of only those areas of the body that require daily bathing to remain clean

passive done for the patient by the nursing assistant

pathogenic causing disease

penis primary male sex organ

perinatal during the birth process

perineal area in the female, the area between the vagina and the anus; in the male, the area between the scrotum and the anus

peripheral vascular disease poor circulation in the extremities

peristalsis rhythmic contractions that assist in moving food through the intestines

perpendicular at a right angle

petit mal seizure type of seizure common in children; does not include convulsions

philosophy search for a general understanding of values

physical needs basic human needs for food, water, oxygen, rest, exercise, and sex

physiology study of how the body functions, how all the body parts work independently and collectively

pituitary gland master gland of the body, which regulates metabolism

planning devising a way of getting a job done

plantar flexion extending the ankle (toward the sole of the foot)

plaque substance that clogs arteries producing atherosclerosis

plasma fluid portion of the blood

platelets cells in the blood that are essential for clotting

PM care assisting the resident with toileting needs, washing face and hands, giving a bedtime nourishment, providing oral hygiene, dressing for bed, and giving a back rub

pneumonia acute infection of the lung

policy describes what is to be done

pons part of the brain through which nerve impulses pass

postnatal after birth

postural drainage physical therapy in which the resident is positioned so that the upper trunk is lower than the rest of the body, forcing secretions from respiratory passages to be coughed up

postural support soft protective device or restraint used to protect a resident from injury

prenatal during pregnancy

presbyopia condition in which the lens of the eye loses its ability to focus clearly due to loss of elasticity

procedure description of how to do a task

procrastination putting off doing something until some other time

prolapse protruding of the uterus into the vagina

prompting a technique used in rehabilitation programs where the staff verbally reminds the resident what to do next

pronation turning palms down

proprietary operated for profit

prostate gland a firm muscular gland which encircles the male's urethra like a donut

prosthesis artifical replacement for a body part such as a limb or eye

protoplasm essential living matter of all animal and plant cells

psychomotor seizure type of seizure that results in temporary impairment of consciousness and abnormal behavior

psychosocial an individual's mental or emotional processes in combination with his ability to interact and relate with others

pulmonic a valve in the heart between the right ventricle and the pulmonary artery

pulse the rhythmic expansion and contraction of the arteries, which can be measured to show how fast the heart is beating

pulse force weak or bounding force of pulse beats

pulse rate number of pulse beats per minute

pulse rhythm regularity of the pulse beats

purulent material liquid inflammation product containing cells and other fluid

Q

quadriplegic person with paralysis of all four extremities

QMRP the qualified mental retardation professional who heads the interdisciplinary team for developmentally disabled clients

R

radial deviation toward the thumb side of the hand

radial pulse pulse felt at the inner aspect of the wrist (radial artery)

range of motion extent to which a joint can be moved before causing pain

reagent   substance used in a chemical reaction to determine the presence of another substance

reality orientation   technique for reducing and eliminating disorientation

rectal   in the rectum

rectum   lowest section of the large intestine adjacent to the outside of the body

reduction   setting a bone in proper position for healing

reflex   automatic response to stimulation

reflux   return flow of urine back into the bladder from a drainage bag

rehabilitation   the restoration of the individual to the fullest physical, mental, social, vocational, and economic capacity of which he or she is capable

rehabilitation philosophy   understanding which promotes independence and recognizes the accomplishment of small, simple goals

reinfection   being infected a second time

reinforcer   a reward

remission   lessening or disappearance of disease symptoms

renal artery   artery that supplies blood to the kidneys

respect   recognition of the worth of another person

respiration   process of inhaling and exhaling

restraint   device that holds back or limits movements; used in reference to postural support or soft protective devices

rheumatoid arthritis   disease characterized by painful, stiff, swollen red joints that eventually become deformed

role   part one plays in relationship to others

rotation   to move a joint in a circular motion around its axis

rounds, making   going to each resident to determine briefly whether they have any immediate needs

S

salivary glands   glands that produce saliva to moisten the mouth and begin the digestion of food

sarcoma   a form of cancer found most often in bone, muscle, cartilage, and lymph systems

scoliosis   s-shaped curving of the spine

scrotum   sac outside the male containing the testes

security needs   basic human needs for physical safety, shelter, and protection

seizure   over-reaction of brain cells; a sudden attack

self-fulfillment   basic human need to reach the highest potential and to accomplish one's life goals

semen   fluid expelled through the penis during ejaculation; contains sperm, water, and nutrients

sensory deprivation   loss or lack of stimulation from the environment

sensory-motor activities   activities designed to improve the thinking of the client

sensory neurons   specialized type of nerve cell

septum   tissue which divides the heart into right and left chambers

setting priorities   looking at all things that need to be done and putting them in the order of importance

sexuality   quality of being male or female

shadowing   a technique of behavior management where the staff member's hands are kept within one inch of the client's hands while he or she performs a task

shallow respiration   breathing with only the upper part of the lungs

shaping   a behavior modification technique used to create a new set of behaviors

shearing   force that occurs when skin moves one way while bone and tissue under the skin move another way

sick role   behavior associated with being sick; dependence, weakness, control by others, decreased responsibility and uselessness

sigmoid colon   lower portion of the large intestine which curves in an 's' shape

slander   a verbal type of defamation of character

smooth muscle tissue   involuntary muscle tissue

social needs   basic human need for approval and acceptance

sodium chloride   table salt

spasm   involuntary contraction of muscle

spasticity   tightening of the muscle with short jerking movements

sperm   male reproductive cells released upon ejaculation

sphincter   type of muscle that contracts to close a body opening

sphygmomanometer   instrument used to measure blood pressure; can be either aneroid (measurer watches a calibrated dial) or mercury type (measurer watches a column of mercury)

spinal cord   long cable of nerves that extends from below the medulla to the second or third lumbar vertebra

spiritual needs   need to find meaning in life

spontaneous breathing   in mouth-to-mouth ventilation, the point at which the victim begins to breathe independently

spontaneous combustion   ignition of burnable materials caused by a chemical reaction

sprain   stretched or torn ligaments or tendons

sputum   mucus from the lungs, usually mixed with saliva

staphylococcus   type of harmful bacteria commonly found in health care institutions; treated by antibiotic drugs

stasis   stoppage of flow

stasis ulcers   open wounds or sores on the legs caused by stoppage of blood flow

status needs   basic human needs for recognition and respect

stem (thermometer)   long narrow portion of a thermometer, opposite from the bulb

sterile   free from all microorganisms

sterilization process of killing all microorganisms

sternum breastbone

stertorous respirations abnormal noises like snoring when breathing

stethoscope instrument that picks up sound when placed against part of the body

stimulus action or agent that causes a response in an organ or organism

stoma an opening

stool solid waste material discharged from the body through the rectum and anus; feces, excreta, excrement, bowel movement, fecal material

streptococcus type of harmful bacteria commonly found in health care institutions; treated by antibiotic drugs

stretch receptors nerve cells in the wall of the bladder that send a message to the brain when the bladder is full

striated muscle tissue type of voluntary muscle tissue

stridor a high-pitched sound produced during airway obstruction

subjective observations individual judgments based on personal feelings

superior toward the head

supination to turn palms up

suppository cone-shaped semisolid medicated substance inserted into the rectum

sweat glands glands that produce moisture to cool the body and excrete waste products

sympathetic nervous system part of the autonomic nervous system that controls response to stress

systolic pressure pressure created when the heart is contracting; highest pressure

T

tact ability to say or do the right thing at the right time

teaching causing to learn by example or experience

tendons elastic cordlike structures that connect muscles to bone

terminal illness serious illness providing life expectancy of six months or less in the end stage of the illness

testes primary male reproductive organs that produce sperm

testosterone male hormone related to sexual activity and reproduction

therapeutic pertaining to or effective in treatment of disease

thrombus blood clot

thymus gland two-lobe ductless gland believed to play a role in the immune system of the body

thyroid gland largest of the endocrine glands; regulates growth and metabolic rate

tissue group of the same type of cells functioning in the same way

tongue-jaw lift in finger sweep procedures, forcing open the mouth and holding the lower jaw and tongue so that the mouth cannot close

tonic phase part of a convulsion in which the muscles become rigid

touch form of communication that conveys friendliness and affection

toxins waste products released by disease-producing organisms

trachea windpipe; the passage that conveys air from the larynx to the bronchi

traction exertion of "pull" by means of weights

transfer to move from one place to another

transfer belt belt placed around the resident's waist to provide a "handle" to hold during transfer

transurethral surgery a procedure that removes some of the prostate tissue

tricuspid valve valve between the right atrium and right ventricle of the heart

trochanter roll a rolled towel or blanket

tuberculosis an infectious disease that commonly attacks the lungs and which is usually spread by contact with the sputum of an infected person

tympanic membrane thin membrane inside the ear that vibrates when struck by sound waves; the eardrum

U

ulcer break in the skin creating an open wound

ulnar deviation away from the thumb side of the hand

unconscious unaware of the surrounding environment

unoccupied bed empty bed

ureterostomy opening into one of the ureters

ureters tubes that extend from the kidneys to the bladder through which urine passes

urethra tube from the bladder to the outside of the body

urgency an immediate need to urinate

urinary incontinence inability to control urination

uterus womb

V

vaginal irrigation or douche introduction of solution into the vaginal canal with immediate return by gravity

vaginitis inflammation of the tissue of the vagina

varicose veins swollen (distended) veins especially prominent in the leg caused by lack of exercise, prolonged standing, and loss of elasticity associated with aging

veins blood vessels that carry blood back to the heart

ventricles thick muscular walls of the heart

venules very tiny veins that carry blood back to the heart

vertebrae bones of the spine

vertebral column column of bones of the spine through which the spinal cord passes; spine; backbone

villi small finger-like projections of the duodenum which absorb digested food particles and release them into the bloodstream

virus microorganisms that can cause infection and disease

vital signs temperature, pulse, blood pressure, and respiration

vulvitis inflammation of the vulva

W

warmth demonstrating concern and affection

well role behaviors associated with being well, i.e., independence, increased responsibility, usefulness, control, and decision making

■ Index

Skin (*cont.*)
  skin care, goals of, 153
  See also Bathing; Warm/cold
    applications
Skin breakdown, risk factors for, 149
Slander, 16
Smell/taste/touch, 139-40
Smooth muscle tissue, 195
Social needs, 70
Soft protective devices, application
    guidelines, 33
Spasms, 276
Spasticity, 214
Sperm, 349
Sphincter muscles, 218
Sphygmomanometer, 119-20
Spinal cord, 271-72
Spinal cord injuries, 275-76
  effects, 276-78
    initial treatment of, 276
    rehabilitation, 279
Spiritual needs of residents, 79-80
Spontaneous combustion, 39
Sprains, 180
Sputum specimens, 313
Stages of dying, 83-88
Standing balance scale, weighing
    residents on, 103
Stasis ulcers, 332
State resident rights, 12-14
Sterilization, 44
Stertorous breathing, 117
Stool specimen, collecting, 243
Stretch-receptor nerve cells, 247
Striated muscle tissue, 195
Strict isolation, 48
Stroke, *See* Cerebral vascular accident
Subjective observations, 96
Supine (face-up) position, 211-12
Surgery, and cancer, 132-33
Sweat glands, 342
Sympathetic nervous system, 272
Systems, 129
Systolic pressure, 119

T

Tact, 23
Temperature:
  conversion, 107
  measuring, *See* Body temperature
    measurements
Tendons, 178
Tes-tape, 347
Testes, 341
Testosterone, 349
Theft/loss, of residents' personal items, 16

Therapeutic diets, 226-29
  enteral feeding, 228-29
Thermometers:
  and indications for use, 107
  methods of temperature measurement,
    108-10
  parts of, 108
  reading, 109-10
  See also specific types
Thrombosis, 279
Thrombus, 334
Thymus gland, 341
Thyroid gland, 341
Tissue, 126-27
Toilet, tranferring residents on/off of, 193
Tongue-jaw lift, 304
Total parenteral nutrition (TPN), 228-29
Toxins, 43
Trachea, 296, 297
Traction, 184
Transfers, 63-64
Transfer techniques, 190-93
  pivot transfer of hemiplegic resident.
    191-93
  training in, 378
  transfer belt, 191-93
Trans-urethral surgery, 351
Tricuspid valve, 318
Trochanter roll, as positioning device,
    210, 211
Tub bath, procedure, 157-58
Tuberculosis, 309-10
  symptoms of, 310

U

Ulcers, 218
Unconscious residents, oral hygiene,
    163-64
Undressing totally dependent residents,
    168-69
Universal precautions, 46, 347
Unoccupied bed, making, 57-58
Ureterostomy, 240-43
Ureters, 247
Urethra, 247, 349
Urinal, offering, 257-58
Urinary drainage bag, emptying, 254
Urinary specimens, 264-65, 347
Urinary system, 245-68
  age-related changes, 248-49
  fluid balance, 249
  fluid imbalance, 250-51
  fluid intake/output, 249-53
  functions of, 246
  kidneys, 247-48
  nursing measures related to, 256-65

and spinal cord injuries, 277
  See also Fluid intake/output
Urinary tract infections, 248-49, 260
Urine testing, for sugar/acetone, 347
Uristix, 347

V

Vaginal douche/irrigation, 352-53
Vaginitis, 352
Varicose veins, 334
Veins, 317, 318
Ventricles, 318
Venules, 318
Verbal aggression, coping with, 76-77
Vertebral column, 271
Viruses, 43
Visitors, dealing with, 23-24
Visual impairment, 141-42
  and diabetes mellitus, 345-46
  See also Blindness; Eyes
Vulvitis, 352

W

Walkers, 207, 379-81
Warm/cold applications, 170-74
  alcohol sponge bath, 173
  Aquamatic K-pad, 171, 172
  guidelines, 173-74
  See also Bathing; Skin
Weight, measuring, 101-5, 381
  with bed scale, 105
  with mechanical lift, 104
  on standing balance scale, 103
Welcoming the resident, 62
Well-balanced diet, 219-23
  See also Diet; Mealtime; Nutrition;
    Therapeutic diets
Well role, 74
Wheelchair:
  of amputee, 336
  position residents in, 209
  transferring resident from, 63-64
Wheeled walker, 207
Whirlpool baths, 381-82
Withdrawal:
  and aphasia, 282-83
  and loss of a loved one, 88
Working environment:
  emergencies/accident prevention, 28-35
  fire safety/disaster preparedness, 36-39
  infection control, 40-46
  isolation techniques, 47-55
  resident's unit, 55-64